Surgical Nursing
Twelfth Edition

Surgical Nursing
Twelfth Edition

Colin Torrance
Professor of Nursing Research and Professional Development, School of Nursing and Midwifery, University of Glamorgan, Pontypridd

and

Eve Serginson
Lecturer in Surgical Nursing, Mid and West Wales College of Nursing, University College of Swansea

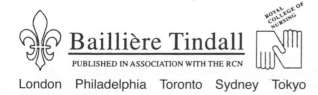

Baillière Tindall
PUBLISHED IN ASSOCIATION WITH THE RCN

London   Philadelphia   Toronto   Sydney   Tokyo

Baillière Tindall   24–28 Oval Road,
London NW1 7DX

The Curtis Centre, Independence Square West,
Philadelphia, PA 19106–3399, USA

Harcourt Brace & Company
55 Horner Avenue, Toronto,
Ontario M8Z 4X6, Canada

Harcourt Brace & Company, Australia
30–52 Smidmore Street, Marrickville,
NSW 2204, Australia

Harcourt Brace & Company, Japan
Ichibancho Central Building, 22–1 Ichibancho
Chiyoda-ku, Tokyo 102, Japan

First published 1938
Eleventh edition 1985

A catalogue record for this book is available from the British Library

ISBN 0–7020–1969–0

Phototypeset by Phoenix Photosetting, Chatham, Kent
Printed and bound in Great Britain by WBC Book Manufacturers Ltd,
Bridgend, Mid Glamorgan

Contents

Section Two   Nursing Care and Management

Preface

Surgical nursing is a major nursing speciality that is currently experiencing many changes. Surgery and surgical nursing are rapidly developing fields. New imaging technologies, innovations in surgical technology and techniques, and in particular the development of day and minimal invasive (keyhole) surgery have resulted in major changes in the organization and delivery of surgical care. Improved surgical and anaesthetic techniques mean that surgery is now practicable on older patients and on those previously considered too ill to risk surgical intervention. In general, surgical patients now spend less time in hospital and much of the preoperative assessment and investigation may take place as an outpatient. For elective surgery the inpatient period may be short with an early discharge and convalescence in the community. For example, in the past cholecystectomy always involved a major surgical incision and deep general anaesthesia, but can now be performed as a laparoscopic procedure taking only 40–90 minutes. Laparoscopic cholecystectomy can be carried out under local anaesthesia as day surgery, although a general anaesthetic is usually used in the UK. Hospitalization rarely exceeds two days and some patients have returned to work within one week (Dubois *et al.*, 1990).

These changes in surgical practice mean that the surgical nurse has relatively little time to assess the patient admitted for routine surgery. Surgical nursing is now concentrated into a relatively short period of intervention, and patient preparation and providing information are likely to be as important as direct 'hands on' care. The traditional surgical nurse's skills of assessment, preoperative preparation, acute postoperative care, and discharge planning are all still required, but must involve the patient and family as much of the recovery period will take place at home.

This book presents a structured review of surgical nursing to help the nurse identify perceived needs and formulate an individualized model of care. It provides an introduction to surgical nursing for the student of nursing and is a useful reference text for the registered nurse embarking on a surgical nursing career. The processes of assessment, identifying potential or actual problems, and planning, implementing, and evaluating interventions are emphasized, but no individual model of nursing care is proposed. The authors concentrate on the principles of care, allowing the readers to apply them using a model of their choice. The approach acknowledges that nursing requires a nursing model of care rather than a medical model, but also recognizes that knowledge previously viewed as 'medical' is also a legitimate part of nursing. Surgical nursing has to be based on an understanding of the general impact of surgery on the individual and of the effects of specific surgical conditions and procedures.

Due to the rapid pace of developments in surgery, this book presents surgical nursing in two sections: section one covers central concepts such as infection control, nutrition, and wound care, and mastery of these core concepts is the basis of safe surgical nursing; section two explores topics related to surgery of specific systems. A clear understanding of the central principles, insight into system-specific needs, and a framework for identifying individual needs will equip the surgical nurse for planning and delivering individualized care and adapting care planning as new surgical approaches are developed for specific conditions.

This text has been inspired and developed from the many editions of *Surgical Nursing* published by Baillière Tindall in the Nursing Aids Series. We have tried to emulate the virtues of readability and practical use that marked those texts, but have increased the range and content to produce a new text that will meet the needs of nursing students undertaking diploma and graduate courses. We hope this text can develop and grow as nursing develops and grows while retaining a firm basis in practical patient care.

Colin Torrance
Eve Serginson

Reference

Dubois F, Icard P, Berthelot G, Levard H (1990) Coelioscope cholecystectomy: preliminary report of 36 cases. *Ann Surg* **211**:60–62.

Publisher's Note
The generally accepted simplification of referring to all patients as he and all nurses as she has been used. No insult is intended and the weakness of the above method is recognized.

Section One
Principles of Surgical Nursing

CONTENTS

Chapter 1
Surgery and Surgical Nursing

CONTENTS

Any surgery can have a profound impact on the physiological and psychosocial well-being of an individual. Even a relatively healthy individual can have serious worries about or reactions to surgery, and the ill or elderly may experience grave consequences. Even minor surgery is seldom viewed as minor by the patient. The surgical nurse has a critical role in assessing the individual undergoing surgery, identifying existing and potential problems and developing appropriate interventions with the patient to avoid or minimize the potential complications of surgery. The surgical nurse is in the privileged position of being able to assist, comfort, and support the patient undergoing surgery. Appropriate advice and education can allow patients to preserve their integrity and make informed decisions. A knowledge of surgical conditions and techniques, general responses to surgery, skilful assessment, vigilant observation, and informed care are central to surgical nursing. Every surgical nurse will formulate an individual model of care based on her conceptualization of the nurse–patient relationship, but a systematic approach acknowledging these key concepts is essential (*Box 1.1*).

The considerable impact of new surgical technologies should not be allowed to overshadow the importance of nursing practice. Malby (1991) studied a surgical ward and reported a significant fall in postoperative complications, reduced length of hospitalization, and increased patient satisfaction, despite no reported changes in medical practice during the study period. Malby attributed these effects to changes in nursing practice, including the introduction of primary nursing.

GENERAL RESPONSES TO SURGERY

Surgery represents a major insult to the body tissues and results in a range of compensatory and adaptive stress responses. Surgery always involves some

---

Box 1.1 A systematic approach to nursing care.

- A nursing process constructs care logically and systematically to meet identified needs.
- Assessment is the key to identifying needs.
- A need will become a problem if it is not met.
- A nursing care plan is designed to meet specific individual needs and by definition individualized nursing care can never be routine care.
- Implicit in a care plan for a patient who will undergo surgery is that the nurse is responsible for the patient's safety and preservation of integrity when the patient is unable to control the environment, for example, when affected by premedication, anaesthesia, and postoperative analgesia.
- Any model of care that provides an adequate framework for identifying needs and planning, implementing, and evaluating care may be used.
- A care plan should be based on individual assessment and, research-based interventions, and evaluated by the extent to which the objectives are achieved.
- Professional responsibility and public accountability are based on communicating and documenting care.
- Care plans are nursing tools that should be the basis for scientific practice. They should be research based, using replicated and validated theory.
- New developments in surgery may require new nursing approaches. These should be tested using appropriate research methods before being accepted as new nursing knowledge.

---

tissue destruction and manipulation, and in most cases there is the additional effect of anaesthesia. The effects of surgery depend on the extent of tissue manipulation and destruction, the depth and length of anaesthesia, and the preoperative condition of the patient. If the patient is relatively healthy and undergoing a minor surgical procedure the effects of surgery are likely to be manageable and day surgery is an option. If the patient has a major underlying pathology or requires extensive surgical intervention the effects may be severe and require extensive postoperative hospitalization, and perhaps even a period of intensive care nursing.

Responses to surgery include alterations in:

- Fluid composition, volume, and distribution.
- Nutrition.
- Oxygenation and respiratory function.
- Temperature regulation.
- Skin and tissue integrity.
- Patterns of elimination.

Potential systemic consequences include:

- Impaired mobility and its complications.
- Altered mood and thought processes.
- Impaired communication and sensory–perceptual function.
- Altered immune function.

Obviously surgical trauma can impact on any system and the range of potential nursing diagnoses is wide. Although many of the responses to surgery are discussed in more detail in subsequent chapters, a general summary is presented below.

Alterations in Fluid Status

Surgical trauma can disrupt body fluid homeostasis, causing changes that cover a range of problems from dehydration to overhydration with effects on fluid volume, distribution, and composition. The effects of surgery are particularly problematic if the patient experiences a significant disruption of body fluid homeostasis in the postoperative period. Blood loss and loss of fluid by evaporation from exposed organs during extensive surgery can lead to dehydration, especially if perioperative and immediate postoperative fluid replacement is inadequate. Continued blood loss, wound drainage, gastrointestinal suction, and fever may contribute to dehydration and electrolyte imbalance postoperatively. Paradoxically surgery may also cause water retention with hyponatraemia and a decreased serum osmolarity. There is a risk of shock with extensive blood loss, infection, and trauma. Nursing vigilance in assessing and monitoring fluid and electrolyte status, cardiovascular parameters, and fluid replacement therapy is critical.

Altered Respiratory Function

Although modern techniques of anaesthesia have greatly reduced the risks, respiratory complications remain the most frequently reported postoperative problem and are the cause of death in about 25% of surgical fatalities (Moossa et al., 1991).

Anaesthesia and surgery cause changes in respiratory function (Risser, 1980), and the central nervous system control of ventilation, the musculoskeletal mechanics of breathing, and lung physiology are all affected. In most cases general anaesthesia involves the use of skeletal muscle relaxants and a period of mechanical ventilation. Muscle relaxants include the short-acting depolarizing muscle relaxants (e.g. suxamethonium) and the longer acting nondepolarizing relaxants (e.g. tubocurarine, pancuronium). The effects of the nondepolarizing muscle relaxants are reversed by administering an anticholinesterase (e.g. neostigmine), but the anticholinesterases are associated with muscarinic side effects, including bradycardia and bronchospasm. The general effects of anaesthesia, mechanical ventilation, and postoperative analgesia depress respiratory function and suppress reflexes such as coughing, periodic deep sighs, and yawning, which normally help clear secretions and expand collapsed alveoli.

The respiratory effects of surgery and anaesthesia include atelectasis and pneumonia, pulmonary aspiration and aspiration pneumonia, pulmonary oedema, immediate postoperative respiratory depression (usually evident in the recovery suite), and acute respiratory failure. Patients will usually be fully recovered before they return to the ward, but it is important to continue monitoring respiratory activity in the immediate postoperative period.

Impaired Skin and Tissue Integrity

Surgery involves tissue destruction and usually some breaching of skin integrity. With a clean surgical incision there should be minimal tissue loss and the wound will heal by primary intention. However, the surgical nurse should be aware of the likely manipulation and loss of tissues from internal structures, which can be extensive. Trauma and the healing process massively increase nutritional and metabolic demands, and a small incision does not necessarily mean that the healing process is minor. Healing of the surface wound is only one part of surgical healing. Wound healing is discussed in more detail in Chapter 9.

Altered Patterns of Elimination

Surgery and anaesthesia will disrupt bladder and bowel function, and depending upon the surgical problem and the extent of trauma, this can range from a transient to a permanent problem.

Postoperative urinary retention is common, but usually self-limiting. However, acute renal failure can develop in patients with postoperative oliguria. It is important to note that surgery and anaesthesia can increase plasma antidiuretic hormone (ADH) concentrations and this effect may be sustained by postoperative pain. The surgical nurse should therefore monitor urine flow and concentration during the immediate postoperative period.

Surgery, particularly of the abdomen, can disrupt gastrointestinal function. Peristalsis may be slow or sluggish, uncoordinated (adynamic ileus), or absent in part or all of the bowel (paralytic ileus). Nausea and vomiting are common after surgery. Wound drains, fistulae, gastrointestinal suction, and diarrhoea can all contribute to altered elimination.

Altered Consciousness and Neurological Function

General anaesthesia is an induced loss of consciousness. This is normally rapidly reversed at the end of anaesthesia, but some patients, particularly the elderly, may be sensitive to anaesthetic agents and recover much more slowly. The surgical patient is likely to experience some fear and anxiety, and postoperative confusion is not uncommon when an elderly patient recovers in strange surroundings. Factors such as sleep deprivation, pain, infection, fever, and dehydration may also contribute to postoperative confusion, psychosis, or delirium. If the surgery involves the brain or spinal cord, trauma can disrupt neurological function. There are few dangers from epidural or spinal anaesthesia provided surgery and perioperative care are managed properly. However, it is important to ensure that full leg movement has returned after anaesthesia and that the patient is excreting satisfactorily.

Altered Body Image

Perception of physical appearance is an important component of the concept of self and can have a major influence on psychosocial functioning. This body image may differ substantially from the individual's actual appearance and can be an important factor in perception of self-worth, sexuality, and self-confidence. Illness and surgery can undermine this body image, and surgery such as amputation, mastectomy, genital surgery, or stoma formation can be a major source of morbidity.

SURGICAL NURSING

Surgical nursing is concerned with supporting patients as they move through all phases of their surgical experience. The surgical patient may require support during the diagnostic process, preoperative preparation, the perioperative period, the immediate postoperative period, and during preparation for discharge and rehabilitation.

Patients require surgery for a wide range of conditions ranging from removal of a sebaceous cyst under local anaesthesia by a general practitioner to conditions requiring major surgery, hours of general anaesthesia, and extensive teams of surgical specialists. However, the basic principles of surgical nursing will apply in all cases and can be used to develop appropriate individualized plans of care. The pattern of care delivered is highly dependent on the individual patient, the nature of the condition, and the surgical interventions. The diagnostic process may be relatively simple or may require days or weeks of extensive investigations. Surgery itself may be on a day basis or require extensive preoperative preparation and postoperative rehabilitation. The role of the surgical nurse therefore varies depending on each individual patient's surgical needs.

Central to effective surgical nursing are assessment, observation, and knowledge. A knowledge of the principles of surgical nursing, disease processes, diagnostic procedures, surgical procedures, and associated risks and complications, combined with assessment of the individual patient are key factors in effective care planning. Nightingale observed the effects of environment on patients' health and suggested that nursing should facilitate 'the body's reparative process' by manipulating environmental factors such as nutrition, hygiene, and sanitation. Today in surgical nursing the emphasis might be on knowledge and education as a way of allowing patients to improve their manipulation of their environment to facilitate the reparative process. However, we would agree with Nightingale in recognizing the importance of basic factors such as hygiene and nutrition.

Box 1.2 **Maslow's hierarchy of needs.**

1 **Physiological needs**
   - Relief from thirst
   - Relief from hunger
   - Sleep
   - Sex
   - Relief from pain
   - Relief from physiological imbalances

2 **Safety needs**
   - Security
   - Protection
   - Freedom from danger
   - Order
   - Predictable future

3 **Love and belonging needs**
   - Friends
   - Companions
   - Family
   - Group identification
   - Intimacy

4 **Esteem needs**
   - Respect
   - Confidence based on good opinion of others
   - Admiration
   - Self-confidence
   - Self-worth
   - Self-acceptance

5 **Self-actualization needs**
   - Fulfil personal capabilities
   - Develop one's potential
   - Do what one's best suited to do
   - Grow and expand metaneeds to discover truth, to create beauty, to produce order, to promote justice

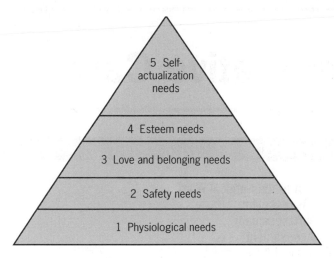

Figure 1.1 Maslow's hierarchy of needs.

Maslow (1970) presented a view of human needs that can be useful for assessing needs and priorities in nursing (Torrance and Jordan, 1995) and proposed a hierarchy of lower and higher needs, with physiological needs forming the broad base of the pyramid and self-actualization as the pinnacle (*Figure 1.1*, *Box 1.2*). Physiological, safety, love and belonging, and esteem needs were classed as deficit needs, and self-actualization as growth needs. Maslow considered that the lower needs took priority over higher needs. The lower needs had to be at least partly satisfied before an individual could be motivated to meet higher needs and move towards self-actualization. In surgical nursing this can be a useful approach. In the surgical setting nursing interventions aim to help with both deficit and growth needs, but ensuring immediate physiological and safety needs is a priority. If the patient–nurse interaction is effective in meeting these basic needs it can then offer assistance in meeting higher needs. If patients do not feel secure in their basic physiological and safety needs they are less likely to trust the nurse to help them to meet higher needs. Surgical nursing must help patients meet physiological and safety deficits before it can be trusted by both patients and families and help with higher order needs.

References

Malby R (1991) Audit audibility in a nursing development unit. *Nurs Times* **87(19)**:35–37.

Maslow A (1970) *Motivation and Personality*, 2nd edition, pp. 17–26. Harper & Row, New York.

Moossa AR, Mayer AD, Lavelle-Jones M (1991) Surgical complications. In *Textbook of Surgery*, 14th edition. Sabiston JD (ed.), pp. 299–316. WB Saunders, Philadephia.

Risser N (1980) Preoperative and postoperative care to prevent postoperative pulmonary complications. *Heart & Lung* **9(1)**:57–67.

Torrance C, Jordan S (1995) Bionursing: putting science into practice. *Nurs Stand* **9(49)**:25–27.

Chapter 2
Preoperative Care

CONTENTS

Patients will present for elective, planned, or emergency surgery. If the surgery is elective the patient will probably have had a range of medical consultations and diagnostic tests. In emergency surgery the patient is likely to have been admitted via the accident and emergency department and to present with acute symptoms and without time for extensive preoperative investigations. Preoperative care can encompass the complete process from first consultation and outpatient investigations to admission and preoperative preparation. However, this chapter will concentrate on the preoperative care of the patient admitted for an elective procedure. The same basic steps will be required for emergency or day surgery, but there is much less time for assessment, patient education, and preoperative preparation.

ADMISSION TO THE SURGICAL WARD

Patients entering hospital, whether as planned or emergency admissions, will have needs that will vary according to their past experiences and knowledge of events to follow. They may be apprehensive and frightened, and it is essential that first impressions are positive. When patients arrive at hospital, the staff should be friendly and welcoming; the unexpected patient for whom no provision has been made should be kept as unaware of this fact as possible. Patients who can move about should be shown facilities such as toilets, bathrooms, day rooms, and the telephone. They should also be shown the fire exits. New patients can be introduced to their neighbours and to the nurses who will care for them during their stay.

Any written information that may have been sent to the patient before admission, may need to be reinforced with further details if necessary, for example any restrictions on visiting hours and smoking. Facilities for locking away personal valuables should be made available, but most hospitals encourage the patient to retain the minimum of valuable property while on the ward. The patient's locker should be furnished with fresh water and a glass if the patient is allowed to drink. Information about the usual meal times, availability of tea and coffee and the times of newspaper rounds should be provided, while adjustment of the radio and call bell should be explained. If possible, the patient should be told when the doctor will visit, what investigations are planned.

Ideally this early introduction to the ward should be carried out by the nurse who will be responsible for making the nursing assessment and supporting the patient during the hospital stay. An identification band bearing the patient's full name, date of birth, and hospital number is placed on the patient's wrist by the admitting nurse and is usually worn throughout the stay in hospital. The patient's partner or family may also appreciate some information about the ward and its routines.

PATIENT ASSESSMENT

When patients have had time to become accustomed to the ward, their psychological, social, and physical state should be assessed by the admitting nurse. It is important to remember that the preoperative patient is likely to be very anxious and may be confused by even the simplest question. Vital signs will be elevated by anxiety. It is better to take the history first, so that the patient can get used to the new environment before measuring vital signs. Reviewing or recapping the answers to the first few questions will allow time for the patient to relax and feel more in control.

The admission process should not be rushed. The patient may need time to answer questions, to express anxieties, and to ask questions. When admitting patients, make sure that they know that you will be available and pleased to clarify any information not previously understood and that they may ask questions that may have arisen subsequent to the admission interview. It may not be possible to obtain the full history in one sitting if the patient is anxious or uncomfortable or if it is interrupted by diagnostic tests or medical consultations. In this case essential information can be obtained and a preliminary assessment to establish priority needs carried out. A more detailed assessment can follow later.

The general information needed when taking the patient's history is as follows:

- Biographical information (e.g. name, age, occupation, religion).
- Reason for admission.
- Current illness and health status (including any medications, symptoms, complaints, and disabilities).

- Previous medical history (including hospitalization, clinics, chronic illness).
- Family medical history.
- Nutritional history (including eating and drinking habits or preferences, food allergies, religious or other dietary preferences, eating problems).

The preoperative assessment is also based on more detailed information to identify factors that may influence surgical risk as follows:

- Cardiovascular and haematological function.
- Respiratory function.
- Neurological status.
- Renal function.
- Gastrointestinal function.
- Endocrine function.
- Nutritional status.
- Hepatic function.
- Immunological status and infection.

Box 2.1 summarizes the general surgical risk factors, but specific types of surgery may involve additional risk factors.

Cardiovascular and Haematological Function

Does the patient have any history of cardiovascular disease? Any disease resulting in a reduced cardiac output is likely to increase the risk of both pre- and postoperative complications, and almost all general anaesthetic agents and adjuncts have effects on the cardiovascular system. The degree of risk will vary and surgery may need to be postponed or the approach to anaesthesia may need revision. It is important to note and report any signs, symptoms, or problems that indicate cardiovascular disease such as hypertension, palpitations, chest pain at rest or on exertion, breathlessness or dyspnoea, lung congestion, oedema, or abdominal tenderness.

Are there any indications of peripheral vascular disease such as cold extremities, claudication, numbness or tingling in the fingers or toes (paraesthesia), poor peripheral pulses, or oedema of the limbs.

Anaemia or coagulation disorders will increase surgical risks. Impaired coagulation in bleeding disorders will increase the risk of peri- and postoperative haemorrhage, haematoma formation, delayed wound healing, and postoperative wound infection. It is also likely to alter the use of anticoagulant prophylaxis for deep venous thrombosis (DVT) and pulmonary embolism (PE) in the pre- and postoperative periods. Conversely any previous history of DVT or venous disease may require a more aggressive approach to DVT prevention. The following preoperative factors (listed in order of significance) were identified by Goldman *et al.* (1977) as being associated with the development of cardiac complications in the postoperative period:

Box 2.1 Operative risk factors.

General and systemic factors
- Aged over 70 years (the very young are also at risk)
- Overall physical status
- Number of concurrent illnesses
- Duration and extent of the operative procedure
- Emergency vs elective procedure
- Extreme weight (i.e. over- or underweight)
- Nutritional deficits
- Hypovolaemia or dehydration
- Electrolyte imbalances
- Infection and sepsis
- Immunological problems

Cardiovascular disease
- Coronary artery disease
- Previous myocardial infarction
- Cardiac arrhthymias
- Cardiac failure
- Hypertension
- Valvular disease
- History of thromboembolism
- Haemorrhagic disorders
- Cerebrovascular disease

Respiratory disease
- Thoracic or upper abdominal surgery
- Chronic obstructive airways disease
- Purulent cough
- Smoking
- Anaesthesia longer than three hours

Renal disease

Endocrine alterations
- Diabetes mellitus
- Adrenal conditions
- Thyroid disease
- Pregnancy

Liver disease

- Jugular vein distension.
- Myocardial infarction in the previous six months.
- Premature atrial contractions or other dysrhythmia.
- 3–5 premature ventricular contractions per minute.
- Aged 70 years plus.
- Significant aortic valve stenosis.
- Poor general medical condition.

Respiratory Function

Factors affecting respiratory function are important for the patient facing surgery. If the patient smokes, a detailed history of the habit is required. How long has the patient smoked? How many cigarettes a day? Has the patient recently stopped smoking? Carbon monoxide in cigarette smoke forms a complex with haemoglobin (carboxyhaemoglobin) that reduces the oxygen-carrying capacity of blood. In addition smoking damages the epithelium lining respiratory structures, impairing protective mechanisms and predisposing to cough and infections. Smoking is a major factor increasing the risk of postoperative pulmonary complications and ideally the smoker should give up smoking for 4–6 weeks, but at least for one week before surgery. Also note any recent respiratory infection, allergic conditions (asthma or hay fever), previous reactions to general anaesthetics, other respiratory disease such as chronic obstructive airways disease (COAD) (e.g. asthma, chronic bronchitis, emphysema). If the patient has a cough, find out more about the type, pattern, and nature of any sputum produced.

It is also important to obtain information on factors that might affect lung expansion and the mechanics of breathing. Is the patient mobile or immobile? Is the patient in pain? Thoracic or abdominal pain can make breathing uncomfortable; shallow breathing limits respiratory movements and is therefore more comfortable, but reduces lung expansion and will increase the risk of postoperative chest infection. Sedatives and postoperative analgesics may also reduce ventilation. Specific risk factors associated with the development of postoperative respiratory problems include:

- Thoracic and upper abdominal surgery.
- A history of cigarette smoking.
- Preoperative history of COAD.
- Preoperative history of productive purulent cough.
- Aged 60 years plus.
- Obesity.
- Poor preoperative nutritional state.
- Duration of anaesthesia longer than three hours.
- An abnormal chest radiograph.
- Abnormal findings on respiratory examination.
- Any symptoms of respiratory disease.

(Houston *et al.*, 1987)

Neurological Status

Record any history of neurological disorders, for example epilepsy ('fits'), Parkinson's disease, multiple sclerosis, or myasthenia gravis. Medications used to treat these conditions might need to be reviewed during the pre- and postoperative period. Generalized indicators of possible neurological disease such as headaches, migraine, paraesthesia, tremors or weakness, gait problems, memory loss, confusion, or perceptual disturbances should be noted. This is critical for discriminating between the complications of surgery or anaesthesia and ongoing or drug-related problems in the postoperative period. Use of other drugs that affect the nervous system, for example sedatives, antidepressants, anxiolytics, and neuroleptics must also be recorded. The use of narcotic drugs or alcohol must be explored, but patients with addictions to drugs or alcohol may try to hide their problem. As the elderly constitute a major proportion of those requiring surgery, a careful assessment is needed to identify any indication of cerebrovascular disease.

Renal Function

The patient's history should establish any current or previous complaints of kidney or bladder dysfunction. If the patient has had renal or bladder problems, when was the last episode? Does the patient experience pain in the back or suprapubic regions that might be connected to the kidneys? Chronic renal disease, the use of incontinence aids, urinary bladder catheterization, or possession of a urostomy should be recorded and considered when preparing the care plan. Urinary infections may be asymptomatic and only detected by urinalysis, and patients are more likely to experience urine retention in the postoperative period if they have prostatic hypertrophy.

It is important to establish whether the patient has any symptoms of urinary tract disease:

- Has the patient noted any change or problem with micturition?
- Is there any change in urgency or frequency of urination?
- Is there any pain or burning sensation on urination?
- Has the patient noticed blood in the urine (haematuria).
- For the male patient in particular, is there any history of urgency, frequency, reduced urine stream or hesitant flow, incomplete emptying of the bladder, or nocturia (more than twice a night)?
- In the female patient are there any indicators of stress incontinence, such as passing urine, on coughing, or laughing.

Improvements in perioperative care and maintenance of appropriate hydration have greatly reduced the risk of major renal complications after surgery, but if there is any history of renal disease, a full preoperative assessment, including appropriate clearance studies, is indicated.

Gastrointestinal Function

Nutritional status is an important factor before surgery and the nurse should ask about the patient's general gastrointestinal function. Nausea, vomiting, diarrhoea, constipation, flatulence, bleeding from the upper or lower gastrointestinal tract, current or previous gastrointestinal ulcers, and inflammatory or diverticular bowel disease can all be significant as all anaesthetics and analgesics affect the gastrointestinal system.

Endocrine Function

A number of endocrine disorders can have an impact on surgical risk. Diabetes mellitus increases the risk of some postoperative complications, for example delayed wound healing and postoperative infection, as well as the risk of postoperative hyper- or hypoglycaemia. The effect of any preoperative investigations (especially if they involve periods of fasting), surgery, and anaesthesia on diabetic control will need to be discussed. Is the patient currently taking glucocorticosteroid drugs or taken them within the last year. Surgery causes a major activation of neuroendocrine mechanisms and additional preoperative tests may be needed if the patient has had or is on glucocorticosteroid therapy. Chronic alcoholism also alters endocrine function and additional pre- and postoperative precautions may be needed. Pregnancy can also complicate surgery and anaesthesia because it has major effects on the maternal endocrine system and physiological reserves.

Nutritional Status

A detailed dietary and clinical history will provide a range of information on estimated food and fluid intake, normal eating habits, food preferences and dislikes, medications, medical conditions, and other factors that may influence the intake, digestion, and absorption of nutrients. Miller and Torrance (1991) identify the following points as important when taking a detailed nutritional history:

- Patients' perceptions of their normal weight and any recent weight loss or gain.
- Changes in appetite and changes in taste or smell.
- Dental problems or problems with badly fitting dentures.
- Food restrictions, whether due to allergies, cultural or ethnic factors, individual choices (e.g. vegetarian), dieting, or general likes and dislikes.
- Food habits.
- Economic or social factors, which might affect food intake (e.g. cooking facilities).
- Medical conditions restricting intake or affecting gastrointestinal function.
- Medications (e.g. laxatives, antibiotics).

- Use of alcohol or drugs.
- Usual physical activity and exercise.

Box 2.2 provides a complete summary of the type of data required from a nutritional history.

Box 2.2 **Data required from a dietary and clinical history (Miller and Torrance, 1991).**

Activity level
- Occupation
- Exercise

Appetite
- Good, poor, recent changes?
- Changes and problems with the sense of taste or smell
- Effects of stress

Factors influencing food habits
- Cultural and ethnic influences
- Religion
- Educational level
- Nutritional knowledge and insight
- Eating patterns and family meal pattern

Gastrointestinal status
- Indigestion, 'heartburn'
- Flatulence, constipation
- Diarrhoea

Medical conditions
- Chronic disease (e.g. diabetes mellitus, ulcerative colitis, coeliac disease)
- Special diet (e.g. diabetic diet, low salt diet, lactose-free diet)

Social drug use
- Alcohol consumption (amount and frequency)
- Smoking
- Other recreational drugs

Economic and social factors
- Income and spending on food
- Social benefits and services
- Cooking facilities and other services (e.g. meals on wheels)

Foods
- Likes and dislikes
- Type and amount

> **Box 2.2** (*continued*)
>
> - Food restrictions (e.g. due to allergies, intolerance)
> - Fluid intake (type, amount, and frequency)
>
> **Medications**
> - Type, dose, frequency
> - Length of treatment
> - Use of laxatives and emetics
> - Vitamins or other supplements
>
> **Other problems**
> - Dental problems, dentures
> - Problems with chewing or swallowing
> - Physical or mental handicap

Hepatic Function

The liver is the main site for metabolizing drugs and nutrients and any impairment of hepatic function will affect the patient's response to anaesthesia and surgery. If the patient has known or suspected liver disease a full range of preoperative liver function tests will be required. If the patient has extensive cirrhosis a lengthy period of preoperative preparation may be needed before surgery, and some factors associated with cirrhosis may preclude any surgery except for immediate life-saving operations (Polk, 1991).

Immunological Status and Infection

It is important that any allergies or hypersensitivity to food, drugs, skin preparations, surgical tapes, and similar agents are recorded. Reactions can range from those that cause minor irritation, to those with fatal consequences. It is also important to find out if the patient has recently suffered or been exposed to infections that might mean that surgery should be postponed. Alerting staff to the presence of specific infections such as hepatitis B or human immunodeficiency virus (HIV) infection will help ensure rigorous precautions are taken to prevent cross-infection. Any local or systemic symptoms of infection should be recorded and reported. Does the patient have a fever, lymph node enlargement, malaise, or rashes? Are there any specific indications of urinary infection, upper or lower respiratory tract infection, or infection near the point of surgical entry (e.g. skin irritation, rashes, boils)? The following factors have been associated with decreased host resistance and an increased risk of postoperative infection by Polk (1991):

- Increasing age.
- Obesity or malnutrition.

- Diabetic ketoacidosis.
- Glucocorticosteroid therapy.
- Immunosuppressive drugs.
- Infection.
- Cancer (some types).
- Radiotherapy.
- Adrenocortical insufficiency.
- Early shaving of operative site.
- Percutaneous foreign bodies.

PHYSICAL ASSESSMENT

A full preoperative physical assessment is required to establish baseline data and to identify factors that may increase the risk of postoperative complications. The physical assessment may be carried out by the doctor or by the nurse admitting the patient depending on hospital practice. In the UK the full physical assessment is normally a medical task, but with the developing extending role of the nurse and the introduction of nurse practitioners this may change. Each of the other phases of the nursing process depends upon the quality of the assessment data for their effectiveness and assessment is a critical element of the nursing process. The admitting nurse will certainly record vital signs and carry out a basic assessment of height, weight, skin condition, and general appearance. If a full physical assessment is carried out by medical staff the admitting nurse should consult the notes to check the results.

Baseline observations are used to assess immediate and continuing postoperative responses. They should include temperature, pulse, respiration rate, blood pressure, weight, and urinalysis, and should be charted and included on charts used in the operating theatre. Any abnormalities should be reported as the operation may need to be postponed for further investigation or to allow relevant treatment to be started.

Any specimens such as urine, sputum, or swabs should be obtained only after the patient has been given clear and specific explanation of how they will be obtained and why they are required. This also applies to any investigations carried out by other staff. Specimens must be clearly labelled and sent for the appropriate investigations. The results of these investigations should be available before the patient goes to the operating theatre.

An assessment of mobility must be included at this time:

- Is the patient able to carry out a normal range of daily activities?
- Can the patient move about freely or are there gait or balance problems?
- Can the patient cope independently with activities such as dressing, hygiene, eating, and elimination, or are mobility aids or help from carers required?

It is important that the patient's own mobility goals are identified and understood by the staff, and that the patient's goals compare with those of the staff. Pugh and Millar (1989) point out that mobility limitations, for example an intravenous infusion, can have a great effect on an individual's postoperative activity (see Chapter 4), and each limitation should be explained during assessment.

In addition to weight and vital signs a comprehensive physical assessment involves a systematic assessment of all body systems using the techniques of inspection, palpation, percussion, and auscultation. Physical assessment also includes a general inspection, assessment of the skin, hair and nails, and a nutritional assessment. Key elements of the physical assessment of surgical patients are discussed below, but the reader is referred to Chapter 14 for a more detailed discussion of the techniques of physical assessment.

Cardiovascular Assessment

Cardiovascular disease, congenital heart disease, coronary heart disease, valve disorders, cardiac arrhythmias, heart failure, peripheral vascular disease, anaemia, and blood disorders increase surgical risk. Even asymptomatic or minor conditions can increase the risk during surgery and the postoperative period. When assessing the surgical patient the nurse should note any signs or symptoms that indicate a reduced cardiac output or peripheral vascular disease (*Box 2.3*). Inspection may reveal pallor or cyanosis. Cold and discoloured extremities may indicate peripheral vascular disease, while finger clubbing can be a sign of cardiac or respiratory problems. Auscultation may reveal a range of

---

Box 2.3 Signs and symptoms of cardiovascular disease.

Decreased cardiac output
- Shortness of breath
- Fatigue on exertion or rest
- Syncope, orthostatic hypotension
- Hypotension
- Arrhythmia
- Irregular pulse
- Oedema

Peripheral vascular disease
- Diminished or absent peripheral pulses
- Pulse asymmetry
- Claudication
- Oedema
- Varicose veins
- Signs of DVT
- Temperature changes

abnormal heart sounds and murmurs. A preoperative electrocardiogram (ECG) is required if any cardiac problems are suspected.

Respiratory Assessment

Any indication of respiratory infection (e.g. coughing or wheezing, nasal discharge, inflammation of the throat or tonsils) should be noted. The neck and chest wall should be observed:

- Are accessory muscles being used?
- Is the chest normal in shape? An abnormal chest shape such as a barrel or pigeon chest may indicate longstanding respiratory disease.
- Is there any intercostal or substernal retraction?
- Is chest wall movement symmetrical?
- Is the patient tachypnoeic or bradypnoeic?
- Is the patient hypoventilating or hyperventilating?
- What is the rhythm or pattern of breathing?
- Inspection, palpation, and auscultation can be used to identify a range of respiratory problems.

Nutritional Assessment

Nutritional status can have a major effect on recovery from surgery. The skills required to obtain a nutritional history and assess nutritional status are not difficult and should become part of the general nursing assessment of a patient (Miller and Torrance, 1991). The nurse needs to be able to assess the general appearance of the patient, carry out some simple anthropometric measurements, and understand the nutritional implications of the results of certain blood tests. Physical signs of malnutrition are often a late manifestation, while a number of factors may suggest malnutrition, but are not definitive indicators. The patient's general appearance, fit of clothes and condition of hair, skin, eyes, mouth, and neurological and musculoskeletal system should be noted. Box 2.4 provides a brief summary of changes to look out for in the physical assessment. These changes are more likely to be seen in the very elderly, in patients with chronic health problems, and in patients suffering from neglect or problems such as chronic alcoholism.

The depth of nutritional assessment required will depend on the individual, the nature of the surgical problem, and the expected postoperative prognosis. If extensive surgery, with a protracted period of postoperative hospitalization and rehabilitation is expected, particularly surgery involving the gastrointestinal tract, a full nutritional assessment involving the dietician will be required. If the surgery is relatively minor, a nutritional history and simple anthropometric measurements such as weight and height may be sufficient. If nutritional problems are identified, for example obesity, undernutrition, or eating disorders, a full nutritional assessment may be indicated.

Box 2.4 Clinical signs of nutritional significance with associated deficiency in parentheses (Miller and Torrance, 1991).

Hair
- Dull or dry (PEM)
- Thin or sparse
- Easily falls out
- Loss of colour
- Alopecia (essential fatty acids)

Face
- Moon face (PEM)
- Enlarged thyroid (iodine)
- Nasolabial seborrhoea (riboflavin, niacin, zinc)
- Seborrhoeic dermatitis

Eyes
- Dryness, softening, inflammation of cornea (vitamin A, vitamin B complex, iron, folate)
- Pale conjunctiva
- Keratomalacia
- Loss of vision or night blindness

Lips
- Angular stomatitis, cheilosis (riboflavin, niacin, iron)

Tongue
- Glossitis, red, swollen (folate, vitamin B complex, iron)

Gums
- Reddened, spongy, receding, bleeding (vitamin C)

Nails
- Spoon shaped (iron)

Skin
- Dryness, petechiae, ecchymoses, oedema, colour changes, texture changes (vitamins A, C, K, niacin)
- Follicular hyperkeratosis
- Pellagrous dermatosis

Musculoskeletal
- Fat and muscle wasting (PEM, vitamin D)
- Fatigue, stiffness, pain

Neurological
- Paraesthesia, sensory loss (B complex, thiamine, PEM)
- Irritability, confusion, depression
- Motor weakness, hyporeflexia

(PEM, protein–energy malnutrition)

The patient's general appearance is assessed as discussed above. Is the patient obviously obese or cachexic? Weight is an essential measurement for all patients and is the most commonly used indicator of nutritional status, but weight and height together may be more informative. Weight and height can be used for comparison with ideal weight for height and sex obtained from standard weight and height tables. Weight and height can also be used to calculate the body mass index (BMI), which provides a simple and useful method of recording changes in nutritional status (see Chapter 6). Weight and height should be recorded on admission. To ensure accuracy, particularly if serial measurements are carried out, the patient should be weighed on the same scales, at the same time each day preferably in the same clothes, and after emptying bladder and bowels. Scales, as with any measurement equipment, have to be regularly checked for accuracy. Additional simple anthropometric measurements that can be routinely used include skinfold thickness and upper arm circumference. Anthropometric and laboratory investigations used to assess and monitor nutritional status are discussed in more detail in Chapter 6.

Gastrointestinal Assessment

Note any abdominal distension. Are gut sounds normal? The history should have identified any problems such as constipation or diarrhoea. Any indication of problems with intestinal motility or peristalsis must be reported because of the risk of nausea, vomiting, and reduced intestinal motility (paralytic ileus) postoperatively.

Urinary System Assessment

It is important to note any signs of urinary tract infection, to monitor urine output, and to carry out a routine urinalysis. The results of urinalysis may suggest an infection or other problems in a patient who is otherwise asymptomatic. Any indication of prostatic hyperplasia should also be reported, as the patient will have a much greater risk of postoperative urine retention.

SOCIAL ASSESSMENT

Information about the patient's social, family, and domestic circumstances are relevant in planning pre- and postoperative care and discharge arrangements. Any information directly relevant to the surgical outcome is essential, for example is there a responsible adult able to help care for the patient immediately after discharge? The *Patient's Charter* (1995) recommends that prior to discharge from hospital, patients should expect a decision to be made about how to meet any continuing needs that they may have. Discharge planning should be commenced before admission for non-emergency cases. If not, the planning should be started at the time of the initial nursing assessment in collaboration with the patient. The social work department may be able to help reassure the patient if there are family or financial worries.

PSYCHOLOGICAL ASSESSMENT

A hospital can cause patients to feel confused and lonely. Many patients have not been in hospital before and do not know what to expect. Patients may be anxious about the effects of the anaesthetic: they may fear not waking up after the operation or that waking up while the operation is still in progress. They may also have a fear of unrelieved pain, or of being restricted after the operation, for example of having to use a bed pan. They may fear distortion of body image and the effect this may have on their relationship with their partner or family. There may be worries about the family, perhaps about children or dependent relatives, and there may be fears about financial problems, particularly if the patient is the sole financial provider for the family.

The nurse must assess how much patients understand about their condition and what is to happen to them. The value of preoperative teaching in relieving anxieties related to uncertainty is discussed later. Fear of pain can be alleviated by explaining the measures that will be taken to control any pain. A pain scale can be introduced to patients at this point to ensure that they understand the significance of the various ranges on the scale. Patient-controlled analgesia can be explained to the patient and used in the immediate postoperative period. An assessment of the emotional state of patients and how they are responding to hospitalization and the impending surgery is important. Many writers empha-size the need for the nurse to explain the experience of surgery and anaesthesia, which requires careful judgement of the patient's readiness for learning (Oakley, 1984; Castledine, 1988; Swindale, 1989).

PREOPERATIVE NURSING CARE

Consent

Explanation and reassurance must be continued throughout the preoperative period. The doctor and the patient will have discussed the procedure and completed a consent form. Jameton (1984) points out that in a conversation where informed consent is sought, the information should cover:

■ The procedure offered.
■ Reasonable alternatives to the procedure.
■ Possible benefits of the procedure to the patient.
■ Risks, inconveniences, and discomforts of the procedure.
■ Answers to all the patient's questions.

The criteria for valid informed consent are given in *Box 2.5*.

Box 2.5 Criteria for informed consent (adapted from Douglas and Larson, 1986).

Voluntary
■ Consent must be given freely without coercion to be valid.

Competent
■ The patient must be competent. Incompetent patients (e.g. those who are comatose or seriously mentally ill) cannot give or withhold consent.

Comprehension
■ Information should be given both verbally and in writing in language that is understandable to the patient. The patient must be offered opportunities to ask questions to explain or expand on the information presented.

Informed
■ Written consent should be obtained identifying that the subject has received and understood:
  ■ An explanation of the surgical procedure.
  ■ An explanation of any risks of the procedure.
  ■ A description of the benefits.
  ■ An opportunity to ask questions.
  ■ An explanation of any deviation from normal protocols.
  ■ An explanation that they have the right to withdraw consent.

The nurse has an important role in ensuring informed consent. The key is that the patient must fully understand what is being consented to and the nurse can reinforce information provided by the doctor and check the level of comprehension. There is a potential for conflict if medical information is withheld or nursing staff feel that the patient's understanding of the procedure is limited. Incomplete information or incomplete understanding undermine the validity of the consent obtained. If the patient is unable to give informed consent it is usual to discuss the surgery with the relatives, but they do not have the legal right to give or withhold consent. In this case the surgeon has to act in the patient's best interests. Relatives also have no legal right to request that information be withheld from a patient. Again the nurses and doctors have to be guided by the patient's best interests. Information about the specific timing of events such as the time the premedication drug will be given and the approximate time the patient will go to the operating theatre and return to the ward may help reduce anxiety.

Relatives and friends who visit the patient must be informed of the approximate time of the operation and what time to telephone for news concerning the patient's immediate postoperative condition. Castledine (1988) emphasizes the value of involving family members or significant others in the patient's preoperative preparation. It is often a family member who will encourage the patient to carry out postoperative exercises and comply with the care plan. Involved relatives may also help the patient understand postoperative events and therefore reduce anxiety.

Preoperative Information Giving and Patient Education

Individuals vary in their response to surgery, but preoperative anxiety and stress linked to uncertainty and 'anticipatory fear' is common. The prospect of surgery can induce a variety of fears: fear of anaesthesia; fear of pain or death; fear of the effects on body image; fear of separation from the familiar and loved; and fear of the unknown. Factors contributing to preoperative anxiety include:

■ Uncertainty about diagnosis and prognosis.
■ An unfamiliar environment and lack of knowledge about ward routine and one's role and behaviour.
■ A lack of experience or knowledge about medical and nursing procedures and what to expect in the pre- and postoperative periods.
■ Loss of control of one's own life and environment.

Ramsay (1972) and Ray (1982), for example, have identified stress associated with surgery under a general anaesthetic, and Volicer and Volicer (1978) have demonstrated that surgical patients have a higher stress score than other patients. People under stress heal more slowly (Kiecolt-Glaser et al., 1995). High levels of preoperative anxiety have been linked with:

■ The need for higher doses of anaesthetic agents (Williams et al., 1972).
■ The need for more postoperative analgesia (Hayward, 1975).
■ A higher frequency of postoperative complications (Janis, 1974).
■ Longer postoperative hospitalization (Egbart et al., 1964).

Preoperative information provision and education can allay anxiety and improve physical and psychological preparation for surgery. Nurses have had a major role in developing effective preoperative teaching strategies that can alleviate stress and improve postoperative healing (Hayward, 1975; Boore 1978; Johnson, 1983). Structured teaching about preoperative procedures, anaesthesia, surgery, and what to expect in the postoperative period has many benefits, including:

■ Better compliance with preoperative breathing exercises.
■ Improved postoperative ventilatory capacity (Lindeman and van Aernam, 1971).
■ Improved compliance with postoperative activities and higher patient satisfaction (Wong and Wong, 1985).
■ Earlier ambulation.

- A reduction in postoperative analgesia.
- A reducion in postoperative hospitalization.

Preoperative education allows the patient to become an active participant in his own care and recovery. Effective teaching strategies are based on assessing a particular patient's needs using individually focused approaches rather than routine repetitive teaching programmes. Bellman (1994) suggests that the surgical nurse should avoid making assumptions about patients' preferences. The nurse should check with the patient about:

- The educational approaches (e.g. group or individual) with which the patient feels most comfortable.
- The timing of teaching.
- The type of information that is required and can be assimilated during the various stages of the surgical experience.

Pre-admission clinics

In modern surgery the period of hospitalization required for even quite major procedures is decreasing rapidly. Patients may be admitted less than 24 hours before surgery and discharged one or two days after surgery. Pre-admission or pre-assessment clinics are developing into an important aspect of preoperative preparation. They allow the patient to be assessed 10–14 days before surgery and the clinics can be staffed by outpatient, surgical, or theatre nurses (Breeze, 1995). In the clinic patients meet hospital staff who will be involved in their care and have the opportunity to ask questions. A full assessment can be carried out and the proposed operation rescheduled if the patient proves to be unfit for surgery. The clinic can be the first stage in discharge planning. Verbal information can be supplemented with written information, and postoperative care can be discussed and planned with the patient. Newton (1996) listed the aims of a pre-admission clinic as follows:

- To minimize cancellations and maximize use of theatre time and inpatient beds.
- To improve admission procedures and assessment.
- To improve discharge planning.
- To allow a full and thorough patient education and preparation for surgery.

Pre-admission clinics were first developed in orthopaedics, but are now used by day surgery units, general surgery, and other specialities. Newton (1996) noted that patients:

- Felt less anxious having met staff and visited the ward.
- Liked having a chance to clarify details such as dates, times, points of contact.
- Were glad of the opportunity to discuss the operation with the doctor.
- Appeciated the opportunity to discuss and plan care with the nurses.

Preoperative education

Risk of chest infection

Chest infections are among the most common postoperative infections. Inhalation anaesthetics irritate the bronchial mucosa and depress the action of the respiratory cilia. Analgesic drugs, particularly the opioid drugs depress respiration, and postoperative pain can also reduce respiratory effort. Irritated respiratory mucosa, shallow breathing, and retained secretions combine to provide an ideal opportunity for a chest infection to develop. This will be even more likely if the patient is a smoker. Preoperative education should focus on explaining the risks to the patient and encouraging the practice of deep breathing and coughing exercises. Deep breathing hyperventilates the alveoli, helping to keep them open and mobilizing secretions trapped in the smaller airways. Coughing exercises mobilize secretions so they can be expelled. Incentive spirometers can be used to encourage deep breathing. If an abdominal incision is planned, the patient can be taught how to support the wound during coughing. *Box 2.6* lists patient guidelines for breathing and coughing exercises. The physiotherapist may be involved in teaching these techniques, but the surgical nurse has an important role in reinforcing learning and encouraging compliance.

Box 2.6 Deep breathing and coughing exercises.

Patient guidelines for deep breathing
- This exercise can be performed while sitting in bed with a pillow behind your head.
- Try to repeat the exercise three times an hour for the first day after your operation and then once an hour until you are moving around normally.
- Place your hands on each side of your chest, inhale slowly, and hold your breath for a count of three. You should be able to feel your ribcage expand under your hands.
- Exhale slowly and completely.

Patient guidelines for coughing exercises
- This exercise can be performed while sitting in bed with a pillow behind your head or sitting on the side of the bed with your feet supported.
- Clasp your hands over the front of your abdomen or place a pillow over your abdomen for support.
- Take a deep slow breath through your nose and hold for a count of three.
- Exhale slowly and repeat three times.
- Inhale and hold your breath for a count of three.
- Exhale coughing three times.
- Inhale again slowly and cough twice immediately.
- Repeat this exercise.
- End the exercise with more deep breathing.

Risk of deep venous thrombosis and pulmonary embolism

Surgery and postoperative inactivity are associated with a risk of DVT and PE. Pulmonary embolism is the major complication resulting from thromboembolism. Thromboembolism occurs most often in the deep veins of the legs. It also occurs less commonly in the subclavian and pelvic veins, when it is associated with a high mortality. Venous thrombosis occurs when there is stasis of blood flow, injury to the venous endothelium, and a state of hypercoagulability (Virchow's triad). In surgery, stasis occurs as the muscle pump is inactivated and distension increases the volume of blood in the lower leg veins by up to 48% (Coleridge Smith *et al.*, 1991). This distension and stasis may also cause endothelial damage. Raised fibrinogen levels after surgery increase the risk of coagulation. Risk factors for the development of DVT in surgical patients are shown in *Box 2.7*. Das (1994) estimated that the incidence of DVT varies from about 10% after inguinal hernia repair and prostatectomy to 75% after surgery of the knee. The incidence of PE varies from 0.8% after abdominal surgery to 5.9% after hip fracture surgery (Das, 1994). The incidence of DVT may be underestimated because as many as 50% of patients with DVT have no local signs or symptoms. PE is most often diagnosed after death as about 60% of deaths occur within 30 minutes of the embolism. Common symptoms include tachypnoea, dyspnoea, chest pain, and hypotension. Haemoptysis, pleuritic pain, and cyanosis may also be reported, and large emboli can cause syncope.

Prevention of DVT and PE is an important goal of pre-, intra-, and postoperative nursing care. Assessment will have identified patients particularly at risk, but DVT prophylaxis will be required by all patients. The two main approaches to prophylaxis are:

■ To reduce venous stasis.
■ To reduce hypercoagulability.

Methods for reducing venous stasis include leg elevation and early ambulation, graduated compression stockings, intermittent pneumatic compression, and

---

Box 2.7 Risk factors for DVT.

■ Age over 40 years
■ Varicose veins
■ Malignancy
■ Pregnancy
■ Myocardial infarction
■ Cerebrovascular accident
■ Oestrogen therapy (including oral contraceptive, hormone replacement therapy)
■ Obesity

■ Immobility (including an extended period in theatre)
■ Trauma or sepsis
■ History of thromboembolism
■ Congestive heart failure
■ Hypercoagulable states (e.g. deficiency of anticoagulant factors such as antithrombin, protein C, protein S)

electrical stimulation of calf muscles. Electrical stimulation is usually reserved for use during the operation, and intermittent pneumatic compression will be discussed under postoperative care. Leg exercises and the use of compression stockings are usually started preoperatively. Graduated compression stockings work by improving venous return and blood flow. They improve the velocity of blood flow, but the patient must be properly assessed and correctly fitted with a stocking of the right size to achieve the desired result. Patients will generally accept the stockings, but it is important to explain the reason for their use because they can be uncomfortable to wear and embarrassing for some men. In addition to stockings, patients should be educated about the value of early ambulation and hourly leg exercises. Regular dorsiflexion of the foot in the postoperative period will activate the calf muscle pump and improve venous blood flow. Deep breathing exercises by increasing intrathoracic pressure also improves venous return. Preoperative teaching should emphasize the importance of carrying out leg and breathing exercises frequently and correctly.

Adequate hydration may help reduce hypercoagulability, but the main prophylactic measure is anticoagulant therapy using low-dose heparin. Low molecular weight heparins that avoid the disadvantages of regular heparin regimens are currently advocated for DVT prevention. These newer forms of heparin can be given as a once daily injection.

Other risks of immobility
Immobility is associated with other problems in addition to chest infection, DVT, and PE. These include paralytic ileus, contracture, and pressure sores. During preoperative preparation the patient should be encouraged to consider the benefits of sitting, turning, leg exercising, and early ambulation:

- Sitting at least once every four hours helps improve venous return, decreases oedema of the dependent areas, and improves circulation. Patients are taught how to turn onto their side, place their palms on the mattress and push themselves into a sitting position as they swing their feet around. Leg dangling for 5–10 minutes may be the first stage in early ambulation.
- Turning: when the patient is unable to sit upright he can turn himself from side to side in bed.
- Leg exercises not only prevent DVT, but also help prevent joint stiffness and contractures. They are detailed in *Box 2.8* and can be taught unless contraindicated by the patient's condition or proposed surgery.

IMMEDIATE PREOPERATIVE PREPARATION

Fasting

It is routine to fast patients for a minimum of four hours before a general anaesthetic to empty the stomach and so avoid peri- or postoperative vomiting

---

Box 2.8 Leg exercises.

A

- This exercise is performed while sitting in bed with your hips aligned.
- Bring one knee up towards your chest, keeping the calf parallel to the bed and the foot flexed.
- Extend your leg and then lower it to the bed.
- Repeat five times for each leg.

B

- Using both feet, point the toes towards the head of the bed.
- Relax your feet.
- Now point the toes of both feet towards the foot of the bed.
- Relax your feet.
- Repeat the exercise five times an hour while in bed.

C

- Using your ankle move your feet with a circular motion in one direction and then in the opposite direction.
- Repeat the exercise five times an hour while in bed.

D

- Place your feet about an inch and a half apart with the heels resting on the bed.
- Point the toes inward, towards each other.
- Then rotate at the hip to point the toes outward.
- Repeat the exercise five times an hour while in bed.

---

or regurgitation, which increase the risk of aspiration and the resulting respiratory complications (Bannister, 1962). Torrance (1991) noted that investigations of preoperative fasting reported times ranging from 5–22 hours. In one study 33% of patients on a morning list had been fasted for ten or more hours and 16% on a morning list for six or more hours (Smith, 1987). Physiological studies suggest that even with a moderately heavy meal including meat, bread, and dairy products, the volume of stomach contents drops to almost zero within four hours and that a fast of more than four hours has no effect on stomach acid volume or pH (Malagelada *et al.*, 1976; Hester and Heath, 1977). Shevde and Trivedi (1991) studied healthy volunteers given 240 ml of fluid (coffee, orange juice, or water) and found that all had gastric volumes of less than 20 ml two hours later. Maltby *et al.* (1991) measured residual gastric volume and pH in patients receiving general anaesthesia and found no significant difference in either volume or pH for patients fasted for 1–3 hours, 3–5 hours, 5–8 hours or more than eight hours. The conclusion from these studies is that extended fasting is not usually required and that most patients can probably have moderate amounts of clear fluids up to

2–3 hours before surgery. Torrance (1991) concluded that many studies indicated that four hours fasting should be more than sufficient except in cases where gastric emptying is delayed (e.g. pregnancy or some gastrointestinal conditions) or when extensive handling of the bowel is anticipated. Fasting patients should be offered facilities for cleaning their teeth or cold water mouth washes to improve oral comfort.

Some drugs have to be continued even when food and fluids are restricted, for example beta blockers and respiratory drugs via an inhaler. Diabetic patients continue to take insulin, but within a prescribed programme, which would include intravenous glucose. Drugs that interfere with clotting such as anti-coagulants and oral contraceptives should be stopped some days before operation. The anaesthetist must be informed about all medication the patient is receiving as it may interact with the drugs used during anaesthesia.

Gastrointestinal Preparation

It is usual to ensure bowel evacuation to prevent defaecation during surgery and to reduce the risk of accidental damage to the colon during abdominal surgery. Aperients, an evacuant suppository, or a small disposable enema may be prescribed. After these treatments, the patient should be allowed to use the toilet (if possible) or a bedside commode rather than a bedpan. Prophylactic antibiotics may also be prescribed for intestinal surgery to reduce intestinal flora. A more rigorous and extensive bowel preparation may be ordered for some operative procedures. However, bowel preparation should not be viewed as routine and is not required for all types of surgery. In some cases a nasogastric or duodenal tube may be required, but it is often possible to delay insertion and pass the tube after induction of anaesthesia.

Skin Preparation

General hygiene is important preoperatively and the patient is encouraged to bath or shower daily. However, many surgeons routinely request some specific form of preoperative skin preparation. Preoperative skin preparation aims to reduce the risk of postoperative wound infection by cleansing and disinfecting the area around the proposed incision. Physical cleansing of the skin and hair and the use of detergents or antiseptic preparations aims to:

- Remove dirt and transient microorganisms from the area.
- Reduce the residential microbial population.

Physical cleansing (i.e. washing the skin using soap or detergent) removes dirt, transient microorganisms, secretions, and loose skin cells, which will reduce the effectiveness of antiseptic washes. An antiseptic wash is used to reduce the population of residential microorganisms. All soap or detergent residues must be washed off as they can inactivate some antiseptics such as the widely used antiseptic chlorhexidine (MacKenzie, 1988). Combined antiseptic detergent preparations can also be used and allow cleansing and disinfection in one wash. Patients should be reminded that the umbilicus is a frequently neglected area and must be clean. Finger nails and toe nails should also be clean and varnish free, and no make up should be worn. Preoperative skin preparation may be undertaken at home if the patient is to be admitted on the day of operation, but the patient will require clear instructions and the appropriate antiseptic solutions.

The true value of ward-based skin preparation has not been conclusively demonstrated by research. Some studies appear to demonstrate a reduction in postoperative infection with the use of detergent chlorhexidine preparations (Cruse and Foord, 1980; Ayliffe *et al.*, 1983). In a large scale randomized double-blind study comparing a chlorhexidine–detergent preparation (two preoperative baths) to a placebo control, Rotter *et al.* (1988) found no significant decrease in wound infections. Hayek *et al.* (1987) reported an increase in the number of viable skin organisms after bathing with a non-medicated soap. It is difficult to compare or combine the findings of research studies because the methodology varies. Llewellyn-Thomas (1990) listed some of the problems involved in assessing research into skin preparation as due to variations in:

■ The methods used.
■ The number of patients studied.
■ Definitions of postoperative wound infection.
■ The number of showers or baths taken.
■ Types of surgery included.
■ The use or type of preoperative shaving.
■ The use of antibiotics.
■ The use and interpretation of statistical evidence.

Until conclusive evidence appears, it is probably best to follow local procedures, although showering is preferable to bathing (Byrne *et al.*, 1990). However, it is worth noting that Rotter *et al.* (1988) suggested that skin preparation might have been directed at eliminating staphylococcal bacteria from irrelevant sites on the wrong people. Surgical staff and not patients are probably the most important reservoirs of infection (see Chapter 8). After showering patients are dressed in a theatre cap and gown, and the beds to which they return must be clean with fresh linen.

Hair Removal

Preoperative removal of body hair is another area of considerable controversy and discussion. Shaving of a large area around the site of operation has been a major element of preoperative routine for many decades. Great effort has been expended in achieving a clean shave. Even areas with no visible hair are meticulously shaved. However, there is considerable evidence suggesting that routine removal of body hair is unnecessary, and that preoperative shaving may significantly increase the risk of postoperative wound infection (Seropian and Reynolds, 1971; Hamilton *et al.*, 1977; Cruse and Foord, 1980; Court-Brown, 1981; Alexander *et al.*, 1983; Hoe and Nambiar, 1985). The reasons suggested by proponents of preoperative hair removal include:

- A reduction of postoperative infection rates.
- A clear field of vision.
- Avoidance of hairs trapping in the incision.

Kovach (1990) maintains that the need to achieve a field of asepsis and to ensure a clear field of vision at the site of operation are still valid reasons for shaving. The three methods of hair removal in use are shaving, clippers, and depilatory creams. Electric clippers are expensive to buy, but cost less than shaving or the use of depilatory creams (Hamilton *et al.*, 1977). However, they require maintenance and the clipper body must be cleaned and the head sterilized between patients. Depilatory creams are the most expensive form of hair removal and can cause a skin reaction in some individuals, but have the advantage of being easy to use and patients can take responsibility for applying the cream.

The main debate, however, is not about hair removal methods, but whether it is necessary at all. Seropian and Reynolds (1971) reported that of 406 clean operations, wound infection developed in 5.6% of shaved cases compared with only 0.6% of those treated with a depilatory cream. The infection rate when there was no preoperative hair removal was also only 0.6%. Cruse and Foord (1980) similarly found that the wound infection rate was lowest when there was no preoperative hair removal: 0.9% with no hair removal, 1.4% using electric clippers, 1.7% when pubic hair was clipped with scissors, and 2.5% for shaved patients. Alexander *et al.* (1983) also found that shaving increased the rate of wound infection when compared to that associated with hair removal using clippers. Using electron microscopy Hamilton *et al.* (1977) demonstrated that shaving and to a lesser extent clipping damaged the skin surface. The evidence suggests that shaving is not only unnecessary, but probably contraindicated unless hair is likely to interfere with the operative field. If shaving is deemed necessary, it is important that it is carried out as close to the time of surgery as possible (Association of Operating Room Nurses, 1987).

Premedication and Final Preoperative Preparation

Any dentures, contact lens, or prostheses are removed before transfer to the operating suite. Jewellery is also removed into safe keeping. If the patient is reluctant to remove a wedding ring, it may be left on but is covered to avoid injury or damage during the operation. If the patient wears a hearing aid it is not removed until after the patient has been anaesthetized and is replaced in the recovery period.

Before any premedication is given, the nurse must ensure that the patient is wearing an identity band and that it is labelled correctly. The consent form is checked: it must be signed by the patient and the doctor. The patient is asked to void urine before going to the operating theatre and the amount is measured and recorded on the preoperative check list. If urinary bladder catherization is necessary it should be performed in the operating suite just before surgery.

The prescribed premedication is given before the patient goes to the operating theatre. Depending on the drugs prescribed, it may be given orally or intramuscularly 30–90 minutes before the anticipated time of operation. If given orally, 15–30 mL of water can be safely given with the drugs. If the operating list is running late the premedication may need to be delayed and given after notification from theatre. Premedications may be used:

- To allay apprehension in the preoperative period.
- To relieve pain or discomfort in the preoperative period.
- To augment the action of drugs used for anaesthesia.
- To reduce bronchial and salivary secretion (antisialagogue).
- To prevent the muscarinic effects of neostigmine.

Some of the drugs used may provide some preoperative amnesia (*British National Formulary*, 1996). Premedication may be omitted for minor procedures and antisialagogues are often given intravenously during the induction of anaesthesia.

The antimuscarinic drugs atropine, hyoscine, and glycopyrronium bromide are used to reduce secretions and to counteract the muscarinic effects when neostigmine is used to reverse non-polarizing muscle relaxants. Atropine is the most commonly used, but must be used with caution in patients with glaucoma, thyrotoxicosis, prostatic hyperplasia, and some types of cardiovascular disease. Glycopyrronium bromide is a more potent and longer acting antisialagogue that causes less bradycardia than atropine. Hyoscine is an effective antisialagogue that also produces a degree of amnesia, but its use is not recommended in the elderly because it may cause excitement, ataxia, hallucinations, behavioural abnormalities and drowsiness (*British National Formulary*, 1996).

Sedation may be prescribed the night before surgery to reduce insomnia or as a preoperative medication. Short-acting oral benzodiazepines (e.g. diazepam, lorazepam, temazepam) are currently favoured, but there is some evidence suggesting that preoperative visits and reassurance from a theatre nurse and an anaesthetist may be as effective in reducing anxiety.

Preoperative analgesia may be required in some cases. Non-opioid analgesics or opioid analgesics can be used depending on the severity of pain. The non-opioid analgesics (e.g. ketorolac trometamol, diclofenac sodium) do not depress respiration, but are inadequate for relieving severe pain. Opioid analgesics (e.g.

fentanyl, papaveretum, pethidine hydrochloride) were once commonly used as premedication, but are now more usually administered intravenously during induction of analgesia. *Box 2.9* lists some common premedications, but the reader is directed to the *British National Formulary* for more information on the use of these drugs.

The reasons for the premedication are explained and the patient is warned that the drugs may cause drowsiness and a dry mouth. Before the premedication is given any last minute questions or anxieties can be discussed. After it has been given the patient is encouraged to rest quietly and to avoid getting out of bed. The call bell must be easily available.

The preoperative check list is completed and checked by the registered nurse, and this list is put into the patient's notes, together with the consent form, laboratory reports, and the nurses' records. These notes together with any radiographs must accompany the patient to theatre. A typical preoperative checklist is presented in *Box 2.10*.

The patient is gently transferred to the operating theatre on his bed or on a theatre trolley. Great care must be taken to ensure that the patient's limbs are not injured in the process. The nurse who has been responsible for preparing the patient should oversee the transfer to the operating theatre and if possible remain until anaesthesia is induced. Ideally a theatre nurse should visit patients before surgery and then be on hand to greet patients when they arrive at the operating suite.

Box 2.9 **Some common premedications used for adults with dose and route of administration given in parentheses. (*British National Formulary*, 1996).**

Antimuscarinic drugs
- Atropine (300–600 μg intramuscularly)
- Hyoscine (200–600 μg intramuscularly)
- Glycopyrronium bromide (200–400 μg intramuscularly)

Benzodiazepine anxiolytics
- Diazepam (5 mg orally)
- Lorazepam (2–4 mg orally)
- Temazepam (20–40 mg (elderly 10–20 mg) orally)

Opioid analgesics
- Papaveretum* (7.7–15.4 mg (elderly 7.7 mg initially) intramuscularly)

(*Papaveretum is a formulation containing three alkaloids: morphine, papaverine, and codeine. It is often given in combination with hyoscine.)

Box 2.10 A typical preoperative checklist.

Date .... Name .... Hospital No. ....

Ward .... Consultant ....

Vital signs: Temperature .... Pulse .... Respiration .... BP ....

Allergies? .... Communication problems? ....

Time of last food or drink .... Premedication given at ....

	Yes	No
Identification band present and correct?	☐	☐
Urine passed before premedication?	☐	☐
Loose teeth, crowns, bridges?	☐	☐
Dentures removed?	☐	☐
Hearing aid?	☐	☐
Contact lenses removed?	☐	☐
Preoperative skin preparation?	☐	☐
Jewellery removed and rings taped?	☐	☐
Valuables securely stored?	☐	☐
Cosmetics and clothing removed?	☐	☐
Theatre gown or pants?	☐	☐
Consent form signed?	☐	☐
Operation site marked?	☐	☐
Case notes accompanying patient?	☐	☐
Radiographs accompanying patient?	☐	☐
Checklist complete	☐	☐

Ward Nurse's Signature .... Theatre Staff Signature ....

References

Alexander W, Fischer JE, Boyajian M, Palmquist J, Morris M (1983) The influence of hair-removal methods on wound infections. *Arch Surg* **118**:347–352.

Association of Operating Room Nurses (1987) Proposed recommended practices: preoperative skin preparation. *AORN J* **46(4)**:719–724.

Ayliffe GAJ, Noy MF, Babb JR, Davies JG, Jackson J (1983) A comparision of pre-operative bathing with chlorhexidine–detergent and non-medicated soap in the prevention of wound infection. *J Hosp Infect* **4**:237–244.

Bannister R (1962) Vomiting and aspiration during anaesthesia. *Anaesthesiology* **23**:251–264.

Bellman L (1994) Principles of educating patients. *Surg Nurse* **7(1)**:7–10.

Boore J (1978) *Prescription for Recovery*, pp. 67–77. Royal College of Nursing, London.

Breeze C (1995) From start to finish. *Nurs Times* **91(40)**:62–64.

British National Formulary (1996) Number 32, p. 523. British Medical Association and Royal Pharmaceutical Society of Great Britain, London.

Byrne DJ, Napier A, Cuschieri A (1990) Rationalizing whole body disinfection. *J Hosp Infect* **15**:183–187.

Castledine G (1988) Preoperative information. *Surg Nurse* **1**:11–13.

Coleridge Smith PD, Hasty JH, Scurr JH (1991) Deep vein thrombosis: effects of graduated compression stockings on distension of the deep veins of the calf. *Br J Surg* **78**:724–726.

Court-Brown CM (1981) Preoperative skin depilation and its effect on postoperative wound infections. *J Roy Coll Edin* **26**:238–241.

Cruse PJE, Foord R (1980) The epidemiology of wound infection – a 10-year prospective study of 62,939 wounds. *Surg Clin North Am* **60**:27–40.

Das SK (1994) Venous thrombosis and pulmonary embolism. *Surgery* **12(10)**:217–223.

Douglas S, Larson E (1986) There's more to informed consent than information. *Focus Crit Care* **13(2)**:43–47.

Egbart LD, Battit GE, Welch CE, Bartlett MD (1964) Reduction of postoperative pain by encouragement and instruction of patients: a study of doctor patient rapport. *New Engl J Med* **270**:822–827.

Goldman L, Caldera DL, Nussbaum SR *et al.* (1977) Multifactorial index of cardiac risk in noncardiac surgical procedures. *N Engl J Med* **297**:845–849.

Hamilton HW, Hamilton KR, Lone FJ (1977) Preoperative hair removal. *Can J Surg* **20**:269–275.

Hayek LJ, Emerson JM, Gardner AMN (1987) A placebo-controlled trial of the effect of two pre-operative baths or showers with chlorhexidine-detergent on post-operative wound infection rates. *J Hosp Infect* **10**:165–172.

Hayward J (1975) *Information: a Prescription against Pain*. Series 2, No. 5, pp. 36–50. Royal College of Nursing, London.

Hester JB, Heath ML (1977) Pulmonary acid aspiration syndrome: should prophylaxis be routine? *Br J Anaesth* **49**:595–599.

Hoe NY, Nambiar R (1985) Is preoperative shaving really necessary? *Ann Acad Med* **14(4)**:700–704.

Houston MC, Ratcliff DG, Hays JT, Gluck FW (1987) Preoperative medical consultation and evaluation of surgical risk. *South Med J* **80**:1385–1397.

Jameton A (1984) *Nursing Practice: the Ethical Issues*. Hemel Hempstead, Prentice Hall. p. 185.

Janis IL (1974) *Psychological Stress: Psychoanalytic and Behavioural Studies of Surgical Patients*, pp. 274–301. New York, Academic Press.

Johnson JE (1983) Preparing patients to cope with stress while hospitalized. In *Patient Teaching*. Wilson-Barnett J (ed.), pp. 19–33. Churchill Livingstone, Edinburgh.

Kiecolt-Glaser JK, Marucha PT, Malarkey WB, Mercado AM, Glaser R (1995) Slowing of wound healing by psychological stress. *Lancet* **346**:1194–1196.

Kovach T (1990) Nip it in the bud. *Todays OR Nurse* **12**:23–26.

Lindeman CA, van Aernam B (1971) Nursing intervention with the pre-surgical patient. *Nursing Res* 20:319–333.

Llewellyn-Thomas A (1990) Preoperative skin preparation. *Surg Nurse* 3(2):24–26.

MacKenzie I (1988) Pre-operative skin preparation and surgical outcome. *J Hosp Infect* **11(Suppl. B)**:27–32.

Malagelada J-R, Longstretch GF, Summerskill WHJ, Go VLW (1976) Measurement of gastric functions during digestion of ordinary solid meals in man. *Gastroenterology* 70:203–210.

Maltby JR, Lewis P, Martin A, Sutherland LR (1991) Gastric fluid volume and pH in elective patients following unrestricted oral fluids until three hours before surgery. *Can J Anaesth* **38(4)**:425–529.

Miller B, Torrance C (1991) Nutritional assessment. *Surg Nurse* 4(5):21–25.

Newton V (1996) Care in pre-admission clinics. *Nurs Times* 92(1):27–28.

Oakley A (1984) The importance of being a nurse. *Nurs Times* 80:24–27.

Patient's Charter (1995) The patient's charter and you. Raising the standard. Leaving hospital. p. 18. Department of Health, London.

Polk HC (1991) Principles of preoperative preparation of the surgical patient. In *Textbook of Surgery*, 14th edition. Sabiston DC (ed.) pp. 77–84. WB Saunders, Philadelphia.

Pugh J, Millar B (1989) Nursing management for mobility: pre-operative phase. *Surg Nurse* **2(3)**:24–27.

Ramsay MAE (1972) A survey of pre-operative fear. *Anaesthesia* 27:396–402.

Ray C (1982) The surgical patient: psychological stress and coping resources. In *Social Psychology and Behavioural Medicine*. Eisser JR (ed.). pp. 483–507. Wiley, Chichester.

Rotter ML, Olesen LS, Cooke EM *et al.* (1988) A comparison of the effects of pre-operative whole-body bathing with detergent alone and with detergent containing chlorhexidine gluconate on the frequency of wound infections after clean surgery. *J Hosp Infect* 11:310–320.

Seropian R, Reynolds BM (1971) Wound infections after pre-operative depilatory versus razor preparation. *Am J Surg* 121:251–254.

Shevde K, Trivedi N (1991) Effects of clear liquids on gastric volume and pH in healthy volunteers. *Anesth Analges* 72:528–531.

Smith SH (1987) *Nil by Mouth*, pp. 65–70. Royal College of Nursing, London.

Swindale J (1989) The nurse's role in giving pre-operative information to reduce anxiety in the patients admitted to hospital for elective minor surgery. *J Ad Nursing* 14:899–905.

Torrance C (1991) Pre-operative nutrition, fasting and the surgical patient. *Surg Nurse* **4(4)**:4–8.

Volicer BJ, Volicer L (1978) Cardiovascular changes associated with stress during hospitalisation. *J Psychosom Res* 22:159–168.

Williams B, Williams JGL, Jones R (1972) The measurement and control of postoperative anxiety. 12th Annual Meeting of the Society for Psychophysiological Research, Abstracts Vol. 10, No. 2, March 1993, p. 200.

Wong J, Wong S (1985) A randomised trial of a new approach to preoperative teaching and patient compliance. *Int J Nurs Studies* **22(2)**:105–115.

Chapter 3

Intraoperative Care

The nurse has many roles and functions within the theatre suite. Depending on the size of the unit there may be specialized anaesthetic nurses, operating room nurses, and recovery nurses. In small units theatre nurses may take on aspects of all roles. For a detailed discussion of theatre nursing the reader is directed to specialized texts, for example *Alexander's Care of the Patient in Surgery* edited by Meeker and Rothrock, 1995. This chapter comprises a general review of anaesthesia and intraoperative care with particular emphasis on the nurse's role in ensuring safety and acting as the patient's advocate. Understanding of anaesthesia and operative experience is critical for informed planning of postoperative nursing care and discharge preparation.

COMMUNICATION IN THEATRE: THE HANDOVER

Arriving in theatre to be greeted by unfamiliar staff and conducted into an unknown environment can increase anxiety within the operating suite (Ashworth, 1980). This may be reduced by effective communication between the theatre nurse and patient. A preoperative visit by the theatre nurse provides the patient with an opportunity to meet the nurse, for the nurse to provide information, and for the patient to express anxieties and ask questions. Preoperative visiting can help to alleviate anxiety and reduce postoperative complications (Boore, 1978; Devine and Cook, 1983). The patient can then be greeted on arrival at the theatre suite by a familiar face. Chesson *et al.* (1980) noted that 'patients who were received into theatre by their nurse were appreciative of this.'

An agreed preoperative checklist must be used to ensure that the right patient is presented for the correct procedure, that all details and information are available, and that preoperative preparation is complete. It is important to ensure that details such as the patient's name, address and hospital number are correct. It must also be ensured that the patient's false teeth have been removed, and that the fasting time and consent form have been checked. However, Allin (1991) recommends a more extensive handover involving the ward nurse, the theatre nurse, and the patient. This would allow more time for additional details and concerns to be addressed. To develop an effective nursing care plan the theatre nurse needs more information than is available on a routine checklist. During the handover the patient is transferred into the clean area and taken into the anaesthetic room.

THE ANAESTHETIC ROOM

A calm efficient atmosphere is important in the anaesthetic room and staff are encouraged to talk quietly and move around as little as possible. The patient's identity is again checked using full name and hospital number from the identity bracelet. An additional check should be made against the theatre list. The consent form should be consulted and should detail the type of operation proposed and the site and side of the body. If possible the site of operation should have been marked with an indelible pencil by a member of the surgical team before the patient arrives in the operating theatre. The anaesthetist will also check the consent form and examine the other records accompanying the patient before giving the anaesthetic. The correct notes and radiographs must accompany the patient into the anaesthetic room.

If the patient is not having a general anaesthetic, the surgeon who performs the operation is responsible for ensuring that the correct patient has been brought for operation and that the correct body area has been identified. If the patient is having general anaesthesic, it is also the surgeon's responsibility to make sure that the accompanying documents relate to the patient before the patient is anaesthetized (Medical Defence Societies, 1988).

A further check is made to ensure that the patient is not wearing any dentures or jewellery, and that the operation site is appropriately prepared. The time from which the patient has fasted is also checked and that the patient does not have any allergies. The patient's blood pressure is recorded and the electrocardiograph (ECG) electrodes are attached to the patient. The anaesthetist explains what is to happen to the patient, inserts a venous cannula, usually into the hand or forearm of the patient, and induces anaesthesia. The patient's gown is then loosened by undoing the tapes, the neck is extended, an oral airway is inserted, and oxygen and nitrous oxide are administered. A patent airway and no risk of gastric contents entering the respiratory system are paramount in any anaesthetic induction. This is achieved by introducing a laryngeal mask or endotracheal tube; oxygen, nitrous oxide, and other anaesthetic gases can then be given by this route. The cuff of the endotracheal tube is inflated and the tube is secured in position with tape. Muscle relaxation must be achieved before passing the endotracheal tube to ensure no damage occurs to the vocal cords. A clear unobstructed view of the cords will ensure that the trachea and not the oesophagus is entered. The anaesthetist will check the patient's respiratory sounds after intubation. Spontaneous respiration will become depressed as the depth of analgesia increases; at this point the anaesthetist squeezes the reservoir bag of the anaesthetic machine to facilitate oxygenation. The diathermy pad is attached to the patient's thigh. The corrugated tube is detached from the anaesthetic machine so that the patient can be removed into the operating theatre. In the theatre, the corrugated tube (black antistatic compliance tubing) is attached to the ventilator and the patient is gently moved onto and carefully positioned on the operating table.

GENERAL ANAESTHESIA AND ANAESTHETICS

Anaesthesia is a reversible state of insensibility induced by drugs. General anaesthesia aims to produce unconsciousness and loss of sensation. Local or regional anaesthesia aims to block pain sensation from the operative site without inducing unconsciousness. The three main objectives of general anaesthesia are:

- Narcosis.
- Suppression of reflex activity and analgesia.
- Muscle relaxation.

In the early days of anaesthesia, single agents such as ether were used to achieve all three objectives, but in modern practice a combination of intravenous drugs and anaesthetic gases are used to produce controlled reversible anaesthesia, analgesia, and muscle relaxation.

Narcosis

Narcosis can be defined as 'the safe controlled depression of the central nervous system (CNS) so that consciousness is lost and, on recovery of consciousness, there is no recall' (Jameson, 1994). Intravenous or inhalation agents can be used to induce and maintain anaesthesia. Intravenous drugs are commonly used to induce anaesthesia, but may be used for maintenance during short procedures. Intravenous anaesthetics are potent, rapidly acting drugs, with most producing their effects in one arm–brain circulation. Intravenous anaesthetics can also cause hypotension and apnoea and should not be used if there is any doubt about maintaining a patent airway. The *British National Formulary* (BNF) (1996a) recommends extreme care if surgery involves the mouth, pharynx, and larynx, and in patients with shock. *Box 3.1* lists the characteristics of an ideal intravenous anaesthetic as identified by Jameson

---

Box 3.1 Characteristics of an 'ideal' intravenous anaesthetic agent (adapted from Jameson, 1994).

Physiochemical
- Water soluble
- Long shelf-life
- Stable to light exposure
- Lipophilic
- Small injection volume
- Nontoxic to tissues
- No pain on injection
- No venous or arterial thrombosis or spasm

Action
- Rapid onset
- Short duration
- Rapid recovery
- Nontoxic metabolites
- Some analgesic effect

Other effects
- Minimal effect on other physiological systems
- Nonemetic
- Nonallergenic
- No release of histamine
- No excitatory phenomena
- No emergence phenomena
- No interference with neuromuscular blockade
- No stimulation of porphyria

(1994). Commonly used intravenous agents, their uses, and associated problems are listed in *Box 3.2*.

Inhalation anaesthetics can be used for induction, but are mainly used for maintenance. They may be volatile liquids or gases. Gaseous anaesthetics may be piped in (via a pipeline that meets all legal criteria) or supplied from gas cylinders attached to the anaesthetic equipment. The volatile liquids are supplied via calibrated vaporizers using carrier gases (air, oxygen, or oxygen–nitrous oxide mixes). *Box 3.3* lists the characteristics of an ideal inhalation anaesthetic. Jameson (1994) notes that newer agents such as sevoflurane and desflurane approach these ideal characteristics more closely, but disadvantages remain. Like intravenous agents inhalation anaesthetics tend to depress respiratory drive by reducing the response to hypoxia or carbon dioxide. *Box 3.4* details the main inhalation anaesthetics, their uses, and associated problems.

Box 3.2 Intravenous anaesthetics (*British National Formulary*, 1996a).

BARBITURATES

Thiopentone sodium
- Produces a rapid smooth induction.
- Rapid recovery from a moderate dose, but sedative effects may last for 24 hours with large or cumulative doses.
- Contraindicated in porphyria.
- Very irritant and can cause tissue damage if the injection leaks from the vein.

Methohexitone sodium
- Hiccup, tremor, and pain on injection may be experienced at induction.
- Recovery is rapid and risk of tissue damage reduced.
- Contraindicated in porphyria.

NON-BARBITURATES

Etomidate
- Used for induction of anaesthesia.
- Rapid recovery with less hypotension than other drugs used for induction.
- Associated with pain on injection and extraneous muscle movement.

Ketamine
- Induction and maintenance of anaesthesia with some analgesic effects.
- Muscle tone is increased and airway is usually well maintained.
- May increase salivation, blood pressure, and heart rate.
- Associated with a high incidence of hallucination.
- Contraindicated in hypertension.
- Particularly used with children, where the adverse effects seem less severe.
- Adverse effects seem less prominent.

Propofol
- Rapid recovery without hangover effect.
- May be some pain on injection.
- Delayed convulsions have been reported after use, so not advised for day surgery.

Analgesia

Although the patient cannot feel 'pain' during surgery there is a need to suppress reflex activity in response to the tissue injury caused by surgery. The nociceptors or pain receptors can still respond and initiate autonomic responses.

Opioid analgesics are commonly used for intraoperative analgesia, often in combination with nitrous oxide and a muscle relaxant. Such intraoperative use needs careful monitoring as repeated doses will depress respiratory drive and

Box 3.3 Characteristics of an ideal inhalation anaesthetic (adapted from Jameson, 1994).

Physiochemical
- Stability, nonflammable, nonexplosive
- Vaporizable at room temperature
- Stable in soda lime, no toxic byproducts
- Environmentally safe
- Nonirritant to the respiratory tract

Action
- Rapid onset
- Rapid recovery
- High potency
- Excreted unchanged, unreactive with other drugs

Other effects
- Minimal effects on other physiological systems
- Economic

this can persist well into the recovery period. Ward nurses need to be alerted if repeated doses of opioids have been given. Opioid analgesics are listed in *Box 3.5*.

Muscle Relaxation

Neuromuscular blocking drugs are used to produce muscle relaxation. Some general anaesthetics can produce muscle relaxation, but the concentrations required are too high for safe use. When anaesthetics are used with muscle relaxants, the abdominal muscles and diaphragm can be sufficiently relaxed using much lower quantities of anaesthetic. Muscle relaxants also relax the vocal cords, which facilitates intubation. Because the respiratory muscles are affected, assisted ventilation is required until the effects of the drugs have been reversed. Only a mild degree of muscle relaxation may be required for superficial or minor operations, but deeper relaxation is necessary for surgery within body cavities (Chung and Lam, 1990).

The two distinct groups of muscle relaxants are depolarizing and non-depolarizing relaxants. Suxamethonium is the only depolarizing drug used in the UK. It provides a rapid and complete relaxation of short duration (about 5 minutes), but causes painful muscle fasciculation and must be given after anaesthesia has been established. Its rapid action makes it ideal for intubation and short procedures, but its use is limited because its action cannot be reversed and it is associated with significant side effects including:

Box 3.4 Inhalation anaesthetics (*British National Formulary* (1996) No. 32, p. 522).

GASES

Nitrous oxide
- Low potency, used for induction and maintenance in combination with other agents at concentrations of 50–70% with oxygen.
- Diffuses readily into air spaces and may cause increased pressure in enclosed air-filled cavities.
- Caution required with pneumothorax, obstructed intestine, air emboli, middle ear obstruction, and after pneumoencephalogram.
- Inactivates vitamin B_{12} causing megaloblastic changes in the bone marrow after sustained use.
- Used at lower concentrations for analgesia.

VOLATILE LIQUIDS

Halothane
- Rapid, smooth induction.
- Nonirritant so little problem with coughing, breathholding, or postoperative vomiting.
- Causes marked cardiopulmonary depression, reduced cardiac output, hypotension, and a tendency for ventricular dysrhythmias.
- Use is declining due to problem of hepatotoxicity

Enflurane
- Less potent than halothane.
- Produces marked cardiopulmonary depression, reduced cardiac output, and hypotension.
- Used to supplement nitrous oxide–oxygen mixes.

Isoflurane
- Moderate potency.
- Irritant and can cause coughing and breathholding.
- Produces respiratory depression, but cardiac effects are minimal. Also produces some hypotension due to vasodilation.
- Causes muscle relaxation and potentiation of muscle relaxants.

Desflurane
- New, rapid acting agent.
- May cause coughing, breathholding, and apnoea.
- Rapid emergence.
- Not recommended for neurosurgery or for children.
- Requires special vaporizer.

> **Box 3.5** Opioid analgesics (*British National Formulary* (1996) No. 32, p. 527).
>
> **Short duration**
> - Alfentanil
> - Fentanyl
> - Nalbuphine hydrochloride
> - Phenoperidine hydrochloride
>
> **Sustained duration**
> - Morphine salts
> - Papaveretum
> - Pethidine hydrochloride

- Arrhthymias and bradycardia.
- Hyperkalaemia.
- Raised intraocular pressure.
- Postoperative muscle pain.
- Increased salivation.
- Anaphylactic reaction.
- Myotonia.
- Malignant hyperthermia.
- Suxamethonium apnoea (Jameson, 1994).

Non-depolarizing muscle relaxants compete with acetylcholine, producing a competitive blockade of the postsynaptic membrane. The paralysis produced has a slower onset and is less complete than that produced by suxamethonium, but can be reversed by using an anticholinesterase drug, usually neostigmine.

The depolarizing muscle relaxants are suitable for maintaining longer duration paralysis. A variety of non-depolarizing muscle relaxants are currently in use (*Box 3.6*). When neostigmine is used to reverse the effects of muscle relaxants, atropine or glycopyrronium should be given as a premedication (or with the neostigmine) to prevent bradycardia, excess salivation, and other muscarinic side effects of neostigmine (*British National Formulary*, 1996b).

SAFETY: MONITORING OF ANAESTHESIA

All anaesthetics have the potential to harm the patient and monitoring of anaesthesia is critical to ensure that:

- The depth of anaesthesia is sufficient to prevent awareness or unconscious perception.
- The side effects of anaesthesia are minimized.

Box 3.6 Non-depolarizing muscle relaxants (*British National Formulary* (1996) No. 32, p. 530).

Rapid acting, short duration
- Atracurium
- Vecuronium
- Mivacurium

Longer onset, longer duration
- Pancuronium
- Tubocurarine

Patients presenting for anaesthesia sometimes seek reassurance that they will really be asleep throughout the operation as there have been a variety of reports of patients being awake and aware during surgery. Awareness is when the patient remains alert during surgery due to inadequate narcosis, but is unable to communicate because of muscle paralysis (Barr and Noble, 1994). It can be particularly distressing if the patient is able to feel the surgical pain. Avoiding awareness depends on adequate monitoring and estimation of the depth of anaesthesia. A related problem is unconscious perception (i.e. that information is processed and stored even though the patient is under deep anaesthesia). Barr and Noble (1994) report conflicting evidence for and against the possibility of unconscious perception during anaesthesia, but recommend that theatre staff are careful about what is said during operations. In anaesthesia there will be:

- An absence of voluntary movement.
- Muscle relaxation.
- Hypoventilation.
- Hypotension.
- Suppressed sweating.
- Loss of lacrimation.
- Miosis.

The agents used to produce anaesthesia are potent drugs with many side effects. It is important to avoid an overdose of these drugs, as this could delay a recovery of consciousness. General anaesthesia can cause cardiopulmonary depression and hypothermia due to anaesthesia-induced vasodilatation, which can result in a fall of core body temperature (Milne, 1988). Careful monitoring of respiratory function, pulse, blood pressure, oxygenation, and body temperature is essential. The complications of general anaesthesia will be considered in more detail in the sections on recovery and postoperative care (see Chapter 4).

During induction of anaesthesia and surgery the whole team has a responsibility for ensuring patients' safety and that their dignity is maintained. Safety and advocacy are critical aspects of the nurse's role in theatre. The theatre nurse needs to be aware of and monitor safety with regard to:

- Safe transfer and positioning.
- Pressure relief.
- Skin preparation.
- Asepsis.
- Diathermy.
- Swabs, needles, and instruments.
- Allergies.
- Psychological care and dignity.

Transfer of the patient and positioning on the operating table must be carried out with extreme care and with regard for any injuries or limitations of joint movement. Limbs will need to be supported at all times to prevent peripheral nerve injuries. Pressure damage is a potential problem in the operating room, particularly with long operations or elderly patients. Specialized pressure-relieving mattresses are available for use with theatre trolleys and tables. Trolley and operation table mattresses must be the recommended thickness and in good repair. Operating-room nurses are responsible for keeping track of instruments, needles, and swabs during the operation and ensuring that all are accounted for at the end of the procedure.

Diathermy is commonly used for cutting or coagulation and diathermy-related burns are a risk for the patient and a source of litigation. Machines can be used to supply bipolar or monopolar diathermy. The theatre nurse has a responsibility to check the forceps, lead, and machine before use. The diathermy pad (indifferent electrode) is positioned under the patient's buttock or thigh to ensure good contact over the entire surface of the pad without tenting or gaps. Poor contact can cause a localization of current that results in a burn. Burns are more likely if the diathermy pad becomes disconnected and the patient is in contact with metal (wedding rings should be covered with tape). Memon (1994) notes that alcohol-based skin preparations that may have collected in the umbilicus and vagina may be ignited by diathermy and cause burns.

RECOVERY CARE

At the end of the operation, the patient is transferred to the recovery room. A full verbal report is given by the operating-room nurse to the recovery nurse. The recovery room is fully equipped with facilities for the patient's recovery to consciousness and contains all the equipment that may be needed to deal with emergency situations such as acute haemorrhage or respiratory or cardiac arrest. It is an integral part of the theatre suite. Anaesthetists are readily available and the operating theatre is immediately accessible if further surgical intervention becomes necessary. Nurses working in the recovery room must be specially trained and ideally work one to a patient. A detailed discussion of immediate postoperative care is beyond the scope of this chapter, but the essential points are:

- Maintenance of the airway.
- Monitoring of vital signs.
- Management of intravenous fluid therapy.
- Observation of wound and drains for signs of haemorrhage.
- Pain relief.

Potential problems in the recovery room include nausea and vomiting, pain, altered mental status, hypoxaemia, hyperventilation, hypotension, hypertension, and cardiac arrhythmias. Many of these problems may also occur after transfer to the ward and are discussed in Chapter 4. Patients are not transferred out of the recovery room until they are:

- Fully conscious.
- Able to breathe without assistance.
- Of good colour and with warm-to-touch skin.
- Observed to have a stable pulse and blood pressure.
- Observed to have no signs of haemorrhage.

The patient should be able to state that he is as comfortable as possible. If further analgesia is given, the patient is retained in the recovery room for 30 minutes to ensure there are no adverse effects. The ward nurse should then be given an oral report of the operation and recovery, a copy of which is included in the patient's notes on transfer from the recovery room to the ward. It is essential for continuity of care that the recovery nurse details any problems encountered in the recovery process and the nursing actions taken.

THE POSTOPERATIVE VISIT

There is ample evidence to support the value of the postoperative visit by the theatre nurse (Ellison, 1975; Chesson et al., 1980; Farmer, 1985). It is an excellent way of evaluating the care given to patients in the operating theatre and it enables the nurse–patient relationship to be continued postoperatively.

REGIONAL ANAESTHESIA

Regional anaesthesia is the injection of a local anaesthetic agent at some point along the distribution of a nerve to block sensation of pain. It may be produced by injecting a small volume of local anaesthetic into the cerebrospinal fluid (CSF) (spinal block), the epidural space (epidural block), or by infiltrating peripheral tissues by injection or topical application (peripheral nerve block). Epidural and spinal anaesthetic techniques are being used with increasing frequency for patients who have to undergo surgery, but whose general condition precludes a general anaesthetic. Peripheral infiltration is used for minor procedures.

The preoperative preparation required for regional anaesthesia is essentially the same as for general anaesthesia. There needs to be careful patient assessment and a premedication may be required. It is recommended that vital signs monitoring is established and maintained throughout the procedure. Theatre care requires the same attention to safety. In addition the psychological needs of the patient who remains conscious during surgery must be addressed. Postoperative care is also similar with careful monitoring, availability of the full range of emergency equipment and drugs, and attention to pain relief and infection control. With regional anaesthesia patients remains conscious and in control of their own airway during surgery.

Commonly used local anaesthetics are listed in *Table 3.1*. Local anaesthetics have surprisingly few local side effects. Most nerve damage results from trauma or infection. However, local anaesthetics can have toxic effects if they enter the systemic circulation. The main targets are within the cardiovascular and central nervous systems. Regional anaesthesia is often used for patients who are too ill to risk general anaesthesia. However, Cook (1992) warns that regional anaesthesia can have major side effects in these patients. A serious potential problem with epidural and spinal anaesthesia in the very sick, is sympathetic block. The thoracic and first two lumbar segments provide the body's major sympathetic outflow. Epidural and spinal anaesthesia block these autonomic nerves. This is not usually a problem in healthy patients, but it can result in severe hypotension in patients with serious hypovolaemia (e.g. patients with dehydration, haemorrhage, or sepsis). To avoid this problem Cook (1992) recommends general anaesthesia for acutely ill patients. Systemic side effects of local anaesthetics include:

Table 3.1 Local anaesthetics (adapted from Irving, 1993).

	Lignocaine hydrochloride	Bupivacaine hydrochloride	Prilocaine hydrochloride
Relative potency	1	4	1
Toxicity			
Central nervous system	+	++	
Cardiovascular system	+	++	
Other			Methaemoglobinaemia
Uses			
Spinal	+	++	+
Epidural	+	+	+
Infiltration	+	+	+
Topical	+	–	–
Intravenous	–	–	+

- The cardiovascular effects of hypotension, bradycardia, heart block, cardiac arrest, and ventricular tachycardia and fibrillation.
- The central nervous system effects of agitation, euphoria, respiratory depression, twitching, convulsions, and sensory disturbances.

Spinal and Epidural Anaesthesia

In spinal or intrathecal anaesthesia a local anaesthetic is injected into the subarachnoid space, where it mixes with the CSF. A spinal needle is inserted below the termination of the spinal cord at the first lumbar vertebra, usually at the third or fourth lumbar space. The local anaesthetic diffuses through the CSF and blocks the cord and nerve roots. It can diffuse both up and down so there is a risk of respiratory muscle paralysis if the needle is inserted too high in the column.

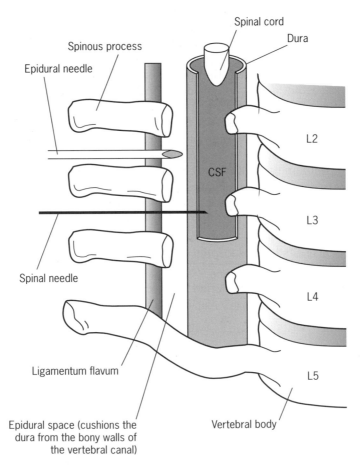

Figure 3.1 Spinal and epidural anaesthesia. (Reproduced from Cook LB (1992) *Surgery* **10(9)**:198 by kind permission of The Medicine Group (Journals) Ltd.)

In epidural anaesthesia (see *Figure 3.1*) a needle or catheter is inserted into the epidural space, which is a potential space containing fat, loose areolar tissue, epidural veins, and traversed by the spinal nerves leaving the vertebral column. Local anaesthetics infiltrate these tissues and block the spinal nerves as they traverse the epidural space.

In caudal anaesthesia the needle is placed in the epidural space via the caudal canal of the sacrum.

Most local anaesthetics cause vasodilation. When used for spinal or epidural blocks they are often administered with adrenaline, which causes vaso-constriction, slowing uptake and prolonging the anaesthetic action. *Table 3.2* provides a comparison of the spinal and epidural approaches.

After surgery under epidural or spinal block the patient requires careful nursing. Pressure areas and superficial nerves are vulnerable to pressure damage and mechanical injury while the patient's limbs are numb. Analgesia should be started early as the block can suddenly wear off. Careful monitoring for indications of cardiovascular or central nervous system side effects is essential. Blood pressure is checked regularly and hypotension is reported: it may be due to hypovolaemia and fluid therapy may need adjusting. Urine retention is common in the immediate postoperative period and may necessitate catheteriz-ation. Nausea and vomiting are not common after local anaesthesia. If they occur they may be due to pain, the side effects of opioid analgesia, or hypovolaemia. They are more likely if the operative procedure involves extensive handling of the viscera. Occasionally the duration of block is prolonged and this will cause the patient some concern. The anaesthetist should be informed, but in most cases the problem resolves naturally and the nurse's main role is in providing

Table 3.2 A comparison of spinal and epidural anaesthesia (after Cook, 1992).

	Spinal anaesthesia	Epidural anaesthesia	Comment
Placement	Lumbar	Lumbar	Epidural is sometimes thoracic
Site of action	CSF	Epidural space	
Needle	Yes	Yes	
Catheter	Uncommon	Common	Epidural catheters are sometimes used for opioid analgesia
Dose of 0.5% bupivacaine (ml)	2–4	10–30	
Success rate by experienced staff (%)	99–100	90–95	
Duration (minutes)	90–120	90–120	Catheter allows top-up
Hypotension	Common	Less common	
High block	Occasional	Occasional	
Urine retention	Common	Common	
Headache	1–5%	No	

reassurance and support. A headache may occur and can be treated with analgesia, rest, and ensuring adequate hydration.

Peripheral Nerve Block

Infiltration by a local anaesthetic can be used to provide blockade for minor surgery to superficial structures. Complications due to the anaesthesia are rare and are usually related to overdose or accidental intravascular injection.

References

Allin K (1991) Preoperative handover. *Surg Nurse* **4(2)**:4–9.

Ashworth P (1980) *Care to Communicate*, pp. 74–90. Royal College of Nursing, London.

Barr J, Noble D (1994) Awareness and unconscious perception during general anaesthesia. *Surgery* **12(3)**:62–63.

British National Formulary (1996a) No. 32, p. 520. British Medical Association and Royal Pharmaceutical Society for Great Britain, London.

British National Formulary (1996b) No. 32, p. 532. British Medical Association and Royal Pharmaceutical Society for Great Britain, London.

Boore JRP (1978) *Prescription for Recovery*, p. 26. Royal College of Nursing, London.

Chesson MM, Reid M, Rumsey JE (1980) Only a pair of eyes. *Nurs Times* (Theatre Nursing Supplement) **76(42)**:3–8.

Chung DC, Lam AM (1990) *Essentials of Anaesthesiology*, 2nd edition, p. 6. WB Saunders Co, Philadelphia.

Cook LB (1992) Spinal and epidural anaesthesia in surgery. *Surgery* **10(9)**:198–201.

Devine EC, Cook TD (1983) A meta-analysis of effects of psycho-educational interventions on length of hospital stay. *Nurs Res* **32(5)**:267–274.

Ellison P (1975) The pre and post operative visit concept. NATN Supplement. *Nurs Times* **71(42)**:4–6.

Farmer G (1985) The role of the anaesthetic nurse. *Natl Br J Theatre Nurs* **22(ii)**:10–12.

Irving CJ (1993) Toxicity of anaesthetic agents. *Surgery* **11(6)**: 413–415.

Jameson P (1994) Principles of general anaesthesia. *Surgery* **12(3)**:58–60.

Medical Defence Societies, Royal College of Nursing, National Association of Theatre Nurses (1988) *Theatre Safeguards*, p. 2.

Meeker MH, Rothrock JC (1995) *Alexander's Care of the Patient in Surgery*, 10th edition. Mosby, St Louis.

Memon MA (1994) Surgical diathermy. *Br J Med* **52(8)**:403–408.

Milne C (1988) Anaesthetics. *Nurs Stand* **2(28)**:22–23.

Shergold L (1986) Epidural and spinal anaesthetics. *Nurs Times* **82(27)**:44–45.

Chapter 4
Postoperative Care

The aim of postoperative care is to facilitate recovery, minimize the development or impact of postoperative complications, and prepare the patient for discharge and continued recovery at home. Postoperative care can be divided into two main phases: immediate recovery and general postoperative care with discharge preparation. Immediate recovery begins in the recovery room and is continued on return to the general surgical ward, or in acute cases, the intensive care unit. In modern surgical practice with early discharge, information-giving and preparation for discharge and recuperation at home are critical aspects of postoperative nursing.

IMMEDIATE POSTOPERATIVE CARE

Observation and assessment are essential skills for surgical nursing and are particularly important in the immediate postoperative period. The need for careful postoperative monitoring can extend from a few hours after procedures under local anaesthesia to days after major procedures. The immediate postoperative period is a potentially dangerous time. Atkinson *et al.* (1982) reported that about 20% of deaths in hospital due to anaesthesia occur within the first 30 minutes after the operation and that almost 50% of deaths during the immediate postoperative period are due to inadequate nursing. Careful assessment is required to identify priority needs in this critical period when the patient is most reliant on nursing care. Care must be systematically planned to meet nursing goals related to the assessed needs. The care plan should encourage progress from a state of patient dependency immediately after the operation to one of independence and eventual self-care, where possible. Until the patient has recovered from the effects of the anaesthetic it is the surgical nurse's responsibility to:

■ Maintain a clear airway.
■ Carry out general observation and monitor vital signs.
■ Alleviate pain and discomfort.
■ Monitor fluid intake and output.
■ Ensure the patient understands the nature of the operation and what to expect.

When the patient returns from theatre the ward nurse must ensure that the notes contain written information about the operation performed, any specific instructions for postoperative care, the type and time of any analgesia, and details of intravenous therapy in progress. The patient should be settled into bed and vital signs and general appearance assessed:

■ What is the colour of the face and extremities?
■ Is the patient cold or sweating excessively?
■ Is the patient sleepy, communicating, restless, disorientated, or in pain?
■ Does the patient have an intravenous infusion in progress, a nasogastric tube, where is the incision located, how is it dressed, is there any bleeding or are there wound drains?

A rapid but thorough assessment is essential to plan priorities of care.

Maintaining a Clear Airway

The receiving nurse should assess the patency of the airway by feeling for expired air and observing the chest movements. Rate, depth, pattern of respiration, and any use of the accessory muscles of respiration should be noted. It is important to listen to the breathing, noting any rhonchi or gurgles, which may indicate secretions gathering in the large airways. If the patient inhales saliva or vomit, an aspiration pneumonia can develop. Suction apparatus must be available at the bedside. The nurse must remember that the patient might vomit, especially if the patient had an emergency-type preparation for surgery or the anaesthetic has not been fully reversed. It should not be assumed that because patients open their eyes and speak in recovery that they have fully regained consciousness. Patients cannot be left unattended until they have a cough reflex. This is necessary to prevent respiratory obstruction, which could be caused by the patient's tongue or secretions blocking the airway. The patient can be placed in the semiprone position (*Figure 4.1*), although this is not always possible after certain types of surgery, for example hip replacement. If necessary the chin can be supported with the neck extended to prevent the tongue obstructing the oropharynx (*Figure 4.2*) or an airway can be inserted. It is essential that the foot of the bed can be elevated, enabling the patient's head to be tipped which facilitates the removal of secretions. Oxygen must be available at the bedside, and airways, face masks, Ambubag, and other resuscitation equipment nearby.

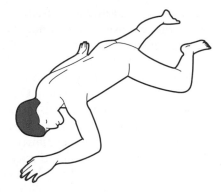

Figure 4.1 The semiprone position.

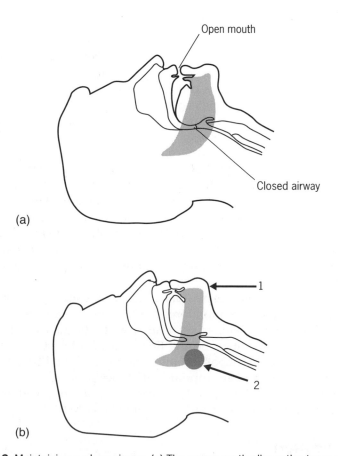

Figure 4.2 Maintaining a clear airway. (a) The open mouth allows the tongue to fall back and block the airway. (b) Gentle pressure exerted by the fingertips in the direction indicated (1) below the chin, closing the mouth or (2) at the angle of the jaw will maintain a clear airway.

The colour of the lips, conjunctiva, skin, and extremities should be observed for signs of central or peripheral cyanosis. Oxygen may be prescribed to relieve hypoxia, and it is important to ensure that oxygen is delivered at the rate prescribed. Some patients with chronic obstructive airways disease (COAD) rely on a low oxygen concentration for their respiratory drive and in such cases an oxygen concentration that is too high can depress ventilation. Oxygen may be delivered via a face mask, nasal cannula, tracheostomy mask, or endotracheal tube if the patient is still intubated. Face masks must be of the correct type and fit to maintain the prescribed oxygen rate. The nurse must explain the need for oxygen and ensure that the face mask is comfortably adjusted. It may be helpful to reassure the patient that oxygen will be needed for only a short time. The usual safety precautions in relation to using oxygen should be followed. The patient should be encouraged to sit up in bed as soon as possible to improve lung expansion.

General Observation and Vital Signs

Regular observation and recording of vital signs, pulse, blood pressure, respiration, and temperature are important during the immediate postoperative period. Systematic observation can reveal early indicators of hypoxia, haemorrhage, shock, and other postoperative complications.

A rising pulse rate and a falling systolic blood pressure may indicate a reduction in the circulating blood volume due to haemorrhage, and the wound site and any drainage tubes should be observed for any signs of bleeding. The patient may also be restless and the skin cold and clammy. Elevating the foot of the bed when appropriate may produce a short term rise in systolic pressure, medical staff must be alerted, and appropriate treatment considered. It may be necessary to return the patient to theatre to ligate bleeding vessels. Oxygen should be administered via a face mask until a medical reassessment has been made. However, pain and the residual effects of anaesthesia may reduce blood flow and the surgical nurse needs to be alert to patterns and changes in the patient's condition. As the pulse rate and blood pressure stabilize, the frequency of recording may be decreased.

The importance of observing respiratory function has already been emphasized. Temperature should also be monitored as prolonged surgery and exposure of the thoracic or abdominal contents may result in a significant loss of body heat. An early rise in temperature may be the first sign of a chest or other postoperative infection. Specimens of both sputum and urine should be collected for culture and sensitivity tests and appropriate antibiotics prescribed.

All observations should be carefully recorded and any medications or activities that might influence the recordings should be noted.

Pain and Discomfort

Pain relief is an essential aspect of immediate postoperative care and can make a major contribution to an uncomplicated recovery from surgery. Carr (1990) emphasizes that while poorly controlled postoperative pain may be 'dull' at rest, when the patient attempts to move it may become severe and 'stabbing.' The patient will be afraid to move, promoting immobility. Immobility increases the risk of deep vein thrombosis (DVT), pressure sores, hypostatic pneumonia, muscle wasting, urinary retention, and constipation. Pain not normally associated with the operation performed should be reported, for example calf pain, which may be a sign of DVT, pleural pain, which may be embolic in origin, and pain at the site of an intravenous infusion. Anxiety, tension, or disorientation will increase the perception of pain. Reassurance and frequent orientation to time and place can help reduce the problem. As the patient becomes more aware, preoperative teaching can be reinforced. The patient will also want to know about the outcome of the surgery and what to expect next. Pain as a postoperative problem is discussed in more detail later in this chapter. Chapter 7 reviews the topic of pain in more detail.

GENERAL POSTOPERATIVE NURSING CARE

As the patient becomes more aware, gentle mobilization, and turning and repositioning in bed (as far as restricting drainage tubes, splints, and dressings allow) can be encouraged. If the patient is unable to move, pressure sore prevention is a priority. Passive movements and exercise can be slowly introduced, but respiratory exercises and coughing should be started as soon as possible. It should be explained to the patient how important these measures are in ensuring a complete recovery. Pain relief should be offered before the patient commences the exercises.

The patient may request a wash and the theatre gown should be changed for usual nightwear. Oral hygiene is important, and the nurse can offer small amounts of fluids if this is permitted. A sputum container should be available, together with tissues and mouthwash solution.

Fluid Balance

Fluid intake and output will be monitored. The surgical patient usually has an intravenous infusion in progress on return from theatre and may have a nasogastric tube. Patient comfort is an important factor in intravenous therapy. The limb containing the intravenous cannula should be comfortably positioned and supported with pillows. It is important to ensure patient safety in relation to intravenous therapy by:

- Maintaining asepsis.
- Ensuring the correct infusion rate.
- Checking all fluids administered against the prescription.
- Observing and looking after the insertion site.

Fluid balance is discussed in more detail in Chapter 5.

Urine output may decrease initially after surgery, but should return to normal within 12–24 hours. Fluid output should be recorded. The patient may have a urinary catheter in place and this is usually removed as soon as possible, but it is important to continue monitoring urinary output in case postoperative oliguria or urinary retention develop. The patient may have difficulty with micturition at first because of fluid loss during surgery or because it is difficult to use a urinal in bed. If the bladder is palpable and the patient is unable to pass urine, ensuring privacy and running adjacent taps might help. It may be possible to get the patient out of bed to use the urinal or to take the patient to the toilet in a wheel-chair. As the patient recovers from the surgery and anaesthetic, bowel sounds will return and oral fluids can be tolerated. The intravenous infusion and nasogastric tube can then be removed.

Nutrition

Malnutrition is a common problem in surgical patients because the trauma associated with surgery increases the need for nutrients and food intake is usually restricted before and after surgery (Moynihan, 1994). The nurse can help the patient recovering after surgery to select an appropriate diet to meet calorific and special needs. If the patient is malnourished there is a danger that his immune system will be impaired, healing of the wound will be delayed, and recovery prolonged. Food intake should be monitored and assistance given when necessary. Food intake may need to be recorded and if there appears to be a deficit between nutrients taken and needed, supplements or alternative approaches to feeding can be used. If oral intake is restricted for more than two days nutritional support such as parenteral feeding will be required. Nutrition and the surgical patient is considered further in Chapter 6.

Suppositories or a mild aperient may be required to initiate bowel movement after surgery. However, as the patient's appetite improves, a normal diet with extra dietary fibre can be introduced to assist normal bowel function.

Mobility

Mobility should be encouraged as soon as the patient's condition allows. Mobility promotes venous return from the lower limbs, preventing venous stasis, DVT, and pulmonary embolism (PE). Lung expansion is easier when the patient is able to get out of bed and move around, and this helps avoid chest complications. The risk of developing pressure sores is lessened when the patient is able to walk about, and urinary tract infection and constipation are less likely to develop if the patient is allowed easier access to the toilet. When the patient attempts to get out of bed for the first time it is important to allow plenty of time. The patient will want to move slowly, taking it in stages and avoiding problems with infusions, drains, and catheters. The patient can sit on the edge of the bed supported by one nurse while another nurse can prepare the chair and clothes to wear while the patient is out of bed. Any infusion or drainage tubes should be adjusted comfortably on the correct side of the bed. When the patient is settled comfortably in the chair, the nurse must make sure that the patient is warm enough and that the call bell is easily available. The patient should be encouraged to continue to do deep breathing and leg exercises in the chair, and periodically should be helped to walk. As the patient's condition improves, he will be encouraged to stay up for longer periods, until he is out of bed for most of the day.

Sleep

Rest and sleep are critical when recovering from surgery. Tiredness and a lack of sleep will adversely affect pain, mobilization, wound healing, and psychological state. Closs (1994) reports that patients say that tiredness makes postoperative pain more nagging and harder to put up with. It may make them feel depressed and give up quicker. Patients observed that when they slept well the pain was not as bad and that they were more relaxed. The link between sleep and wound healing is discussed by Torrance (1990).

Psychological Care

In the postoperative period the nurse can build on the relationship established during preoperative preparation to help the patient cope with any fears or anxieties about the surgery, and its consequences. Postoperative dependency and the need for assistance with basic activities such as excretion and hygiene may cause embarrassment and a reduction in self-esteem. An efficient matter-of-fact approach will help the patient accept these necessities. Embarrassment may be more acute if the surgery involved the urogenital system. The effects of surgery and the restrictions imposed by infusions, drains, and catheters in the postoperative period may affect coordination and movement, making the patient awkward or clumsy. By anticipating these problems and offering assistance in advance the nurse can help reduce any embarrassment about loss of function. However, help should not encourage dependency and there is a need to frequently reassess the assistance required.

Some surgery may be disfiguring or have profound effects on body image and sexuality, for example amputation, mastectomy, or ostomies. The patient may experience very mixed emotions including relief that the condition has been treated and the symptoms have been relieved, and grief, denial, anger, and depression about the loss or change in body image. Relief may be tempered by fear that the condition will recur or worries about follow-up treatment (e.g. chemotherapy or radiotherapy). The nurse will need to assess patients' behaviour and allow time for them to express and work out their feelings. Some may accept things readily, others may take some time to come to terms with their feelings. Information-giving and teaching are key activities at this time. The information given should be sufficient and relevant: sufficient for the patient to develop insight and make informed decisions, but not so much that the patient is swamped and unable to take it in. Preoperative assessment and teaching should provide a framework that can be reinforced and developed in the postoperative period.

POSTOPERATIVE COMPLICATIONS

Postoperative complications may be general, associated with anaesthesia and surgery, or specific to a particular operative procedure or treatment. With appropriate preoperative assessment and planning, the risk of postoperative complications can be reduced. Many postoperative problems originate in the operating room and prevention is clearly better than cure. Attention to patient safety and comfort, asepsis, gentle surgical technique, and expert anaesthetic care will help reduce the risk of postoperative complications. General postoperative complications include:

- Haemorrhage.
- Shock.
- Pulmonary complications.
- Urinary tract infection (UTI).
- Wound infection.
- Dehydration.
- Overhydration.
- Low urine output.
- Nausea and vomiting.
- Paralytic ileus.
- Pain.
- DVT and PE.

It is important to note that on a surgical ward postoperative infection represents not only an individual hazard, but also carries the risk of cross-infection. Patients may require antibiotic treatment, but overuse or abuse of antibiotic therapy may contribute to the development of antibiotic-resistant strains.

Haemorrhage

Haemorrhage can be a problem during or after surgery. Inadequate haemostasis is the commonest cause of postoperative haemorrhage. Blood vessels damaged during surgery can be sealed by diathermy, clipping, or ligatures. Postoperative bleeding may require a return to theatre for wound exploration and ligation of the bleeding vessel.

Patients with coagulation disorders have a higher risk of postoperative haemorrhage, but this should have been identified in the preoperative preparation. For patients with a recognized bleeding disorder it is important to ensure that the deficient factor is available in sufficient quantities. Bleeding times will be monitored in the postoperative period. Coagulation problems may arise in patients with congenital disease (e.g. haemophilia and von Willebrand's disease) and platelet disorders, and in those receiving anticoagulant therapy (e.g. heparin or warfarin). Disseminated intravascular coagulation (DIC) is a systemic problem that leads to generalized coagulation in small blood vessels. It may develop as a consequence of severe trauma, sepsis (endotoxic shock), and hypoxia, and is also a complication of transfusion reactions.

Shock

Shock can be defined as a clinical condition in which the metabolic needs of the body cannot be met because of inadequate tissue perfusion due to a reduction in cardiac output. The main clinical manifestation of shock is low blood pressure with the signs and symptoms that accompany hypotension. The consequences of untreated shock can be serious and are sometimes fatal.

Inadequate perfusion of metabolically active tissues can cause profound lactic acidosis, which results in breathlessness due to respiratory compensation (Montgomery and Jenkins, 1995). Acidaemia will also tend to depress myocardial contractility, and this contributes to further hypotension.

Low perfusion pressure of certain organs may lead to specific organ failure. Inadequate cerebral perfusion may present as agitation or confusion and eventually unconsciousness. The kidneys are particularly affected by low perfusion pressure. The immediate effect is a sharp fall in urinary output. If shock persists, acute renal failure rapidly develops. Early fluid resuscitation can prevent further kidney damage, but acute tubular necrosis can occur if hypoperfusion continues.

In severe shock inadequate perfusion of the gut can led to ischaemic damage to the mucosa and altered absorption. Bacterial toxins may enter the portal circulation, further reducing blood pressure. This abnormal uptake of bacterial products may contribute to endotoxaemia and the high incidence of systemic sepsis associated with severe shock (Baker et al., 1988; Wilmore et al., 1988). Holcroft and Blaisdell (1991) identify three primary causes of shock as:

- Inadequate circulating blood volume.
- Loss of autonomic control of blood vessels.
- Impaired cardiac function.

Table 4.1 identifies the main types of shock, the underlying mechanisms, and some examples of clinical causes. It is essential that the surgical nurse is alert to the signs of shock and regularly monitors vital signs. Dressings or wound drains must be checked for evidence of continued bleeding. Postoperative haemorrhage may be sudden or gradual. As the patient recovers from anaesthesia and surgery blood pressure will rise and there is a risk of a reactionary haemorrhage with sudden and substantial blood loss, usually within the first 24 hours. However, hypovolaemic shock may also develop gradually due to slow haemorrhage from leaking blood vessels. If bleeding is internal or hypovolaemia is due to sequestration of fluid in the gastrointestinal tract, shock may be less obvious in the early stages. Careful observation and checking of vital signs is essential. General indicators in the early stages of shock include:

- Pale, sweaty, clammy skin.
- Peripheral cyanosis.
- Restlessness or agitation.
- Reduced urine output.
- Tachycardia and slight elevation of blood pressure.

As compensatory mechanisms fail and shock progresses features include:

- Cold, pale, sweaty skin.

Table 4.1 Types of shock (adapted from Holcroft & Blaisdell, 1991).

Type of shock	Mechanism	Clinical examples
Inadequate circulating volume		

Hypovolaemic shock	Haemorrhage
	Dehydration or third spacing
	  (loss of fluid into the gut)
		Haemorrhage
		Vomiting, diarrhoea,
		  obstructed bowel

Traumatic shock	External haemorrhage or
	  plasma loss plus internal
	  losses
		Trauma and burns

Septic shock	Loss of plasma into the
	  tissues and cutaneous
	  vasodilation
		Systemic sepsis

Loss of autonomic control of vasculature		

Neurogenic shock	Pooling of blood in veins
	  and nonessential vascular
	  beds
		Regional anaesthesia,
		  spinal cord injury

Impaired cardiac function		

Cardiac compressive
  shock
	Compression of the heart
	  or great vessels
		Pericardial tamponade,
		  tension pneumothorax

Cardiogenic shock	Intrinsic cardiac dysfunction	Arrhythmias, congenital
		  abnormalities, myocardial
		  ischaemia

Cardiac obstructive
  shock
	Obstruction of pulmonary
	  or systemic circulation
		Pulmonary embolism,
		  mechanical ventilation

- Central cyanosis.
- Agitation; and confusion, progressing to drowsiness and coma.
- Oliguria (less than 30 mL^{-1}).
- Tachycardia.
- Hypotension.

Table 4.2 summarizes the additional signs and treatment of hypovolaemic, septic, cardiogenic, and neurogenic shock.

Pulmonary Complications

Respiratory infections are the commonest cause of fever in the immediate postoperative period. Pulmonary complications are likely to develop if the

Table 4.2 Signs and treatment of shock (adapted from Holcroft & Blaisdell, 1991).

Signs	Treatment
Hypovolaemic shock	
Pale, cool skin	Restore blood or fluid loss, crystalloids,
Slow capillary refill	treat haemorrhage or source of fluid
Agitation, restlessness	loss
Low cardiac output	
High peripheral vascular resistance	
Low central venous pressure (usually)	
Septic shock	
Flushed, warm (early sign)	Fluid resuscitation, antibiotic therapy,
Confused	may require diuretics and vasoactive
Depressed sensorium (later sign)	drug therapy, may require surgery
High cardiac output (in early stages)	(e.g. drainage or excision)
Low peripheral vascular resistance	
Low central venous pressure (usually)	
Cardiogenic shock	
Pale, cool skin	Fluid volume support, treat causes
Slow capillary refill	
May be quiet or agitated	
Low cardiac output	
High peripheral vascular pressure	
Neurogenic shock	
Skin colour, temperature, and capillary refill usually normal	Exclude other causes of shock, volume support, possibly vasoconstrictive
Variety of effects on mental state, but often unaffected	drugs
May be high cardiac output and low peripheral vascular resistance	
Low central venous pressure with normal circulating volume	

patient had previous pulmonary disease, prolonged mechanical ventilation, or inadequate ventilation. Atelectasis, collapse of the alveoli, is often the first problem. This can be prevented or resolved by deep breathing and coughing exercises as taught in the preoperative period. If atelectasis does not rapidly resolve, pneumonia can develop. Careful preoperative instruction and postoperative encouragement in carrying out breathing exercises will help reduce the incidence of pulmonary complications.

The risk of developing a respiratory complication is increased by abdominal distension, postoperative pain, oversedation, and a history of chronic respiratory disease. Pain, particularly from an abdominal wound, may encourage rapid shallow breathing that fails to ventilate the whole lung adequately. Effective postoperative analgesia and teaching the patient how to support the wound during coughing and deep breathing will encourage better ventilation. The surgical patient will benefit from chest physiotherapy, but breathing exercises should be reinforced by the nurse.

Urinary Tract Infection

After respiratory infections, UTIs are the second most common hospital-acquired infection (Meers *et al.*, 1980). UTI is a probable cause of fever presenting in the first 3–6 postoperative days. Two factors may contribute to the development of UTI in the surgical patient:

- The patient may have been catheterized before or during surgery and the catheter may be left in place in the immediate postoperative period. Indwelling catheters provide a ready route for ascending infection.
- Postoperative pain can contribute by causing patients to incompletely empty the bladder. Residual urine presents an ideal medium for bacterial growth.

Pre-existing bladder problems or obstruction will also increase the risk. Appropriate pain control, encouraging complete voiding of the bladder, and early removal of urinary catheters will all help reduce the risk. If UTI does develop, appropriate antibiotic therapy will be required.

Instrumentation or catheterization of the urinary tract increases the risk of infection and Stucke (1993) identifies several risk factors. Intrinsic risk factors are not amenable to alteration. Older people are more likely to develop UTI than younger patients, and women more than men. The severity and nature of the patient's condition can also influence the risk. However, other risk factors (i.e. extrinsic risk factors) can be altered. Consideration should be given to:

- Using alternatives to catheterization.
- Suprapubic versus urethral catheterization.
- Selection of an appropriate size and type of catheter.
- Reducing the length of time the catheter is *in situ*.

- Reducing the number of times catheterization takes place.
- Use and maintenance of closed drainage systems.
- Aseptic techniques when collecting catheter specimens of urine.
- Appropriate catheter care.

Figure 4.3 identifies the main points where bacteria can enter the drainage system. Stucke (1993) makes the following additional practical recommendations for reducing the risk of catheter-related UTI:

- If possible keep some space between catheterized patients.
- Keep patients with UTI away from other catheterized patients.
- Wash and dry hands carefully before handling any part of the system.
- Secure the drainage bag to avoid traction of the catheter.
- Avoid twisting or flattening the tubing.
- Never raise the drainage bag above bladder level.
- Avoid spigots.
- Avoid bladder irrigation if possible and use a three-way Foley catheter if irrigation is essential.
- Use a sterile syringe, needle, and sampling sleeve to obtain specimens.
- Take care not to contaminate the system when emptying the drainage bag, do not let the tap touch the floor or container, use disposable or sterilizable containers.

Wound Infection

Wound infection is another common hospital-acquired infection. It may be suspected if the patient develops a spiking temperature or has any local signs of infection and inflammation such as redness, warmth, tenderness, increased discharge or drainage, dehiscence, or cellulitis. Wound infections often develop between postoperative days 5–8. In modern surgery patients are often discharged within 2–3 days of surgery and they will require information on how to

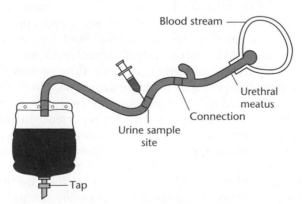

Figure 4.3 Entry points for bacteria in a urinary drainage system (from Stucke, 1993).

identify possible wound infection and who to contact if they suspect it is developing. Treatment may range from improving drainage to full surgical debridement under general anaesthesia. Antibiotics have a role in treating wound infections, but additional measures such as improving drainage or debridement are generally required. Surgical wounds and wound infection are considered in more detail in Chapter 9.

Dehydration

Dehydration can be a problem in the postoperative period. Blood and body fluids may be lost during surgery. In addition fluid may be sequestered at the site of operation or within the gastrointestinal system (so-called third-spacing). Although not lost from the body this fluid represents a hidden loss from the effective circulating volume. If this loss is not recognized dehydration may develop despite fluid support therapy. Tachycardia, postural (orthostatic) hypotension, and oliguria may suggest dehydration. The patient may complain of a dry mouth and thirst. Treatment is simply by rehydration, increasing oral or intravenous intake. Fluid regimens will need to be carefully monitored and adjusted. Diuresis may occur around postoperative days 3–4 as the body mobilizes sequestered fluids back into the circulating volume.

Overhydration

Conversely overhydration is also a risk, especially for patients with impaired cardiac, pulmonary, or renal function. For these patients careful monitoring of fluid intake and output and daily weighing can be invaluable. Intravenous therapy will need to be carefully regulated.

Low Urine Output

A reduced urinary output is not uncommon in postoperative surgical patients. Montgomery et al. (1995) emphasize that the causes of a low urine output are complex, the consequences are potentially disastrous, and inappropriate use of potent diuretics may make the situation worse. Normal fluid balance is discussed in Chapter 5. It is important that the nurse carefully monitors urine output in the postoperative period. Oliguria is defined as a urine flow of less than 17 mL h^{-1} (400 mL day^{-1}). Anuria should strictly mean no urine flow, but is often used when output is less than 100 mL day^{-1}. Low output may be due to prerenal, renal, or postrenal causes. Prerenal causes are of particular importance in the surgical ward when the most common cause is reduced renal perfusion due to reduced circulating volume (see section on shock, p. 63). A single episode of hypotension can result in acute tubular necrosis and oliguria of renal origin (Montgomery et al., 1995). Renal and postrenal problems should have been identified by the preoperative assessment, but acute urinary retention can occasionally occur. Less commonly antidiuretic hormone (ADH) concentration may rise due to the stress response to surgery and there is a resulting oliguria. Contrast agents and some drugs (e.g. gentamicin, nonsteroidal anti-inflammatory drugs) may also precipitate oliguria.

Pain

Postoperative pain will increase postoperative stress and have a negative impact on healing. The patient in pain will find movement and exercise more difficult. This may affect breathing and coughing exercises, DVT prevention, and early ambulation. Sleep will be disturbed and appetite may be poor. Closs (1992) found that pain was one of the main causes of poor sleep in the surgical patient. Pain may also encourage incomplete emptying of the urinary bladder with the problems associated with residual urine. Pain control is essential after surgery. The pain-free patient will be less anxious, able to breath more easily and deeply, and tolerate earlier mobilization. Pain assessment and appropriate analgesia must be used to ensure that the postoperative patient is pain-free. Weis *et al.* (1983) studied the knowledge and attitudes of hospital staff to postoperative analgesic care. They found that many of the doctors and nurses studied believed that patients received adequate pain relief. However, Melzack *et al.* (1987) suggest that postoperative pain is poorly controlled.

A numerical rating scale marked 0–10 is useful for quickly assessing the severity of a patient's pain. However, if not articulated, pain may be apparent from systemic signs such as a reduced blood pressure and raised pulse rate. The patient may appear tense, anxious, pale, and sweating; he may adopt a rigid position and his breathing may be shallow in an attempt to 'splint' the surgical incision by reducing respiratory movement. An important method of overcoming postoperative pain is the use of patient-controlled analgesia. One of the advantages of this is its ability to accommodate the wide variation in individual analgesic requirements. A more even drug concentration and a steady level of analgesia is achieved when patients take analgesia as they require it. The patient can take analgesia at peak periods of pain, such as occurs when physiotherapy is given. The patient is given a degree of independence and control, which underlines his importance as a partner in his own care (Clark, 1992).

It is important to remember that there are other pain-relieving measures that can be used in conjunction with analgesia. These include careful positioning, as the patient will gradually sit up after the operation and must be supported comfortably. Pressure-relieving mattresses and aids are very useful, and it must be ensured that the patient is not too cold or too warm. Quiet conversation and the ability to listen are invaluable nursing aids to pain relief. Pain is a critical topic for surgical nursing and Chapter 7 presents a fuller consideration of postoperative pain.

Nausea and Vomiting

Vomiting that occurs as the patient recovers from anaesthesia is often an attempt to relieve the stomach of saliva and mucus swallowed during the anaesthetic period. Other causes of postoperative vomiting include an accumulation of fluid in the stomach, or ingestion of food or fluid before peristalsis returns. It is very important, therefore, that the patient receives correct preoperative information to reduce the possibility of vomiting after anaesthesia. Following any indication of nausea, the patient should be turned onto one side to facilitate mouth drainage. Prochlorperazine may be prescribed intramuscularly or intravenously to reduce nausea (*British National Formulary*, 1996). Fluids should be withheld for 3 to 4 hours and the patient offered a freshwater mouth-wash (Brunner and Suddarth, 1992).

Paralytic Ileus

Functional paralytic ileus following abdominal surgery may last for 12–36 hours. Food and fluids must be withheld until normal peristalsis returns which is indicated by bowel sounds. Nasogastric aspiration will help relieve the abdominal distension. Fluids must be administered intravenously.

Deep Vein Thrombosis and Pulmonary Embolism

DVT is a common complication in surgery and 80–90% of PEs result from a DVT. The deep veins of the lower leg are the main sites for DVT. As with other postoperative complications the best treatment is prevention, and DVT prevention starts with preoperative preparation (see Chapter 2). DVT prophylaxis may be based on mechanical or pharmacological methods. Simple mechanical methods include early mobilization and compression stockings; for higher risk patients, pneumatic intermittent calf compression may be required. Pre- and postoperative heparin therapy is the mainstay of the pharmacological approach. As with any anticoagulant therapy, the patient on heparin should be observed for signs of bleeding. Compression stockings should be worn because they promote venous flow and reduce stasis. The velocity of the flow is increased not only in the legs, but in the pelvic veins and inferior vena cava. In order to achieve this the stockings must be able to provide a graduated compression from the ankle to the mid-thigh; they must therefore be seamless and contoured to the limbs (Drinkwater, 1989).

DVT classically presents with calf or thigh pain, tenderness, oedema, and calf pain on dorsiflexion of the foot (Homan's sign). However, many patients develop DVT without these signs. If part of the thrombosis breaks away it may lodge in the pulmonary arteries causing a PE. Pulmonary embolism results in decreased cardiac output, hypertension, impaired oxygenation, and bronchospasm, and is one of the commonest causes of sudden death in hospital.

DISCHARGE PLANNING

Discharge planning aims to facilitate a smooth transition from hospital care to community service and family care. With modern practice patients may be discharged within 2–3 days of relatively major surgery. It is generally desirable to discharge patients as soon as possible after surgery, and patients are usually keen to go home. It is widely accepted that care in the community is preferable to protracted stays in hospital (Malby, 1992). However, with early discharge it is possible for postoperative complications to develop at home and unplanned discharge can result in readmission. Poor discharge planning may be a factor in delayed recovery at home (Wilson-Barnett and Fordham, 1982).

Arenth and Mamon (1985) argue that two aspects of discharge planning are crucial: an accurate nursing assessment of the patient's needs and the extent to which the patient and his family are involved in the process. However, involvement of the community team in the discharge process may also be important for patients requiring nursing care. Assessment of needs to identify physical, pyschosocial, or knowledge deficits that might influence recovery at home is essential. Discharge planning can start on admission. The admission interview can provide information regarding worries and concerns about the surgery and ability to cope after the operation. Relatives may be involved in preoperative teaching so that they are better able to deal with the patient after surgery. The patient and family must be assessed to establish that they have the knowledge and physical, emotional, and financial resources to cope.

Before discharge, patients need information about carrying out daily activities in addition to how to care for their wound. In a study by Vaughan and Taylor (1988) about discharged patients, it was found there were deficiencies with regard to:

- Bathing. Some patients did not know when they could safely bath or shower, and some had difficulty getting in and out of the bath, mainly due to weakness, pain, or fear.
- Dressing. Some patients had difficulty getting dressed, the main cause being getting clothes on over the feet and restriction over the wound.
- Eating. Although the majority of people returned to their normal eating habits within a few days, some were not sure if their diet was appropriate for aiding their recovery. Problems included poor appetite, nausea, and indigestion.
- Bowels. Difficulty with bowel function was experienced by some people who then resorted to home remedies or altered their diet.
- Sexual activity. There is evidence of a considerable lack of advice about sexual matters, for example when sexual activity can be safely resumed.

There also appears to be a lack of information about how the patient may feel. Smith (1992) emphasized that there is a gulf between being well in hospital and being well enough to resume one's normal life. Information should include a reminder that to avoid feeling exhausted and possible depression, it is important to resume normal activities gradually and to obtain adequate rest. It is important for the nurse to consider the individual patient's lifestyle and the short- and long-term consequences of surgery and treatment before discussing how best to proceed with their convalescence.

Particular care must be taken in planning discharge arrangements for some patients, for example:

- Patients who live alone, are frail or elderly.
- Those whose principal carer is frail, disabled, or elderly.
- Patients with serious illness.
- The terminally ill.
- Patients with special needs (e.g. incontinence).
- Patients requiring care from the community nursing service.
- The homeless or those in hostel accommodation.

The discharge plan should be compiled by the nurse primarily responsible for the patient's care, together with the patient. A comprehensive assessment should be made of the patient's home circumstances and the support likely to be available, and it should be ensured that any support, help or equipment required to enable the patient and carer to cope at home is available by the time the patient leaves hospital. It is important that the patient, and with their consent, relative or carers, are consulted throughout the time discharge arrangements are being made. The patient should know the expected date of discharge as early as possible, and at least 48 hours notice should be given to the patient's general practitioner, community nursing services if needed, ambulance service, and carers. For some patients it may be appropriate to use a voluntary care service driver or a taxi. For frail or elderly patients living alone or with frail or elderly carers arrangements must be made through the hospital social worker. The home has to be heated and food provided, and there must be safe access to the stairs and toilet. The patient will require suitable clothing to travel home and must be able to gain entry on arrival.

The patient or carers will need to be aware of any dietary arrangements or any other aspects of self care, including the provision of any dressings or medicine for at least 72 hours. An outpatient appointment should be given and the nurse must ensure the patient knows where to attend. If the patient agrees, voluntary organizations can be contacted, for example the Ileostomy Association, the Mastectomy Association, Age Concern.

An important aspect of discharge care is ensuring appropriate communication between the hospital and community services. As Fares (1993) points out, there is an important role for liaison between community and hospital nurses to ensure that individuals receive appropriate assessment, advice, and information about their care before their discharge from hospital. A liaison nurse from the community team may visit the patient in hospital to plan the discharge with the patient and ward staff.

References

Atkinson RS, Rushman GB, Lee JA (1982) *A Synopsis of Anaesthesia*, 9th edition, pp. 572–618. John Wright, Bristol.

Arenth LM, Mamon JA (1985) Determining patients needs after discharge. *Nurs Management* **16(9)**:22–24.

Baker JW, Deitch EA, Berg RD *et al.* (1988) Hemorrhagic shock induces bacterial translocation from the gut. *J Trauma* **28**:896–906.

British National Formulary (1996) No. 32, p. 185. British Medical Association and the Royal Pharmaceutical Society of Great Britain.

Brunner LS, Suddarth DS (1992) *Textbook of Adult Nursing*, Chapter 2, p. 123. Chapman & Hall, London.

Carr EC (1990) Post operative pain: patients' expectations and experiences. *J Adv Nurs* **15**:89–100.

Clark EC (1992) Postoperative patient-controlled analgesia. *Surg Nurse* **5(3)**:20–21.

Closs SJ (1992) Patients' night-time pain, analgesic provision and sleep after surgery. *Int J Nurs Stud* **29(4)**:381–392.

Closs SJ (1994) Sleep. In *Nursing Practice: Hospital and Home. The Adult*. Alexander MF, Fawcett JN, Runciman PC (eds). pp. 743–756. Churchill Livingstone, Edinburgh.

Drinkwater K. (1989) Management of deep vein thrombosis. *Surg Nurse* **2**: 224–226.

Fares S (1993) A smooth path home. *Nurs Times* **89(21)**:48–50.

Holcroft JW, Blaisdell FW (1991) Shock causes and management of circulatory collapse. In *Textbook of Surgery*. Sabiston DC (ed.). pp. 34–56. WB Saunders, Philadelphia.

Malby R (1992) Discharge planning. *Surg Nurse* **5(1)**:4–8.

Meers PD, Ayliffe GAJ, Emmerson AM *et al.* (1980) Report of the National Survey on infections in hospital. *J Hosp Infect* **2**(Suppl. 2): 23–28.

Melzack R, Abbott FV, Zackon W, Mulder DS, Davis MWL (1987) Pain on a surgical ward: a survey of the duration and intensity of pain and the effectiveness of medication. *Pain* **29**:67–72.

Montgomery H, Jenkins DP (1995) Shock: physiology and practical management for surgeons. *Surgery* **13(9)**:213–216.

Montgomery H, Jenkins DP, Miller C (1995) Management of low urine output. *Surgery* **13(11)**:249–252.

Moynihan P (1994) Special needs of the surgical patient. *Nurs Times* **9(51)**:40–41.

Smith S (1992) Tiresome healing. *Nurs Times* **88(36)**:24–26.

Stucke VA (1993) *Microbiology For Nurses*, pp. 372–378. Baillière Tindall, London.

Torrance C (1990) Sleep and wound healing. *Surg Nurse* **3(2)**:12–14.

Vaughan B, Taylor K (1988) Homeward bound. *Nurs Times* **84(15)**:28–31.

Weis OF, Sriwatanakul K, Alloza JL, Weintraub M, Lasagna L (1993) Attitude of patients, housestaff and nurses towards post operative analgesia care. *Anaesth Analg* **62**:70–74.

Wilson-Barnett J, Fordham F (1982) *Recovery from Illness*. Wiley, Chichester. pp. 88–102.

Wilmore DW, Smith RJ, O'Dwyer ST, Jacobs DO, Ziegler TR, Wang XD (1988) The gut: A central organ after surgical stress. *Surgery* **104**:917.

Chapter 5
Fluids and Electrolytes in Surgery

Surgical patients have a risk of fluid and electrolyte imbalance, but with appropriate assessment and intervention the effects of surgery can be controlled. Nursing intervention begins with preoperative assessment. Management of potential or existing problems starts with preoperative preparation and continues through to discharge. This chapter reviews the normal composition and distribution of body fluids. It then presents a discussion of disorders of body fluids affecting the surgical patient. Finally the nursing interventions required are described, including those for intravenous fluid therapy and blood transfusion.

OVERVIEW OF FLUIDS AND ELECTROLYTES

A knowledge of the composition and distribution of body fluids and electrolytes is essential for understanding fluid balance and planning appropriate interventions. Human tissues contain varying amounts of water, ranging from less than 10% in fat to 83% for blood; overall water accounts for about 60% of total body weight (TBW) or 42 L in an average 70 kg man. The exact percentage of water varies between individuals and depends on factors such as age, build, and sex. On average women have more fat than men and TBW is about 50% of body weight or 35 L for a 70 kg woman. Body water is fairly constant at 71–72% for lean body mass (body weight minus fat). Differences in TBW occur due to loss of lean mass or an increase in fatty tissue. With increasing age there is a relative decline in lean body mass and TBW decreases as a percentage of body weight.

Body water is distributed between the two major fluid compartments: water inside cells (intracellular fluid, ICF) and the extracellular fluid (ECF) surrounding cells. The cell membrane is the barrier separating the two fluid compartments. *Figure 5.1* illustrates the distribution of body water. ECF is subdivided into:

- Plasma (intravascular) fluid.
- Interstitial (extravascular) fluid.
- Transcellular fluid.

Transcellular fluid is the specialized fluid found in body spaces or cavities and includes pleural fluid, synovial fluid, saliva, gastric juice, intestinal fluid, pancreatic fluid, bile, and cerebrospinal fluid (CSF). Total transcellular fluid volume is variable, but low at about 1 L. However, turnover of transcellular fluid within

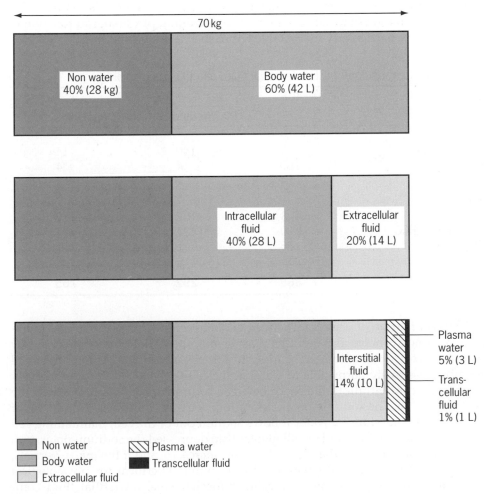

Figure 5.1 Distribution of body water in a standard 70 kg man.

the gastrointestinal (GI) tract is large at 5–8 L day^{-1} and can be as high as 20 L day^{-1}. Because of this high turnover anything that precipitates fluid loss from the GI tract (e.g. vomiting, diarrhoea, fistula) will have profound effects on fluid and electrolyte balance.

Gobbi and Torrance (1994) note that body fluids cannot be simply equated with water; they also contain electrolytes and non-electrolytes (e.g. glucose and urea) in solution and larger molecules in suspension. Typical values for major electrolytes in ICF, plasma, and interstitial fluid are presented in *Table 5.1*. Sodium is the main cation in ECF; potassium, magnesium, and calcium ions are present at lower concentrations, but have important physiological roles. Chloride and bicarbonate are the main anions in ECF. Potassium is the major cation inside the cell, where anions include phosphate and sulphate. Large proteins within the cell also act as negatively charged anions. The cell membrane separates ICF and ECF and regulates movement of ions between the two fluids. Maintaining this uneven distribution of ions is essential for maintaining physiological function in all tissues, but particularly in excitable tissue such as nerve and muscle.

Table 5.1 Composition of ICF, interstitial fluid, and plasma (mmol L^{-1}).

	ICF	ECF	
		Plasma and serum	**Interstitial fluid**
Cations			
Sodium (Na$^+$)	10	140	14
Potassium (K$^+$)	160	4	4
Others	14	2	2
Anions			
Chloride (Cl$^-$)	3	102	117
Bicarbonate (HCO$_3^-$)	10	27	27
Phosphate (PO$_4^{2-}$) and others	106	1	1
Protein	65	16	0
Total	**368**	**292**	**165**

The distribution of water and movement between the intracellular and extra-cellular compartments and between plasma and interstitial fluid is governed by osmotic forces acting across the semipermeable cell membrane. Although the cell membrane is freely permeable to water at the cellular level, ion pumps actively maintain a concentration difference between sodium and potassium across the cell membrane. The sodium–potassium pump actively transports sodium out of the cell and potassium in; water follows sodium out of the cell, maintaining cell volume. If the cell is injured or cell metabolism depressed the sodium–potassium pump fails, water enters the cell, cell volume increases, and if the injury persists, the cell eventually dies. Regulation of cell volume is critical for physiological function. Volume is regulated by cellular mechanisms, interstitial fluid composition, and osmolality, which in turn is controlled by the regulation of plasma osmolality. Maintaining plasma osmolality within a narrow physiological range is essential for maintaining fluid and electrolyte balance.

At the level of the blood vessel the endothelial cells form a semipermeable membrane. Plasma proteins, especially albumin, are trapped inside the vessel, but water, electrolytes, and non-electrolytes can cross the barrier. The plasma proteins provide the osmotic pressure holding fluid within the capillary (i.e. colloid or oncotic pressure). *Figure 5.2* illustrates the forces working across the capillary wall and how they influence fluid movement. The capillary wall is in fact a 'leaky' membrane and some protein does escape. The lymphatic system has a critical role in 'mopping up' plasma proteins and excess interstitial fluid and returning them to the circulation. Oedema occurs when excess fluid accumulates in the interstitial spaces.

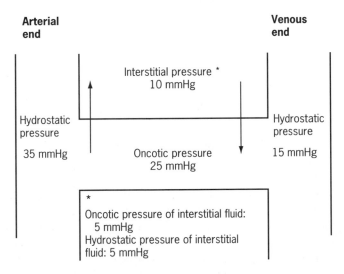

Figure 5.2 Fluid exchange at the capillary.

Fluid Intake and Output

In health fluid intake and output are in a working balance. Water is normally lost through the skin, in the moisture content of exhaled air, by urinary excretion, and in the faeces. Water is absorbed from food and drink, and a smaller amount is produced by metabolic reactions in the body. Taking the example of a 70 kg man the net losses are 2.5–3 L, 120–140 mmol sodium, and 70 mmol of potassium a day, and these deficits are easily replaced by a normal diet (Swaminathan, 1994). Sensible fluid loss via urine and the intestinal tract is measurable, or in the case of sweating observable. Insensible losses from the lungs and evaporation through the skin are more difficult to detect and quantify. Normal fluid balance over 24 hours is summarized in *Table 5.2*. In general, measurement of the fluid intake and urine output is sufficient to monitor water balance, but if losses are

Table 5.2 24-hour fluid balance in an average man (adapted from Metheny, 1992).

Intake (mL)		Output (mL)	
Water in food	900	Urine	1500
Ingested water	1400	Faeces	200
Metabolic water	300	Respiratory	400
		Skin	500
Total	2600	**Total**	2600

excessive careful monitoring and estimation of insensible losses are required. Daily weighing may also be necessary.

Tonicity

Terms such as isotonic, hypotonic, or hypertonic are often used to describe fluids for intravenous infusion:

- Isotonic solutions, for example 0.9% sodium chloride, have the same osmolality as plasma.
- Hypotonic solutions have a lower osmolality than plasma.
- Hypertonic solutions are hyperosmotic compared to plasma.

Tonicity describes the reaction of the red blood cell. In an isotonic solution there is no net movement of solutes or water and the red cell volume is maintained. In hypotonic solutions water is drawn into the cell and it will eventually swell and burst. In hypertonic solution water moves out of the red cell causing the cell to shrink. In practice, infusion fluids rapidly mix with the blood and these extreme effects are not seen. Infusion of an isotonic fluid expands the intravascular volume without altering intercellular or interstitial fluids. However, although 5% dextrose is isotonic when infused, it effectively adds free water to the circulation because the glucose is rapidly removed from the blood. Hypotonic fluids reduce plasma osmolality, and water will be shifted from the circulation to the interstitial and intracellular fluids. Hypertonic fluids increase plasma osmolality and favour movement of interstitial fluid into the blood.

REGULATION OF FLUIDS AND ELECTROLYTES

Fluid intake and output needs to be regulated to maintain homeostasis, and in health daily variations in TBW are less than 0.2%. The kidney has a central function in the retention and excretion of water and maintaining consistency within the ECF, but fluid balance is essentially determined by plasma osmolality. Osmoreceptors in the hypothalamus monitor plasma osmolality and initiate the appropriate physiological mechanisms required to rectify any changes. Sodium is the main factor in plasma osmolality, and at a simple level regulation of total body water can be equated with regulating plasma sodium concentration. The osmoreceptors are sensitive, responding to changes as small as ± 3 milliosmoles (mOsm), keeping plasma osmolality within the normal range of 280–290 mOsm kg^{-1} water.

Osmoreceptors control water intake and excretion by influencing thirst and secretion of antidiuretic hormone (ADH). ADH is secreted by the posterior pituitary gland and acts on the nephron, increasing tubular permeability to water. A rise in plasma osmolality stimulates ADH secretion, and reabsorption of water from the renal collecting tubules is increased. Thirst is also stimulated, promoting water ingestion. A fall in plasma osmolality inhibits ADH secretion, tubular permeability is decreased, and water excretion increases, making the urine more dilute. The kidneys are able to control body fluid and electrolyte status because of their high blood flow. Although plasma volume is only about 3 L the glomerular filtration rate (GFR) is about 125 mL min^{-1} or 180 L day^{-1}: this equates with the plasma being filtered and reabsorbed 60 times a day. With this enormous throughput the kidney is able to regulate not only body water and osmolality, but also electrolyte balance and pH.

ADH is not, however, the only hormone involved: the mineralocorticoid hormone aldosterone is also essential. Aldosterone has a permissive role in sodium reabsorption. In the absence of aldosterone, sodium reabsorption does not occur, but a high concentration of aldosterone results in excess sodium retention. Aldosterone is also important in hydrogen–potassium ion exchange in the kidney. The renin–angiotensin system also influences ADH and aldosterone release. In addition to osmoreceptors, changes in circulating volume are detected by volume receptors located in the glomerular arterioles, the aortic arch, and carotid sinus. Stimulation of the volume receptors activates the sympathetic nervous system (with effects on blood vessels and blood flow) and the renin–angiotensin system (with effects on aldosterone). Atrial natriuretic peptide (ANP) is a hormone released by the heart that may also directly influence sodium reabsorption.

In addition to control of TBW it is important to understand the mechanisms that regulate the concentrations of individual electrolytes. Gobbi and Torrance (1994) present a brief review of control mechanisms and the effects of electrolyte deficits or excess, and the reader is directed to Porth (1994) and Metheny (1992) for a fuller discussion of fluids and electrolytes.

REGULATION OF ACID–BASE BALANCE

Regulation of the acid–base balance means regulating the hydrogen ion concentration in the body fluids. The hydrogen ion concentration or pH of blood is approximately 7.40, while that of body fluids generally ranges from 7.36–7.44. Optimal activity of many of the enzymes controlling physiological processes depends on the pH remaining within the normal range. Variations in pH outside the range can rapidly result in severe injury or death. In health the body does not have to cope with large rapid changes of pH, but rapid changes can occur in disease. Persistent vomiting is an example of a condition causing a sudden loss of fluid and hydrogen ions (gastric acid) that can rapidly alter acid–base balance. The higher the pH value, the lower the hydrogen ion concentration, and the lower the pH value, the higher the hydrogen ion concentration. The pH scale is logarithmic, so small changes in pH represent quite large changes in hydrogen ion concentration. A pH of 7 is neutral, 7.36 slightly acidic, 7.44 slightly alkaline. Acidaemia is a blood pH less than 7.36, while alkalaemia is a blood pH greater than 7.44. Three mechanisms operate to maintain the pH of the ECF and blood:

- An immediate mechanism involving chemical buffering.
- A delayed mechanism involving a respiratory response.
- A slow responding renal response.

Buffering provides an immediate level of control for pH changes. Intracellular proteins including haemoglobin account for more than 50% of buffering activity within the body. The extracellular buffer is bicarbonate, but phosphate and sulphate compounds in the ECF have some buffering activity. The bicarbonate–carbonic acid buffering reaction is extremely effective because its endproduct is carbon dioxide, which is excreted from the body. Effectively this reaction converts excess hydrogen ions into carbon dioxide, and the lungs then increase ventilation to remove the excess carbon dioxide from the body. The kidneys provide a route for excreting hydrogen ions but also make bicarbonate to replenish the buffering system. The three mechanisms work together to ensure a stable pH as follows:

- Bicarbonate buffers against immediate changes.
- The lungs remove excess carbon dioxide.
- The kidneys restore long-term balance by replenishing bicarbonate.

Respiratory or renal disease can interfere with pH regulation. *Table 5.3* summarizes the causes of acidosis and alkalosis.

NURSING MANAGEMENT

The admission history and preoperative physical assessment of the patient should establish any existing problems with fluid and electrolyte status. Using admission information and knowledge of the likely consequences of general anaesthesia and surgical procedures, postoperative interventions to maintain fluid and electrolyte balance can be planned and discussed with the patient. For short procedures that do not involve the GI tract there may be no need for intravenous therapy in the postoperative period. For other procedures the patient

Table 5.3 Causes of acidosis and alkalosis.

Acidosis	Alkalosis
Metabolic acidosis	**Metabolic alkalosis**
Diabetic ketoacidosis	Loss of hydrogen ions (e.g. through vomiting)
Renal failure	Excess intake of sodium bicarbonate (e.g. injudicious use of antacids)
Hypoxia	
Respiratory acidosis	**Respiratory alkalosis**
Primary disorders of the respiratory tract (e.g. asthma, bronchitis)	Hyperventilation (e.g. as in an anxiety attack)
Conditions affecting the respiratory centre (e.g. drug overdose)	
Fault in the management of artificial ventilation	

may return to the ward with an intravenous infusion *in situ*, but intravenous therapy can be discontinued within a few hours, usually after the patient has managed to tolerate oral fluids. However, with lengthy procedures, especially those involving the GI tract, intravenous therapy may be necessary for several hours or days after surgery. It can be helpful to consider fluid therapy for the surgical patient in terms of:

- Maintenance fluids.
- Replacement fluids.

Maintenance fluids represent the fluids and electrolytes required to replace normal losses. These are readily available in a normal diet. If the patient's oral intake is restricted for any reason maintenance fluids may need to be supplied by intravenous therapy. Replacement fluids are additional to maintenance needs and replace any abnormal losses due to the pathology or the consequences of surgery (e.g. fistula, wound drainage, fever, vomiting and diarrhoea). Karanjia *et al.* (1992) emphasize that the general rule with replacement fluids is 'replace like with like'. In this section the role of the surgical nurse in assessing fluid and electrolyte status, re-introducing oral intake, and managing intravenous therapy will be reviewed.

Assessing Hydration and Electrolyte Status

Assessment is aimed at identifying fluid volume deficits (dehydration) or excess (overhydration) or problems with excess or deficits of specific electrolytes. In practice, however, 'free water' losses are rare and water is usually lost in conjunction with sodium (Gobbi and Torrance, 1994). *Box 5.1* summarizes causes and the

Box 5.1   Dehydration in the surgical patient.

Causes

Decreased intake
- Elderly
- Very young
- Unconscious (unable to express thirst, control intake)
- Oral trauma
- Dysphasia
- Fluid restriction
- Nausea

Increased losses
- Vomiting and diarrhoea
- Wound, fistula, and other drainage
- Gastrointestinal suction
- Diuretic therapy
- Osmotic diuresis (glucose)
- Adrenal insufficiency
- Diabetes insipidus
- Fever (increased insensible loss)
- Respiratory infection

Third space losses
- Oedema
- Intestinal obstruction
- Ascites
- Burns

Symptoms
- Thirst
- Weakness
- Apathy
- Fatigue
- Postural dizziness (hypotension)
- Syncope
- Muscle cramps

Signs
- Dry skin and mucous membranes
- Reduced skin turgor
- Dry, cracked tongue
- Acute weight loss
- Oliguria
- Decreased salivation

- Decreased lacrimation
- Weak thready pulse, tachycardia
- Raised body temperature
- Reduced ocular pressure

Laboratory findings
- High urine osmolality and specific gravity
- Low urine sodium concentration
- Increased serum osmolality
- Raised haematocrit
- Increased plasma urea concentration
- Raised plasma urea/creatinine ratio

clinical signs and symptoms of fluid deficit or dehydration in the surgical patient. *Box 5.2* lists the causes and signs and symptoms of overhydration. The extent and effects of changes seen in fluid or electrolyte imbalance depend on the volume and rate of fluid and electrolyte loss or gain. One problem is that significant changes can occur before they are detected by clinical measurements such as blood and central venous pressure (CVP) (Gobbi and Torrance, 1994). The surgical nurse should be alert to symptoms reported by the patient and observe skin and mucous membranes carefully. The state of the buccal mucosa is a useful indicator of hydration, but if the patient is a mouthbreather, having oxygen, or receiving certain drugs (i.e. hyoscine hydrobromide), the mucosa may appear dry. The mucosa in the area between the cheek and gums is usually moist, indicating adequate hydration. The veins of the hand provide another quick, noninvasive gauge of fluid status. If the hand is elevated or lowered the veins should empty or fill within 3–5 seconds. When assessing fluid and electrolyte status it is essential to consult the medical notes for details of a recent physical examination and the results of the most recent laboratory tests (urine and serum electrolytes, haematocrit).

Dehydration is perhaps more common in surgical patients than overhydration. Early recognition of volume depletion can be difficult as the signs and symptoms may be subtle or contradictory (Beckwith and Carriere, 1985). It is important to identify the problem early as hypovolaemia in the critically ill patient can rapidly result in irreversible changes (Maier and Carrico, 1986). The relevant North American Diagnostic Association (NANDA) diagnosis is 'fluid volume deficit related to active isotonic loss.' Gershan *et al.* (1990) investigated factors that could be used as critical indicators of fluid volume deficit and these included:

- Negative fluid balance.
- Low CVP.
- Raised urine osmolality.
- Postural hypotension.
- Thready pulse.
- Decreased pulse volume and pressure.

Box 5.2 **Overhydration in the surgical patient.**

Causes

Increased intake
- Intravenous overload
- Bladder irrigation

Decreased excretion
- Renal disease
- Congestive heart failure
- Liver cirrhosis
- Drugs (e.g. cyclophosphamide carbamazepine, chlorpropamide)
- Stress (postoperative)
- Respiratory disease
- Central nervous system disease

Symptoms
- Polyuria
- Oedema (e.g. swollen ankles, puffy eyes)
- Dyspnoea
- Shortness of breath
- Cough

Signs
- Acute weight gain
- Pitting oedema
- Full pulse
- Venous distension
- Crepitations
- Pulmonary oedema (if severe)

Laboratory findings
- Decreased haematocrit
- Decreased blood urea nitrogen (BUN)
- Decreased plasma sodium

- Dry mucous membranes.
- Decreased urine output.
- Weight loss.
- Decreased blood pressure.
- Tachycardia.
- Raised haematocrit.
- Decreased venous filling.
- Poor skin turgor.

Monitoring Fluid Balance

Monitoring fluid balance is a central nursing activity and the two simplest, but most important elements are:

- Recording fluid intake and output.
- Regular recording of body weight.

Rapid fluctuations in body weight are usually due to acute fluid loss or gain. Acute weight gain in excess of 5% of body weight suggests overhydration. Acute loss of 2% indicates a mild fluid deficit, of 2–5%, a moderate fluid deficit, and of 6% or more, serious dehydration. For accurate daily monitoring it is critical that body weight is measured at the same time of day, using the same scales and under the same conditions.

Recording fluid balance requires careful measurement and estimation of fluid losses and gains. Oral, enteral, or intravenous fluid intake is easily measured; the water content of food should be estimated, but is often ignored. Fluid loss through urine and the GI tract, and from fistulae and drains can also be measured. Insensible losses and exudate from wounds may have to be estimated. Standard values for insensible loss can be applied, but adjustments may be required for the following factors influencing insensible loss (Gobbi and Torrance, 1994):

- Body temperature.
- Ambient temperature.
- Basal metabolic rate.
- Respiratory rate.
- Respiratory assistance (oxygen, humidification, artificial ventilation).
- Fluid content of faeces.
- Wound or burns exudate.
- Other pathologies.

Pflaum (1979) has argued that fluid balance charts are often unreliable and that daily weights may be more accurate. The acceptable margin of error will depend on the condition of the patient. In a relatively fit person small errors may not be important, but in the critically ill or vulnerable patient even small errors can be significant. Problems with fluid balance charting include:

- Reliance on estimation not measurement.
- Measurement errors (e.g. using a high volume jug to measure a low volume of urine).
- Arithmetical error.
- Omission and duplication of items.
- Inaccurate transfer between theatre and ward fluid charts.
- Shift change errors (when and who completes the 24-hour balance).
- Confusion between intravenous fluid prescription chart and fluid balance chart (i.e. confusion between fluid prescribed, in progress, and completed).
- Failure to recognize or act on patterns emerging from consecutive 24-hour balances.

Managing Oral Intake

The oral route is the safest and most physiological route for both maintenance and replacement fluids. To facilitate oral intake the nurse should assess physical and mental fitness, identify preferred fluids, and make them available to the patient in acceptable volumes. It is essential that any vague instructions such as 'restrict fluids' or 'encourage fluids', 'push fluids' or 'sips only' are clarified to establish the total volume allowed or desired for a 24-hour period and the rate or volume permitted; 30 mL per hour is a more useful instruction than 'sips only'. Oral care is critical if oral intake is partially or completely restricted. Mouth rinses, lip salves, and complete oral hygiene can be used to maintain oral hydration and comfort. After some types of surgery oral fluids are reintroduced gradually when bowel sounds indicate motility has returned. Usually 15–30 mL is given hourly, and if tolerated the volume is increased gradually over 1–2 days. Once the patient can tolerate fluid without nausea or distension, and peristalsis is established with the passage of flatus or faeces, a light diet may be resumed. Protein–calorie supplements are required if the patient is not tolerating a diet with a minimum protein content of 45–55 g (Moghissi and Boore, 1983). This approach is based on clinical experience rather than clear research and there is little evidence recommending any particular regimen for the reintroduction of oral fluids.

Managing Intravenous Therapy

Preoperative evaluation of fluid and electrolytes status and correction of existing problems is an essential aspect of surgical care. If the patient is unable to tolerate sufficient oral intake to maintain fluid balance or correct deficits then intravenous therapy will be required. Parenteral fluid therapy is common in the postoperative period. Intravenous fluid may be given as a temporary measure for a few hours after return to the ward until oral intake is established or may be necessary for several days after surgery. Volume deficits are common after surgical trauma and even an experienced surgeon may underestimate operative blood loss by 15–40% (Jenkins and Beck, 1963). After GI surgery the risk of peristaltic inhibition (paralytic ileus) will delay the introduction of oral fluids and intravenous therapy is essential. Other situations that might require intravenous therapy have been identified by Smith (1980) as follows:

- Dehydration.
- Vomiting or diarrhoea.
- Excessive insensible losses (e.g. sweating).
- Pre- and postoperative hydration.
- Hypercatabolism as in severe burns.
- Unconscious patient.

Intravenous therapy is a potential cause of overhydration in the postoperative patient. Intravenous fluids can supply volume (water) and a variety of electrolytes (e.g. sodium) and non-electrolytes (e.g. glucose). In addition to crystalloid solutions, 'clear fluids', colloidal solutions, blood and blood components, and plasma and plasma substitutes can be infused. Intravenous infusion can also be used for drug administration, for example postoperative analgesia or anti-microbials. Transfusion of blood and blood products is discussed later in this chapter. *Table 5.4* lists some common intravenous fluids and their uses. Over a 24-hour period a regimen alternating the type of fluid will be prescribed. The type and volume of electrolyte solution used will depend on specific deficits or metabolic disorders requiring treatment and the maintenance requirements of the individual patient. *Table 5.5* presents a typical 24-hour regimen for main-tenance fluids in a 70 kg man. If some oral fluids are permitted the intravenous regimen would need to be adjusted accordingly.

Care of the intravenous line

The patient should be given an explanation of the purpose of the infusion before the procedure begins. It is important to ask the patient which arm is convenient to have the cannula sited; usually the nondominant arm is used. The patient's arm in the region of the cannula site may need to be shaved. The limb containing the cannula and infusion line should be supported, and the patient must be assisted to maintain a comfortable position at all times; personal possessions should be within easy reach.

Care of an intravenous infusion line is an important nursing function. All relevant information regarding the infusion, type of cannula, date and time started, time for infusion sets to be changed, and patient care generally, needs to be documented. Intravenous fluid prescription charts should be clearly written, fluid containers must be checked carefully for defects, and the nurse must ensure that the fluid to be infused is clear and free from particles. A container should not be hung for longer than 24 hours, and in the case of some solutions such as blood, no longer than eight hours. Handling the infusion line should be kept to a minimum and the line should be carefully secured to avoid traction. If drugs or supplements are to be added to the infusion fluid this should be carried out in aseptic conditions and the nurse must have a knowledge of the drug's dose, action, compatibilities, and side effects. No supplements should be added to blood or blood products. All treatment must be recorded on the prescription chart, fluid chart, and nursing notes. It is essential that staff can easily identify when a fluid pack in progress was started and when it should be completed. The basic principles of care of intravenous infusion are:

- Asepsis.
- Wash hands.
- Maintain a closed system.
- Ensure fluids do not hang longer than recommended (some solutions deteriorate in bright sunlight).
- Inspect insertion site for signs of complications.
- Keep cannula site clean and dry.
- Ensure cannula is secure.

Table 5.4 Some common intravenous fluids.*

Infusion fluid	Constituents	Comments
Sodium chloride 0.9% (500 mL, 1000 mL packs)	Sodium chloride 9 g L^{-1} Na^+ 150 mmol L^{-1}, Cl^- 150 mmol L^{-1} Isotonic	Replacement fluid for sodium depletion. There is a risk of sodium retention and oedema, so it is not used for routine maintenance. Monitor the lung bases for crepitations. 0.45% sodium chloride is hypotonic and may be used to deliver free water with some sodium replacement
Hartmann's solution (Ringer lactate, sodium lactate) 500 mL, 1000 mL packs	Sodium chloride 0.6%, sodium lactate 0.25%, potassium chloride 0.04%, calcium chloride 0.027% Na^+ 131 mmol L^{-1}, K^+ 5 mmol L^{-1}, Ca^{2+} 2 mmol L^{-1}, Cl^- 111 mmol L^{-1}, HCO_3^- 29 mmol L^{-1} as lactate Isotonic	Useful replacement fluid in absence of gross deficits of specific electrolytes. Supplies a range of electrolytes, but not magnesium or phosphate. Lactate is used because it is more stable than bicarbonate in solution
Glucose 5% 500 mL, 1000 mL packs	50 g dextrose monohydrate in 1 L water Isotonic	Maintenance and replacement fluid for free water. Also provides energy (780 kJ L^{-1})
Potassium chloride 0.3% and glucose 5% 500 mL, 1000 mL packs	Potassium chloride 3 g L^{-1}, dextrose monohydrate 50 g L^{-1} K^+ 40 mmol L^{-1}, Cl^- 40 mmol L^{-1}	Hypokalaemia. Concentrated potassium solution 1.5 g or 20 mmol in 10 mL can be added to 500 mL packs of sodium chloride (0.9%) or glucose (5%) to give 40 mmol L^{-1}, but must be mixed extremely well before the bag is attached to administration set to avoid giving a bolus injection
Potassium chloride 0.3% and sodium chloride 0.9%	Potassium chloride 3 g L^{-1}, sodium chloride 9 g L^{-1} K^+ 40 mmol L^{-1}, Na^+ 150 mmol L^{-1}, Cl^- 190 mmol L^{-1}	

*Intravenous solutions commonly used after or during surgery are listed, but a large range of specific fluids (e.g. sodium bicarbonate, sodium lactate) or combination fluids may be prescribed for specific electrolyte or clinical disorders.

Table 5.5 Typical maintenance fluid regimen for a 70 kg male.

Solution	Volume (L)	Infusion time (h)	Sodium and chloride (mmol)	Potassium (mmol)	Energy (kJ)
Dextrose 5%	1	8	–	+27	780
Sodium chloride 0.9%	1	8	150 and 150	+27	–
Dextrose 5%	1	8	–	+27	780
Total	3	24	150 and 150	81	1560

- Ensure infusion rates are accurate.
- Resite and change infusion set according to local policy.

Selecting site, cannula, and infusion sets
Selecting the appropriate site, cannula, and infusion set is important in avoiding complications. An intravenous cannula may be inserted into a peripheral vein by medical staff or nurses with appropriate training. If the cannula is sited at the wrist or antecubital fossa a splint may be required to prevent flexion. Site selection will be influenced by a number of practical considerations including:

- Ease of access and patency of peripheral veins (otherwise venous cutdown may be required).
- Anticipated duration of therapy.
- Type of fluids infused.
- Type of needle or cannula to be used.
- Patient compliance, mobility, and comfort.
- Staff expertise.

Dougherty (1992) maintains that nurses need to be familiar with the range of devices available for this procedure. Traditional steel needles, butterfly or scalp vein needles (*Figure 5.3*), and a variety of plastic cannula can be used. The steel needle is seldom used other than for very short-term infusion. Butterfly needles and plastic cannulae are more suitable for longer duration of use. It is recommended that peripheral infusions should be resited after 48 hours and never left *in situ* more than 72 hours (Centers for Disease Control, 1982). Nightingale and Bradshaw (1982) suggest using a small narrow gauge cannula that allows blood flow around the cannula tip and reduces the risk of occlusion and phlebitis. Cannula selection will depend on:

- Anticipated duration of therapy.
- Type of fluids infused.
- Availability, size, and condition of veins.
- Site and means of securing the cannula.

A variety of infusion sets are available from a number of manufacturers. Those most commonly used are of the macro- or microdrip type. Sets may come with built-in filters or a filter device may be added if required. All sets will have some

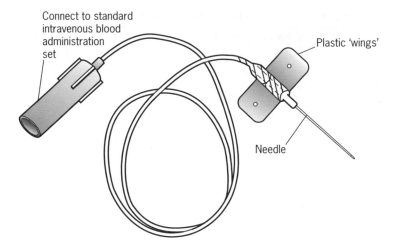

Figure 5.3 A butterfly or scalp vein cannula.

sort of valve mechanism designed to close off the set and prevent air entry if the infusion fluid runs out. Drop size varies with regular macrodrip sets and it is important to read the manufacturer's information to ensure the correct drop size is used when calculating drip rates. Macrodrip sets usually give about 15 drops for every one mL of fluid. Microdrip or paediatric sets usually incorporate an additional graduated chamber and deliver 60 drops for every one mL of fluid. These rates are approximate because the number of drops per ml will depend on the viscosity of the fluid infused. Protheroe and Auty (1986) found that addition of a Vitalipid to an infusion fluid increased drop size by 50%. Manufacturer's instructions must be consulted, especially when using unfamiliar infusion sets. The choice of infusion set will be largely determined by the type and volume of fluid infused and desired flow rate. Macrodrip sets are adequate for general use, but if small volumes or more precise control of flow rate is required a microdrip set may be preferred. If infusion control pumps are used the device may dictate the type of administration set. Blood and blood products are usually given using blood administration sets, which are changed immediately after use.

Flow control
The intravenous fluid prescription chart will state the type of fluid, volume, and infusion time, for example 5% dextrose, 500 ml over four hours. The nurse needs to calculate the flow rate and ensure that the correct rate is maintained. To calculate flow rate it is essential to know the number of drops per mL delivered by the infusion set with crystalloid or colloidal fluids. The formula below is used to calculate the required number of drops per minute to deliver the correct flow rate.

- $$\text{Drops min}^{-1} = \frac{\text{Total volume (mL)} \times \text{drops mL}^{-1}}{\text{Total infusion time (min)}}$$

Taking an example of 500 mL over four hours using an administration set delivering 60 drops mL^{-1} the calculation would be:

■ $\dfrac{\text{Total volume 500 mL} \times 60 \text{ drops mL}^{-1}}{\text{Total infusion time 240 min}} = \dfrac{30\,000}{240} = 125 \text{ drops min}^{-1}$

Careful recording is essential for monitoring and maintaining flow rates. Intravenous fluids are administered by gravity flow unless an infusion pump is used. After setting the flow rate the infusion needs to be checked regularly as a variety of factors may affect the flow rate causing it to slow, increase, or perhaps stop. Factors to consider include:

■ Cannula position, patency, or movement.
■ Local complications of venous spasm, infiltration, phlebitis, or thrombophlebitis.
■ Infusion equipment problems affecting the cannula, air vent (blocked), height of fluid container, volume in container, kinked tubing, blocked filters.
■ Infusion fluid factors such as viscosity, temperature, surface tension, or specific gravity.

If a cannula is not sufficiently secure or patient movement affects the insertion site the cannula tip may be pushed against the wall of the vein, blocking flow. When this happens it may be reported that the infusion is 'positional'. The patient can be asked to minimize movement affecting the infusion and the cannula can be resecured and the site redressed. Infusion is by gravity, so raising or lowering the height of the infusion bag will alter the flow rate. Raising or lowering the bed will have a similar effect. Complications at the insertion site, venous spasm, or clotting within the cannula all slow the infusion rate. The use of saline or heparinized saline flush can help prevent this problem. Gentle aspiration can be tried to remove a clot, but care must be taken to avoid dislodging the clot into the blood flow. If a rigid fluid container is used blockage of the air vent stops air entry and this will slow and eventually stop the flow.

If gravity flow is judged insufficiently accurate or unreliable, an infusion pump or controller may be used. A controller relies on gravity to infuse the fluid, but the electronic sensors monitor drop rate and provide a warning if the flow rate varies from the pre-set limits. An infusion pump uses positive pressure to ensure fluid delivery within pre-set pressure limits. Volumetric or drip-rate pumps are particularly useful for total parenteral nutrition (TPN) or when potent drugs requiring precise infusion rate control are added to the intravenous fluid. Syringe drivers are used to deliver small controlled volumes when accuracy is essential, for example intravenous delivery of an opioid analgesic. Pumps can be used with central or peripheral lines, controllers are more suitable for peripheral lines. Although these devices will help in controlling the rate of infusion they cannot replace careful nursing care and observation. It is also essential that the nurse knows exactly how to use the device, its compatability with different administration sets or filters, and any special operating characteristics or problems. Pumps and controllers are safe and effective in knowledgeable hands, but can create their own problems if used improperly.

Prevention of infection

An intravenous line provides a direct portal of entry into the blood and scrupulous infection control is essential to protect both the patient and nurse. Wilkinson (1991) stated that contamination may occur at many places or stages of the intravenous process, and may be intrinsic and present before use or extrinsic and introduced during use (*Figure 5.4*). Asepsis must be maintained. All solutions and equipment must be sterile and handwashing before handling intravenous lines is mandatory. Preparation of the injection site is important. Contaminated skin will need careful cleaning with detergent and antiseptic solutions. Rubbing the area with a swab impregnated with isopropyl alcohol (70%) is often recommended for cleaning the skin. The site should be allowed to dry before puncture and the skin should not be repalpated after preparation. Adherence to aseptic procedures when setting up or removing intravenous cannulae, fluid packs, and administration sets is important. For peripheral infusion, administration sets are changed every 48 hours. Maki (1977) identified a steady rise in the incidence of infection of cannulae, from 0% on the day of insertion to 2.9% after four days; resiting after 48–72 hours is recommended (Centers for Disease Control, 1982). Maintaining a closed system, avoiding the use of additional stopcocks, connections or extensions, and minimizing handling of the system will help reduce the opportunity for contamination. A semi-occlusive transparent dressing is useful to enable frequent inspection of the insertion site for redness or swelling. The patient should be asked if there is any pain in the area of the infusion. A patient receiving intravenous therapy should be monitored for signs of local or systemic infection.

Complications of intravenous therapy

Intravenous therapy is not without risks. Fluids can be infused via peripheral or central veins. The basic management is similar, but there are additional complications associated with central lines and these are discussed in more detail below. Complications are more likely when the fluid infused is non-isotonic or concentrated or intravenous additives are used. Local complications of intravenous infusion identified by Speechley and Toovey (1987) include:

- Infiltration and extravasation.
- Infection at the insertion site.
- Inflammation and phlebitis.
- Thrombophlebitis.

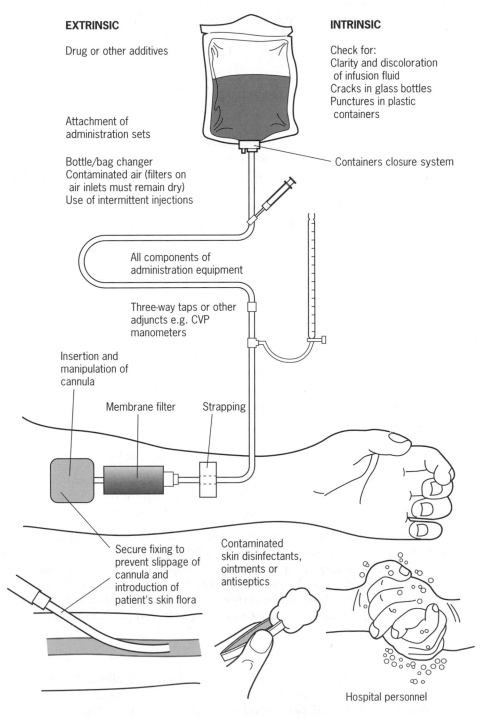

Figure 5.4 Sources of contamination of intravenous systems.

Systemic complications (Speechley and Toovey, 1987) include:

- Septicaemia and bacteraemia.
- Emboli.
- Circulatory overload.
- Allergic reaction to drugs or infusion fluid.

Infiltration and extravasation

If an intravenous cannula or needle becomes displaced fluid will leak into the tissue. Cessation or reduction of flow suggest infiltration; oedema will occur, but may only be evident if the site is compared with the same area on the opposite limb. The skin around the site may feel cooler than surrounding skin and the patient might complain of pain. The extent of pain depends on the volume and nature of the fluid infused. Hypotonic solutions and potassium-containing fluids can cause extensive pain and vasospasm. If infiltration of irritant fluid is not identified early tissue destruction can be extensive. Patient education, ensuring the cannula is adequately anchored, appropriate selection of insertion site, careful insertion technique, and minimal handling of the cannula and site dressings will help minimize the risk of infiltration. If infiltration is suspected Metheny (1992) suggests the following procedure:

- Locate the vein being used.
- Place two fingers on the vein, 3–4 inches above the insertion site.
- Press on the vein while observing the drip chamber: if flow stops the cannula is in place; if the drops keep forming fluid is being infused into subcutaneous tissues so discontinue the infusion.

Phlebitis and thrombophlebitis

Inflammation of the vein is called phlebitis and may be due to:

- Chemical causes (e.g. infusion of fluid with nonphysiological pH or drugs).
- Mechanical causes (e.g. movement of the cannula within the vein).
- Infection (e.g. due to contamination of equipment or fluids).

Using additional filters may reduce the risk of chemical or infectious phlebitis. In thrombophlebitis, inflammation is complicated by the formation of a clot within the vein. As with infiltration, phlebitis and thrombophlebitis can be minimized by careful attention to technique. In addition the use of a small cannula will maximize mixing of infusate with blood, and as large a vein as possible should be selected. Thrombophlebitis is associated with a risk of emboli, and pulmonary embolism can occur.

Air emboli

Air can enter an intravenous infusion if the fluid chamber is allowed to empty or connections loosen. The volume of air required to cause a lethal air embolism has been estimated at 70–150 mL per second (Ordway, 1974). Air emboli in peripheral lines are relatively rare, but are more common in central lines and are associated with a high level of morbidity and mortality (Kashuk and Penn, 1984; McConnell, 1986). Yeakel (1969) reported a fatality after an accidental intravenous infusion of 100 mL of air.

Central venous lines
Central venous catheters, for example Hickman catheters, are commonly used for long-term venous access as in TPN. They may also be used for administering concentrated hyperosmolar solutions that are too irritant for peripheral infusion or when it is essential to monitor CVP. Central lines and TPN are considered in more detail in Chapter 6, and CVP measurement is outlined in *Figure 5.5*.

Blood, blood products and plasma substitutes
Box 5.3 lists the main blood products in common use. There are four main categories: red cell products, platelets, plasma, and plasma fractions. Platelets

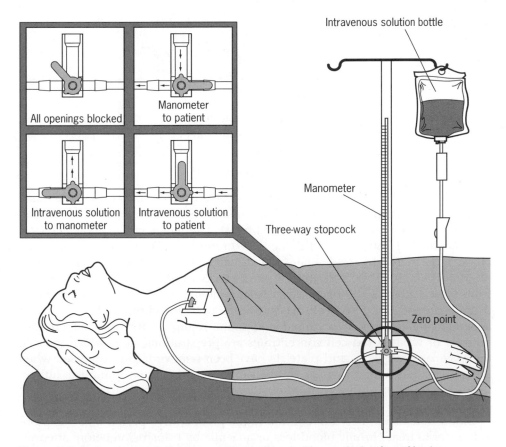

Figure 5.5 Measuring central venous pressure. (Used with permission from *Nursing Procedures*, 2nd edn, © 1996 Springhouse Corporation. All rights reserved.)

Box 5.3 Blood products and plasma substitutes.

Red cells
Whole blood
Red cell concentrate
Filtered red cell concentrate
Washed red cell concentrate

Platelets and granulocyte concentrates

Plasma and plasma products
Fresh frozen plasma
Human albumin solutions
Plasma protein solution

Plasma substitutes
Dextran
Gelatin
Etherified starch

Plasma fractions

and plasma fractions are used for specific pathologies and deficiency states and will not be considered here. Red cell preparations and plasma preparations are more generally used in surgical practice.

Blood transfusion
Whole blood is not routinely used, but may be requested to treat acute massive haemorrhage. A unit of whole blood has an approximate volume of 510 mL (i.e. 450 mL of donor blood, 60 mL of additives). The haemocrit is about 35–45%. The *Handbook of Transfusion Medicine* (1989) recommends that the use of whole blood is restricted to cases where red cell and plasma protein replacement is required. A unit of red cell concentrate consists of about 200 mL of red cells from which most of the plasma has been removed, the packed cell volume is usually around 65%. Red cell concentrate is used for chronic blood loss and anaemia or in addition to colloid and saline regimens for acute blood loss. Filtered or washed red cell concentrates are preparations from which most of the plasma, white cells, and platelets have been removed. They are used when the patient has had previous transfusion reactions or to minimize human leukocyte antigen (HLA) immunization when repeated transfusions are required.

Blood transfusion may be required in the preoperative period and it is probably safer to treat chronic blood loss or anaemia by transfusion before attempting surgery. Any anaemia requiring transfusion is likely to need two or more units of blood. One unit of blood will provide an increase of 10 g L^{-1} (1 g dL^{-1}) of haemoglobin (Davies and Brozovic, 1992). Blood transfusion may also be necessary during surgery and in the postoperative period.

Transfusion of donor blood has significant immunological and infectious risks to the surgical patient and to avoid these risks autologous blood transfusion is becoming increasingly common. Autologous transfusion is use of the patient's own blood to replace losses incurred during surgery. Autologous transfusion may use pre-deposited blood donated several weeks before the scheduled surgery or blood recovered or 'salvaged' from losses during surgery. Autologous transfusion has the twin advantages of reducing transfusion risks and conserving donor stocks.

Use of donor blood requires careful typing and crossmatching to ensure ABO and Rhesus compatibility between the recipient and the donor blood. A severe haemolytic transfusion reaction can occur if a transfusion error occurs and a patient receives incompatible blood. To avoid errors all samples sent for crossmatching must be correctly and clearly labelled and the details of the donor unit must be carefully checked for compatibility before administration. Blood must be stored carefully in specially designated refrigerators with alarms. After removal from the refrigerator transfusion must start within 30 minutes or the unit will have to be discarded. The rate of transfusion will vary depending upon why the blood is being given, but transfusion of a single unit should be completed within four hours. Blood requires a special blood administration set with 170 micrometre filters. Other types of administration set are not suitable, and drugs or additives must never be added to blood. Blood does not generally require warming, but if large volumes are to be given over a short period of time a blood warmer can be used. Blood must never be warmed up in a sink or basin of hot water or on a heater or radiator. *Box 5.4* details the key steps for ensuring safe blood transfusion.

During transfusion, the nurse must monitor the patient's pulse rate, blood pressure, and temperature, and observe the patient carefully. A nurse should stay with the patient for the first 5–10 minutes after a unit has been started, observing closely for an unexpected reaction. Vital signs are recorded every 30 minutes, and CVP measurement may be requested for elderly or severely ill patients. The nurse must be alert for:

- An increase in temperature of more than $1°C$, chills or rigor.
- Allergic reactions (e.g. flushing, sudden rash, urticaria).
- Sudden chest or back pain.
- Tachycardia.
- Hypotension.
- Dyspnoea.
- Oliguria and haematuria.

If there is any indication of a transfusion reaction, the transfusion is halted and a doctor is informed. If the patient passes any urine it should be saved for investigation: haemoglobinuria is an early feature of a haemolytic transfusion reaction.

Box 5.4 Key steps for ensuring safe blood transfusion (Elcock, 1994).

- Correct blood grouping and crossmatching.

- Correct storage of prepared blood.

- Use of appropriate blood administration set.

- Careful pre-transfusion checks.
  1 Time of arrival of blood on the ward.
  2 Ensure blood is not discoloured and bag is not leaking
  3 Check that the expiry date of the blood has not passed
  4 Confirm full name and age of the patient with the patient's identity band.
  5 Ensure that ABO and Rhesus groups, type of blood component (whole, packed cells), and donor number on the blood bag compare with the patient's prescription chart and with the details from the transfusion department.

- Ensure that the patient is comfortable and understands the reason for the transfusion, how long the transfusion is likely to take, the possible reactions that may occur and what observations will need to be taken during the transfusion.

- Take baseline observations of temperature, pulse, respirations, and blood pressure before commencing the transfusion. These observations must be repeated five minutes after starting the transfusion and thereafter as often as local policy dictates.

- Ask the patient to inform the nurse if any unusual symptoms such as pain in the loins or chest, breathlessness, or itching occur. These may indicate a reaction to the transfusion. If the patient is unable to do this, the patient must be frequently observed by the nurse throughout the transfusion.

- Examine the patient's cannula site frequently for signs of inflammation or swelling and ask the patient to report any pain in the site.

- Complete the patient's intake and output chart with the amount of fluid taken in and passed out by the patient. Record the details of the substance transfused on the chart.

- On completing the transfusion, document the transfusion department details in the patient's notes in case of delayed reaction. Empty blood bags are dealt with according to local policy.

Hospital policy for dealing with a transfusion reaction must be followed. Adverse reactions affect 2–5% of transfusions, *Box 5.5* summarizes the acute and delayed complications associated with blood transfusion.

Box 5.5 Complications of blood transfusion (adapted from Elcock, 1994).

Acute haemolytic reaction
- ABO incompatibility can occur with the first 10–15 mL of blood. Group A blood into a Group O patient transfusion is the most severe. This is usually due to a transfusion error. It causes one death per 34,000 patients transfused.
- Signs and symptoms are pyrexia, rigors, tachypnoea, dyspnoea, hypotension, flushing. Pain occurs in the head, lumbar region and chest. It can cause disseminated intravascular coagulation (DIC) and renal failure.
- Treatment includes stopping the transfusion and replacing with saline. Contact medical staff, check all details and send blood for check of crossmatching. Test urine for haematuria. Arrange full blood count, coagulation, and urea and electrolytes. Retain blood bag and giving set for further investigation.

Delayed haemolytic reaction
- Due to previous immunization to foreign antigen, usually due to pregnancy or previous transfusions. Occurs 2–10 days after transfusion and frequency is about one in 500 transfusions. It is seldom fatal.
- Signs and symptoms are an unexplained fall in haemoglobin, jaundice, and renal failure.
- Treatment includes testing the urine for haemoglobin and sending the blood to the transfusion department for further testing.

Non-haemolytic febrile reaction
- Due to a reaction to donor white cells.
- Signs and symptoms are rigors, flushing, pyrexia.
- Treatment includes stopping the transfusion and contacting medical staff. Chlorpheniramine 10–20 mg may be administered intravenously. If the symptoms settle then start next unit for transfusion after 20–30 minutes, using a filter.

Anaphylaxis
- Due to antibody reaction to IgA.
- Signs and symptoms are urticaria and fever.
- Treatment includes stopping the transfusion. Adrenalin, hydrocortisone, amino-phylline may be prescribed. Chlorpheniramine and oxygen may also be prescribed.

Box 5.5 (continued)

Urticaria
- Due to reaction of antibodies to infused plasma proteins.
- Sign and symptom is a rash.
- Treatment includes stopping the infusion, and giving chlorpheniramine as prescribed.

Circulatory overload
- Due to fluid being administered too quickly.
- Signs and symptoms are dyspnoea, cyanosis, tachycardia, restlessness and coughing.
- Treatment includes stopping the transfusion and then administering a diuretic and oxygen.

Infection
- Due to the transfusion of infected blood containing bacteria, parasites or viruses. Infection can also be introduced during cannulation or blood-giving set changes.
- Signs and symptoms are fever, nausea, vomiting, hypotension, diarrhoea and abdominal cramp.
- Treatment includes stopping the transfusion and giving oxygen. Blood cultures should be taken and the prescribed antibiotics administered.

Iron overload
- One unit of red cells contains 250 mg of iron and therefore accumulation is likely over a long course of transfusion.
- Signs and symptoms are pigmentation, hepatic cirrhosis, arrhythmias and cardiac failure.
- Iron chelation therapy should be instituted to prevent or delay this problem.

Plasma, plasma products, and substitutes

Fresh frozen plasma is supplied in packs of 200–250 mL volume. Crossmatching is necessary. Fresh frozen plasma is not generally required in surgical practice, but is used to treat patients with multiple clotting disorders due to liver disease or massive transfusion. Isotonic human albumin solution and plasma protein solution are used as volume expanders and plasma replacements in trauma and burns and to treat complications of surgery. However, albumin solutions are expensive and there is some doubt that they are any more effective than less expensive substitutes. Dextran, gelatin (Gelofusine, Haemaccel), and etherified starch preparations (Hepsan, Pentaspan, Elohes) are slowly metabolized macro-molecules used as plasma substitutes. They are used for short-term volume expansion in the early treatment of shock due to burns or septicaemia. Dextran may interfere with crossmatching and some electrolyte measurements. Blood samples for crossmatching and electrolyte estimation must be taken before dextran infusion (*British National Formulary*, 1996).

References

Beckwith N, Carriere S (1985) Fluid resuscitation: an update. *J Emerg Nurs* **11**:293–299.

British National Formulary No 32 (1996) British Medical Association and Royal Pharmaceutical Society for Great Britain, London.

Centers for Disease Control (1982) Guidelines for prevention of intravascular infection. *Hosp Infect Control, Atlanta* **9(2)**:17–28.

Davies SC, Brozovic M (1992) Transfusion of red cells. In *ABC of Transfusion*, 2nd edition. Contreras M (ed.), p. 11. British Medical Journal Publishing, London.

Dougherty L (1992) Intravenous therapy. *Surg Nurse* **5(2)**:10–13.

Elcock K (1994) Understanding blood transfusions. *Surg Nurse* **7(5)**:20–24.

Gershan JA, Freeman CM, Ross MC *et al.* (1990) Fluid volume deficit: validating the indicators. *Heart Lung* **19(2)**:152–156.

Gobbi M, Torrance C (1994) Fluids and electrolytes. In *Nursing Practice: Hospital and Home. The Adult*, pp. 637–656. Alexander MF, Fawcett JN, Runciman PC (eds). Churchill Livingstone, Edinburgh.

Handbook of Transfusion Medicine (1989) pp. 7–25. HMSO, London.

Jenkins MT, Beck GP (1963) Differential diagnosis of hypotension occurring during anaesthesia and surgery. *Clin Anesth* **3**:106.

Karanjia ND, Walker A, Rees M (1992) Fluids and electrolytes in surgery. *Surgery* **10(6)**:121–128.

Kashuk JL, Penn I (1984) Airway embolism after central venous catheterization. *Surg Gynecol Obstet* **159**:249.

Maier RV, Carrico JC (1986) Developments in resuscitation of critically ill surgical patients. *Adv Surg* **19**:271–319.

Maki DG, Weise CE, Sarafin HW (1977) A semi-quantitative culture method for identifying intravenous catheter related infection. *N Engl J Med* **296**:1305–1309.

McConnell E (1986) Preventing air embolism in patients with central venous catheters. *Nurs Life* **6**:47–49.

Metheny NM (1992) *Fluid and Electrolyte Balance. Nursing Considerations*, 2nd edition, pp. 12–131. Lippincott, Philadelphia.

Moghissi K, Boore J (1983) *Parenteral and Enteral Nutrition for Nurses*, pp. 93–95. Heinemann Medical Books Ltd, London.

Moynihan P (1994) Special nutritional needs of surgical patients. *Nurs Times* **90(51)**:40–41.

Nightingale KW, Bradshaw EG (1982) A review of peripheral cannulae. *Br J Intraven Ther* **3(4)**:14–23.

Ordway C (1974) Air embolism via CVP catheter without positive pressure. *Ann Surg* **179**:479–481.

Pflaum S (1979) Investigation of intake–output as a means of assessing body fluid balance. *Heart Lung* **8**:495–498.

Porth CM (1994) *Pathophysiology. Concepts of Altered Health States*, 4th edition, pp. 591–627. JB Lippincott, Philadelphia.

Protheroe D, Auty B (1986) Drip controllers and drip rate pumps. *Care Critic Ill* **2(1)**:32–33.

Smith K (1980) *Fluids and Electrolytes, a Conceptual Approach*, pp. 148–169. Churchill Livingstone, NY.

Speechley V, Toovey J (1987) Problems in intravenous therapy. *Prof Nurse* **2(8)**:240–242.

Swaminathan R (1994) Normal distribution and composition of body fluids. *Surgery* **12(4)**:77–79.

Wilkinson R (1991) The challenge of intravenous therapy. *Nurs Stand* **5**:24–27.

Yeakel AE (1969) Lethal air embolism from plastic blood storage containers. *JAMA* **204**:175–177.

Chapter 6
Nutrition and Surgical Care

Surgery and trauma can have a major impact on metabolic function and ensuring adequate nutrition is an important aspect of pre- and postoperative nursing care. The trauma of surgery initiates a complex neuroendocrine response that increases metabolic rate and fuel use. Nightingale (1859) recognized the importance of nutrition and included two chapters on the subject in her famous *Notes on Nursing*, while Henderson (1960) stated that 'There is no more important an element in the preparation for nursing than the study of nutrition.' Changes in the organization of health care delivery combined with a more rapid turnover in surgical wards may have de-emphasized the role of the surgical nurse in ensuring adequate nutrition. However, nutritional status influences the patient's response to trauma, rate of wound healing, and immune function, and nutritional care remains a central nursing function.

Most patients presenting for elective surgery are well nourished and able to cope with a short period of pre- and postoperative starvation, but there is evidence of a surprising level of malnourishment in surgical, medical, and elderly hospitalized patients. Bistrian *et al.* (1974, 1976) reported that protein–energy malnutrition was common in surgical and medical patients, while Hill *et al.* (1977) found a significant reduction in nutritional status among 105 surgical patients compared with that of controls. However, comments about nutritional status were recorded in the notes of only 22 of the 105 patients studied by Hill *et al.* (1977) and less that 20% of the patients had been weighed. Todd *et al.* (1984) investigated food intake on medical, surgical, and orthopaedic wards and found that nearly 25% of the patients had a food intake below the level predicted by their basal metabolic rate, and 16% were consuming below the recommended daily intake of protein. Nightingale wrote in 1859 'Every careful observer of the sick will agree in this, that thousands of patients are annually starved in the midst of plenty from want of attention to the ways which alone make it possible for them to take food.' It may be that this comment is just as accurate today. Fearon (1995) has identified the following factors that adversely affect the nutritional status of hospitalized patients:

- Problems with chewing and swallowing.
- Refusing food.
- Malfunction of the gut.
- Long periods without food for medical reasons.
- Dependence on others.
- Physical difficulties.
- Missed meals.
- Inadequate nutritional content of meals.

Fearon (1995) suggests that nurses are in a prime position to improve the nutritional care of hospitalized patients.

In this chapter we discuss nutritional status and response to surgery, nutritional assessment, normal nutrition, and the provision of nutritional support, and review the nursing management of meals and enteral and parenteral feeding. Surgical nurses are ideally placed to ensure the patient is not 'starved in the midst of plenty from want of attention to the ways which alone make it possible for them to take food.'

NUTRITIONAL STATUS AND RESPONSE TO SURGERY

The trauma of surgery initiates a coordinated response involving cardiovascular, respiratory, and neuroendocrine mechanisms. The response is intended to conserve plasma volume, to maintain tissue perfusion, and to ensure the delivery of oxygen and nutrients to vital tissues. It is essential as the stress response and emotional stress such as preoperative anxiety may exacerbate hypovolaemia. *Figure 6.1* illustrates the main phases of the response.

Neuroendocrine Activation

Emotional stress can cause hypothalamic–pituitary and sympathetic activation before surgery has begun. Pituitary hormones – adrenocorticotrophic hormone (ACTH), growth hormone, antidiuretic hormone (ADH), prolactin – are stimulated and the sympathetic branch of autonomic nervous system is activated (Torrance, 1991). ACTH release and sympathetic activation increase the secretion of catecholamines and glucocorticosteroids from the adrenal gland. The

Response to surgical trauma

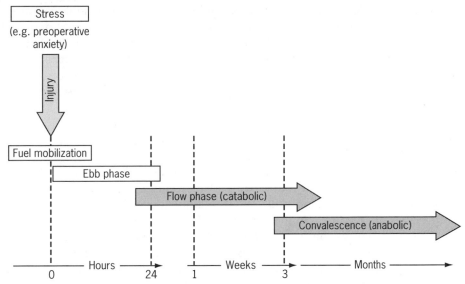

Figure 6.1 Response to surgical trauma. The phases are variable in length and the duration times are approximate. The phases are not discrete, and there will be some overlap. Adapted from Frayn KN (1986). Hormonal control of metabolism in trauma and sepsis. *Clin Endocrinol* **24**:577–599, by Torrance C (1992) *Surg Nurse* (Oxford) p.6. (Reproduced with kind permission of *British Journal of Nursing*, Mark Allen Publishing Ltd.)

main metabolic effect of this neuroendocrine activation is mobilization of body fuels.

Ebb Phase

The next step is called the ebb phase and lasts 12–24 hours. There is continued mobilization of glycogen and triglycerides to provide energy; however, this is not accompanied by a marked increase in metabolic rate. Increased adrenal activation is the dominant feature of this phase and the rise in catecholamines is linked to the severity or extent of injury (Frayn *et al.*, 1985). Adrenaline and noradrenaline stimulate release of liver glycogen, resulting in an increased blood glucose concentration (hyperglycaemia). Glycogenolysis and incomplete utilization of glucose results in an increased lactic acid concentration with possible alkalaemia.

Flow Phase

In this phase there is a marked increase in metabolic rate reflected in a rise in core temperature and increased heart rate. The net effect of this phase is catabolic: protein (mainly muscle protein) is broken down and renal excretion of urea (nitrogen), creatine, and creatinine increases. However, although muscle bulk may be lost, water retention may cause an increase in body weight. Fats are used as an energy source as the body's glucose stores have been rapidly depleted. In this phase fats contribute 70–80% of the energy required, while protein catabolism contributes about 20% (Duke *et al.*, 1970; Lee, 1978). In addition to hypothalamic–pituitary, sympathetic, and adrenal activation, other factors, including prostaglandins, monokines, and lymphokines released from the site of injury play an important role (Frayn, 1986).

Convalescence

Malnutrition reduces the body's ability to cope with surgical stress and is associated with increased morbidity and mortality in the postoperative period (Mullen *et al.*, 1980; Nazari *et al.*, 1982). Malnutrition is particularly linked with infectious complications in the postoperative period. The link between nutrition and immunodepression is clear, and tests of immune function (skin testing or total lymphocyte count) are used as nutritional indicators. Preoperative nutritional support can help reduce postoperative complications (Mullen *et al.*, 1980; Muller *et al.*, 1986; Bellatone *et al.*, 1988).

Preoperative nutritional assessment and support are essential if the patient is clearly malnourished, but may require extensive preoperative preparation. Meguid *et al.* (1990) investigated the impact of total parenteral nutrition (TPN) in the perioperative period. They found no improvement if TPN was delivered for 2–3 days preoperatively, but there was a significant reduction in postoperative complications and mortality if it was continued for 7–10 days.

NUTRITIONAL ASSESSMENT

Nutritional assessment represents the first stage in planning nutritional care. Keithly (1985) stated that a detailed assessment of nutritional status including dietary history and anthropometric and biochemical measurements is required to identify patients at risk. The value of obtaining a detailed nutritional history as part of the preoperative assessment process is discussed in Chapter 2. Unfortunately a lack of data on dietary history and nutritional status is a common finding of nursing audits (Fearon and Goldstone, 1995).

Anthropometric Evaluation and Laboratory Investigations

Anthropometric measurements provide an objective assessment of nutritional status, are relatively simple, can be quickly performed after suitable training, and can be easily incorporated into the physical examination, but form only part of the nutritional assessment. The results must be evaluated with data from the history and general examination. Commonly used anthropometric measurements include:

- Weight.
- Height.
- Skinfold thickness.
- Midarm circumference.

Weight and height

Weight is recorded on admission and should be monitored regularly if there are any problems with fluid balance or nutrition. To obtain accurate and consistent serial measurements it is important that the patient is weighed after emptying bladder and bowels at the same time of day using the same scales and in the same state of dress. Weighing scales should be regularly maintained and calibrated. Serial measurement can help identify weight loss. Rapid weight loss of 10% indicates mild malnutrition, while rapid weight losses of 20% and 30% indicate moderate and severe malnutrition, respectively (Studley, 1936). However, fluid status must be considered with any rapid weight loss or gain; check for dehydration or oedema.

Height is another important, but sometimes neglected measurement. Using height, body weight can be compared with standard tables of ideal weight for height, sex, and build. Height and weight can also be used to calculate the body mass index (BMI), which is the ratio of body weight in kilograms divided by height in metres squared:

$$BMI = \frac{weight\ (kg)}{height\ (m)^2}$$

A normal BMI is 20–25; 25–30 suggests that the patient is overweight; over 30 indicates obesity; under 20 suggests nutritional problems. BMI is an easily calculated 'rule of thumb' measure that allows monitoring of changes in nutritional status. It must, however, be used in conjunction with an assessment of the complete picture. A body builder, for example, may have a high BMI, but will not be obese.

Skinfold thickness

Skinfold thickness measurements can provide an estimate of body fat and allow dietary regimens to be calculated for lean body mass rather than total weight. A number of sites can be used, but the triceps is the most common. The triceps skinfold is conveniently accessible and measurements are reproducible if performed with care. Skinfold callipers such as the Holtain or Harpenden callipers are used. Measurements are made on the posterior aspect of the nondominant arm midway between the elbow (olecranon of the ulna) and shoulder (acromion of the scapula). The skinfold is gently grasped and the callipers applied while the arm is relaxed. An average of three readings is compared with the value from standard tables. Less than 60% of standard value indicates severe malnutrition, while less than 90% suggests moderate malnutrition. Triceps skinfold measurements are useful, but training is needed to use the callipers. Also the callipers must be accurate and the measurements are not accurate if there is oedema. Midarm circumference measurements are recommended for routine use by less skilled personnel.

Midarm circumference

Measurement of midarm circumference can be used to estimate muscle mass and monitor changes. The nondominant arm is bent at right angles to the body and the circumference is measured at a point midway between the olecranon and acromion. A skin pencil can be used to mark the point for serial measurements. The value is compared with standard tables. Midarm muscle circumference can be calculated if the triceps skinfold thickness is known and provides a better estimate of muscle mass than arm circumference alone.

Laboratory investigations

A variety of biochemical parameters and tests of immune function can provide additional information of nutritional status. An investigation of various tissues including blood, plasma, hair, liver, and bone can be used to assess protein, fat, vitamin, and mineral status (Miller and Torrance, 1991). However, biochemical parameters are influenced by a wide range of factors including disease and drugs, in addition to nutritional status. Laboratory results must be considered along with data from the physical assessment and nutritional history. Malnutrition cannot be accurately diagnosed from laboratory data alone. *Box 6.1* summarizes laboratory investigations of nutritional significance.

NORMAL NUTRITION

A healthy diet provides all the essential nutrients in sufficient quantity to meet nutritional needs but avoids excess and the problems of obesity. The diet must provide a balanced supply of:

- Protein.
- Carbohydrate.

Box 6.1 Laboratory investigations of nutritional value.

Creatinine–height index (CHI)
Nitrogen balance
Serum proteins
Serum cholesterol, triglycerides or lipoproteins
Specific vitamins, e.g. vitamins C, D, B_1
Minerals, e.g. iron, zinc
Tests of immune function, e.g. total lymphocyte count

- Fat.
- Vitamins.
- Minerals.
- Fibre.
- Water.

For health, nutrient intake should balance nutrient use. If protein, carbohydrate, or fat intake exceeds use the excess is stored as fat, leading to obesity and its risks (*Figure 6.2*). If intake falls below use the problems of undernutrition begin to develop. In developed countries the gross effects of undernutrition are less evident than obesity and its adverse effects, which represent a major health problem. Lack of single nutrients, usually minerals or vitamins, can cause specific deficiency states (see *Box 2.4*, p. 22). Individual requirements vary

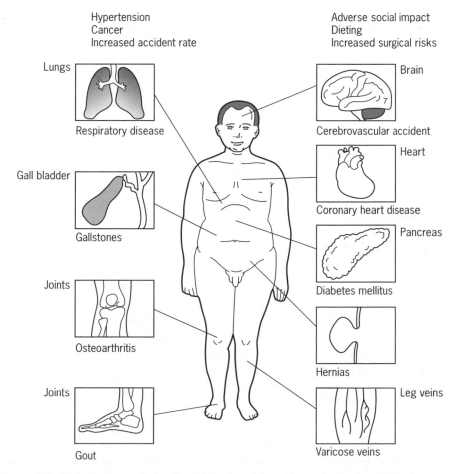

Hypertension
Cancer
Increased accident rate

Adverse social impact
Dieting
Increased surgical risks

Lungs — Respiratory disease

Gall bladder — Gallstones

Joints — Osteoarthritis

Joints — Gout

Brain — Cerebrovascular accident

Heart — Coronary heart disease

Pancreas — Diabetes mellitus

Hernias

Leg veins — Varicose veins

Figure 6.2 Complications of obesity. (Reproduced from Alexander, Fawcett, Runciman (1994) *Nursing Practice, Hospital and Home – The Adult.* Churchill Livingstone, Edinburgh.)

depending on factors such as age, sex, employment, activity level, and general health. For a more detailed review of nutrition the reader is directed to *Human Nutrition and Dietetics* (Garrow and James, 1993) and for recent European recommendations for daily intake of a range of nutrients to the Scientific Committee for Food for the European Community, 1993 editorial.

NUTRITIONAL NURSING

Eating is a biological need, but also has great psychological and social significance. In Roper *et al.*'s (1985) model of living, eating and drinking was one of the twelve essential activities of daily living. In helping patients meet their nutritional needs the surgical nurse must be aware of the wider significance of food and eating, and the impact illness, disability, or surgery can have on it. Torrance and Gobbi (1994) have emphasized that 'Presenting a well-balanced meal is of little value if the patient is unable or unwilling to eat.' Nutritional nursing involves both the art and science of nursing. Calculating appropriate major and minor nutrients and energy requirements requires nutritional knowledge, but assessment of individual likes and dislikes, abilities and disabilities is essential to support dignity and enjoyment of meals and ensure nutrient intake. The surgical nurse may need to consider physical, psychosocial, cultural, and religious factors when planning individualized nutritional care. Dieticians, occupational therapists, and other specialists such as the TPN team can have a major role in nutritional care, but the general nurse is ideally placed to coordinate care and help patients manage their nutritional needs, both in hospital and on return home.

ORAL FEEDING

Managing Oral Intake

Oral intake is the natural and preferred method of feeding. The process of savouring, chewing, and swallowing food increases enjoyment of eating, and mechanical and enzymatic digestion of food starts in the mouth. A patient's ability and motivation to eat enough to meet daily requirements will be influenced by a range of individual, environmental, and organizational factors. In hospital the nurse will be able to order special diets or feeding aids, but these may not be readily available after discharge. If the patient has problems with nutrition, and particularly if the surgery has short- or long-term implications for nutrition, the surgical nurse should consider:

■ Does the patient have adequate knowledge and economic resources to make appropriate informed choices about nutrition?
■ Is the patient physically able to maintain nutritional independence or is help required with shopping, feeding, and cooking?
■ Are adequate facilities available, and can the patient use them safely?

To eat and enjoy food and drink normally requires coordination of the motor and sensory systems. The sight, smell, taste, and texture of food are important in stimulating appetite and enjoyment. Many conditions can affect the ability to enjoy food. Respiratory infections may reduce the ability to detect odours, while anosmia may develop after head injury or with an intracranial tumour, and some types of cancer alter gustation and olfaction. The sight and texture of food is important: poorly presented, overcooked food is unlikely to stimulate a sick person's appetite. Oral health involving the condition of the teeth and mouth can also influence eating behaviour and affect food choice: dry, inflamed, or infected oral mucosa and gums may make eating painful and interfere with taste and enjoyment of food, while healthy teeth and gums make it easier to chew food. If the patient has dentures these should be clean and fit well. Patients with chewing or swallowing difficulties may require softer food or food cut into small pieces. For a few patients maintaining oral intake involves a purely mashed, minced, or liquidized diet, but this is exceptional. Edentulous patients may have a poorer diet due to their inability to chew effectively. Davidson *et al.* (1962) found that protein intake was inversely correlated with chewing ability in healthy individuals. Motor function is also important. Adults usually expect to feed themselves and loss of the mobility or fine muscle coordination may limit access to food or the ability to feed oneself. Loss of independence in eating can have an equally negative impact on confidence and self-perception as loss of independence in meeting the need to excrete.

Food preferences, nutritional needs, motor and sensory deficits, and the social meaning of meals to the individual patient are assessed and interventions planned to maximize the patient's enjoyment and independence when eating. The impact of physical factors influencing eating (*Box 6.2*) can be minimized by manipulation of the diet, presentation of food, and the environment during mealtimes. Managing mealtimes for a patient with feeding problems can be much more challenging than simply presenting a liquid diet or a feeding cup. If nutritional deficits are identified it will be important to maintain an accurate record of food intake. For a patient with eating problems the nurse should consider how to:

■ Organize mealtimes (social setting, timing, and place).
■ Present food (type of food, visual appeal, portion size, temperature).
■ Assist the patient (special feeding aids, help with eating).

Reintroducing Feeding

After some types of surgery it may be considered necessary to reintroduce oral intake slowly. Initially intake will be limited to small volumes of water (usually 30 ml hourly), and if tolerated and if bowel sounds and motility return, the volume is increased gradually over the next few days. A light diet can be resumed once the patient can tolerate fluid without nausea or distension, and

Box 6.2 Physical factors influencing eating (Torrance and Gobbi, 1994).

Oral cavity
- Congenital abnormalities (e.g. cleft lip and palate)
- Dentition (natural teeth, dentures, edentulous)
- Oral health (xerostomia, gingivitis, stomatitis, mouth ulcers, pain)
- Sensory (temperature sensation, taste, smell)

Chewing and swallowing
- Age
- Dentition
- Dysphagia
- Achalasia

Dexterity and mobility
- Perceptual problems
- Upper limb function
- Mobility
- Positioning

Others
- Dyspnoea
- Pain

peristalsis is established with the passage of flatus and faeces. Protein–calorie supplements are required if the patient is not tolerating a diet with a minimum protein content of 45–55 g (Moghissi and Boore, 1983).

ENTERAL NUTRITION

Enteral or tube feeding is the delivery of food directly to the stomach or small intestine. Enteral feeding involves the gut and represents a more physiological route than parenteral (intravenous) feeding. However, enteral feeding is artificial and intrusive. A feeding tube has to be inserted and it bypasses the mouth, so there is no chewing or tasting of the food. Enteral feeding may meet nutritional needs, but it cannot fulfil the nonnutritional aspects of eating. A number of approaches can be used in tube feeding:

- In the short term, nasoenteral feeding can be used. A tube is passed via the nose to the stomach (nasogastric), duodenum (nasoduodenal), or jejunum (nasojejunal). Less commonly the tube may be inserted through the mouth (orogastric).

■ If tube feeding is likely to be of long duration or permanent a surgically-inserted tube is used i.e. an enterostomy). The commonest approach is to insert the tube through the body wall into the stomach (gastrostomy), but tubes may also be inserted into the oesophagus (oesophagostomy) or jejunum (jejunostomy). If tube feeding is anticipated the tube may be inserted during surgery. Percutaneous endoscopic gastrostomy (PEG) is the endoscopic placement of a gastrostomy and can be carried out under local anaesthesia.

Enteral feeding is considered if the patient is unable to meet nutritional needs by the normal route. It can be used to supplement the oral diet or as the sole route for food and fluid ingestion. For enteral feeding to succeed there must be adequate absorption from the small intestine, and the route of access must be accessible and the tube well tolerated. Tube feeding is not indicated for major surgery of the upper gastrointestinal (GI) tract, paralytic ileus, intestinal obstruction, and some cases of malabsorption, or if there is persistent vomiting. It can be used for the unconscious patient, but parenteral feeding will be preferable if the patient has serious respiratory disease or lacks a gag reflex. Indications for enteral feeding are presented in *Box 6.3*

Nasoenteral Feeding

The nasal route is indicated for short-term feeding and to supplement oral intake because it does not interfere with oral function. Large-bore tubes such as the Ryle's tube intended for GI drainage can be used, but are uncomfortable and poorly tolerated. This type of tube can cause trauma and pressure necrosis to the nares and oropharynx, and may also increase the risk of cardiac sphincter incompetence, gastric reflux, and aspiration (Silk, 1980; Janes, 1982). Modern feeding tubes are smaller, softer, and more flexible, but may be more difficult to pass, and due to the narrower lumen, are more prone to blockage. These fine silicon or polyurethane tubes are essential if nasoenteral feeding is required for more than a day or two. These tubes may pass into the trachea without causing respiratory distress, so positioning must be checked by radiography as aspiration is difficult with these collapsible small-bore tubes. The position of a large-bore tube can be checked by aspiration. It is important to explain the purpose and care of the nasoenteral tube to the patient. The tubes are secured, but can be easily displaced or removed. A spigot may be needed to close the end of the tube between feeds. The tube may be flushed with a small volume of water before and after feeding. Feeding may be by bolus feeds or by continuous drip feeding. For safety, the ports and connections on nasoenteral tubes must not be compatible with intravenous infusion equipment.

Enterostomies

A gastrostomy or jejunostomy tube may be used if the nasoenteral route is obstructed (e.g. due to oesophageal obstruction). Enterostomy tubes can be kept

Box 6.3 Indications for enteral feeding (Torrance and Gobbi, 1994).

Increased nutritional needs
- Protein–energy malnutrition
- Persistent anorexia
- Hypercatabolic states (burns, major sepsis, severe trauma)

Compromised oral access to GI tract
- Facial and oral surgery
- Head and neck surgery
- Oesophageal stricture, surgery, fistula
- Carcinoma of the mouth or upper alimentary structures
- Functional or mechanical obstructions

Inability to eat
- Unconscious
- Confused or uncooperative

Unwillingness to eat
- Odynophagia (mucositis, pharyngitis, oesophagitis)
- Persistent anorexia (e.g. related to chemotherapy or radiotherapy)
- Psychiatric disorders resulting in a refusal to eat (anorexia nervosa)
- Cancer cachexia or anorexia
- Persistent nausea and vomiting

Danger of aspiration
- Dysphagia
- Neurological disorders with loss of cough reflex

GI disorders
- Fistula
- Short bowel syndrome
- Malabsorption syndromes
- Inflammatory bowel disease

in place by a retention balloon or may be sutured in position. Liddle and Yuill (1995) have reviewed the use of PEG. After insertion of the tube a dressing is not generally required and feeding can begin when bowel sounds return. The tube stoma requires daily cleansing and the tube is flushed before and after feeding with about 30 ml of water. The stoma site is monitored for any indication of inflammation or infection. Traditional gastrostomy tubes were quite bulky, but PEG systems are less obtrusive, and a button gastrostomy tube is very discrete, with only a small external fixator visible. Gastrostomy tubes need to be replaced at between six months to two years depending on the type of tube used. As with nasoenteral tubes, blockage is the major problem, but there is also a continual risk of infection.

Enteral Feeding

Once the nasogastric tube, gastrostomy tube, or jejunostomy tube is in position, the patient's metabolic requirements are reviewed and the relevant nutrient solutions are prescribed. Continuous regular-rate drip feeding, preferably using an enteral feeding pump, is better than bolus feeding because it reduces the risk of diarrhoea. The feed should be at room temperature, and the tube flushed daily with a little clear water to maintain patency. Bolus feeding is sometimes used for gastrostomy feeding, and should be given slowly and at room temperature. Oral hygiene is essential and the patient's mouth must be kept clean and moist.

A variety of commercially prepared enteral feeds are available and provide a sterile feed designed for tube administration and of known nutritional content. Liquidized meals can be used with large-bore tubes, but are generally not suitable for modern small-bore nasoenteral tubes. Asepsis is essential in the preparation and delivery of enteral feeds. Prescription of tube feeds is based on a careful assessment of nutritional needs as commercial feeds vary in composition, osmolality, viscosity, the nutrient sources, and the balance between fats, protein, and carbohydrate. Many of the feeds are hyposmolar and may cause a GI disturbance when first used or if they are infused too quickly. The complications of enteral feeding with appropriate patient selection and monitoring (*Table 6.1*) can be reduced.

PARENTERAL NUTRITION

Parenteral nutrition can be used to supplement oral intake or as the only method of feeding if GI tract function is delayed for more than seven days. Total parenteral nutrition (TPN) may be used to 'rest' the bowel and facilitate wound healing after major intestinal surgery or if there is insufficient small bowel to allow for adequate absorption of nutrients.

Parenteral nutrition can be delivered via a peripheral or central vein. However, peripheral veins are only suitable for very short term use or for administering limited nutrition as the solutions used for TPN are often hypertonic, irritant, or too viscous for small peripheral veins. Central veins are more commonly used: a catheter such as a Hickman's catheter is inserted into a major vein and eased up the vein until the catheter tip is lodged in the superior vena cava. The superior vena cava is the usual site, but with care the inferior vena cava may also be used. The catheter may be inserted using a simple cutdown technique or a tunnelling procedure. Tunnelling results in separation between the point where the catheter enters the skin and the point where it punctures the vein, reducing the risk of contamination. Typically the subclavian vein using an

Table 6.1 Mechanical and infectious complications of enteral feeding (adapted from Torrance and Gobbi, 1994).

Complication	Intervention
Mechanical	
Tube blockage	Flush tube with water after feed
	Maintain continuous flow
	Use correct tube/nutrient solution
Misplacement	Insert tube with patient upright
	Use correct type/length of tube
	Aspirate and pH or X-ray
	Particular care needed if patient lacks gag reflex
Displacement	Secure tube firmly
	Check position of tube daily
Aspiration	Elevate head of bed during feeding
	Correct placement of tube
	Check position of tube before starting feed
Discomfort	Ensure hydration
	Provide regular oral care
Contamination	Avoid nonsterile feeds
	Change equipment regularly
Metabolic	
Hyperkalaemia	Use lower potassium feed
Hyponatraemia	Restrict water
Hypophosphataemia	Phosphate supplements
Hyperglycaemia	Reduce infusion rate
	Administer insulin
Uraemia	Deal with dehydration
	Correct protein imbalance
Overhydration	Reduce flow rate
Dehydration	Additional water
Gastrointestinal	
Nausea and vomiting	Reduce infusion rate
	Dilute feeds
Diarrhoea	Dilute feeds
	Change to lactose-free feeds
	Check for contamination
Cramps	Reduce infusion rate
	Change to lactose-free feed
	Dilute formula
Constipation	Extra fluid and bulking agents

infraclavicular approach is used for access, although internal and external jugular and brachiocephalic veins can be used for TPN. Occasionally a peripheral vein may be cannulated using a longer catheter. Radio-opaque catheters are used and the position of the catheter tip is checked by X-ray.

Indications for TPN

The benefits of TPN must be considered against the risks and costs. Disadvantages of TPN include:

- Mechanical complications.
- Infection complications associated with the intravenous route.
- Metabolic problems.
- Cost.

The complications of TPN are summarized in *Box 6.4*. Contamination of TPN fluids, administration equipment, or catheter can lead to serious systemic infections. If the GI system is functional, alternatives to TPN may be considered, but TPN is the only choice when the GI system is malfunctioning or obstructed. The efficacy of TPN has been demonstrated as:

- Primary therapy for acute burns, short bowel syndrome, hepatic failure, renal failure, and GI fistula.
- Supportive therapy for major preoperative weight loss, prolonged paralytic ileus, acute radiation enteritis, and chemotherapy toxicity.

Box 6.4 **Complications of TPN.**

Infection
- Contamination of TPN fluids
- Contamination of administration equipment
- Catheter infection
- Insertion site infection
- Septicaemia and bacteraemia
- Septic thrombosis

Mechanical complications
- During insertion: pneumothorax, arterial laceration, haemothorax, hydrothorax, air embolism
- General: catheter displacement, accidental withdrawal, catheter fracture and embolus, catheter blockage, thrombosis

Metabolic complications
- Trace element deficiencies
- Plasma electrolyte imbalance
- Essential fatty acid deficiency
- Hypoglycaemia
- Hyperglycaemia
- Altered liver function

TPN is also considered as a primary and supportive therapy for inflammatory bowel disease, anorexia nervosa, and malignancy, although its efficacy is not as clearly demonstrated in these situations.

TPN Solutions

After detailed assessment of the patient's nutritional and metabolic needs a TPN regimen will be prescribed and must supply all the required nutrients including protein, energy, fats, vitamins, minerals, trace elements, and water. The four main types of TPN fluids are:

- Amino acid solutions.
- Lipid preparations.
- Carbohydrate–electrolyte solutions.
- Nutrient additives.

Individual regimens will be constructed using commercially prepared solutions, which may provide different proportions of amino acids, electrolytes, and energy sources. Amino acids are provided to replace protein. Various preparations are available and provide varying proportions of essential and nonessential amino acids, nitrogen, and electrolytes (e.g. Aminoplasmal and Aminoplex). Lipid preparations are generally based on soya oil (e.g. Intralipid and Ivelip), but are available in formulations providing 4430–8520 kJ L^{-1}. There are many carbohydrate–electrolyte preparations available that provide energy and electrolytes (e.g. Plasma-Lyte with dextrose and Glucoplex 1600). Nutrient additives provide additional vitamins, electrolytes, minerals, or trace elements, for example Additrace (electrolytes and trace elements), Multibionta (vitamins), and Vitlipid N (fat-soluble vitamins).

Nursing Management

Careful assessment and monitoring is required to ensure that the patient receives adequate nutrition and to reduce the complications of TPN. Essential areas for nursing consideration are:

- Flow control and minimizing mechanical complications.
- Infection control.
- Meeting metabolic needs.
- Physical and psychological support.

With TPN it is essential to maintain the correct rate of flow. It is usual to use an electronic infusion pump, although burettes can be used. Administration sets should have Luer locks and inline filters may be required. The external part of the catheter must be secured and the site adequately dressed: clear film dressings have been developed for this purpose. Catheters and tubing should be checked for leaks or loose connections. The number of connections or extensions should be kept to the minimum. Drugs and blood products should not be administered via a TPN line.

Strict asepsis is essential when handling any component of the TPN system. A strict protocol for insertion and management of catheters, insertion site, and equipment is essential.

Careful monitoring will aid early identification of complications. Precise intake–output recording, daily weight, regular physical and anthropometric assessment, and checking of biochemical parameters (urinary and blood) can identify nutritional progress or metabolic complications. Rapid weight gain is often due to fluid retention: observe for signs of peripheral or pulmonary oedema. Monitoring of vital signs (pulse, blood pressure, temperature, and respiration) is advisable.

Patients receiving TPN are usually unable to eat. Oral hygiene is important and the patient may need help or encouragement to maintain mobility. The nurse should also be aware of the psychological impact of TPN. The patient can rapidly become detached from the normal drives and sensations associated with the physical and social aspects of eating. If TPN is to be long term or permanent the whole family may require support and education. The patient may also require extensive support to re-establish normal eating once TPN is stopped. TPN is gradually supplemented by enteral or oral feeding, at this stage the patient may experience problems with nausea, vomiting, constipation, diarrhoea, and loss of appetite.

References

Bistrian BR, Blackburn GL, Hallowell E, Heddle R (1974) Protein status of general surgical patients. *JAMA* **230**:856–860.

Bistrian BR, Blackburn GL, Vitale J, Cochran D, Naylor J (1976) Prevalence of malnutrition in general medical patients. *JAMA* **235**:1567–1570.

Bellatone R, Doglietto G-B, Bossola M *et al.* (1988) Preoperative parenteral nutrition of malnourished surgical patients. *Acta Chir Scand* **154**:249–251.

Davidson CS, Livermore J, Anderson P, Kaufman S (1962) The nutrition of a group of apparently healthy aging persons. *Am J Clin Nutr* **10**:181–199.

Duke JH, Jorgensen SB, Broell JR, Long CL, Kinney JM (1970) Contribution of protein to calorific expenditure following injury. *Surgery* **68**:168–174.

Fearon M (1995) Nutritional care – changing practice with audit. *Surg Nurse* **8(3)**:19–23.

Fearon MM, Goldstone LA (1995) *Monitor 2000: An Audit of the Quality of Care for Medical and Surgical Wards*, pp. 164–173. Unique Business Services Ltd, Newcastle upon Tyne.

Frayn KN, Little RA, Maycock PF, Stoner HB (1985) The relationship of plasma catecholamines to acute metabolic and hormonal responses to injury in man. *Circ Shock* **16**:229–240.

Frayn KN (1986) Hormonal control of metabolism in trauma and sepsis. *Clin Endocrinol* **24**:577–599.

Garrow JS, James WPT (eds) (1993) *Human Nutrition and Dietetics*. Churchill Livingstone, Edinburgh.

Henderson V (1960) *Basic Principles of Nursing Care*, p. 21. International Council of Nurses, Geneva.

Hill GL, Pickford GA, Young CJ, *et al*. (1977) Malnutrition in surgical patients. An unrecognised problem. *Lancet* i:689–692.

Janes EMH (1982) Nursing aspects of tube feeding. *Nursing* **2(4)**:101–104.

Keithly JK (1985) Nutritional assessment of the patient undergoing surgery. *Heart Lung* **14**:449–455.

Lee HA (1978) Parental nutrition. In *Nutrition in the Clinical Management of Disease*. Dickerson JWT, Lee HA (eds), pp. 349–376. Edward Arnold, London.

Liddle K (1995) Making sense of percutaneous endoscopic gastrostomy. *Nurs Times* **91(18)**:32–33.

Liddle K, Yuill R (1995) Making sense of percutaneous endoscopic gastrostomy. *Nurs Times* **91(18)**:32–33.

Meguid MM, Campos AC, Hammond WG (1990) Nutritional support in surgical practice: Part I & II. *Am J Surg* **159**:345–358, 427–443.

Miller B, Torrance C (1991) Nutritional assessment. *Surg Nurse* **4(5)**:21–25.

Moghissi K, Boore J (1983) *Parenteral and Enteral Nutrition for Nurses*, pp. 161–167. Heinemann Medical Books Ltd, London.

Muller JM, Keller HW, Brenner U, Walter M, Holzmuller W (1986) Indications and effect of preoperative parenteral nutrition. *World J Surg* **10**:53–63.

Mullen JL, Buzby GP, Matthews DC, Smale BF, Rosato EF (1980) Reduction of operative morbidity and mortality by combined preoperative and postoperative nutritional support. *Ann Surg* **192**:604–613.

Nazari S, Dionigi R, Comodi I, Campani M (1982) Preoperative prediction and qualification of septic risk caused by malnutrition. *Arch Surg* **117**:266–270.

Nightingale F (1859) *Notes on Nursing* (1952 edition), Chaps VI and VII, pp. 73–85. Duckworth, London.

Roper N, Logan WW, Tierney AJ (1985) Eating and drinking. *The Elements of Nursing* 2nd edition, Chap. 10, pp. 158–182. Churchill Livingstone, Edinburgh.

Scientific Committee for Food for the European Community (1993) Report on proposed nutrient and energy intakes for the European Community. *Nutr Rev* **51(7)**:209–212.

Silk DBA (1980) Enteral nutrition. *Hosp Update* **8**:761–776.

Studley HO (1936) Percentage of weight loss: basic indicator of surgical risk in patients with chronic peptic ulcer. *JAMA* **106**:6458–6460.

Todd EA, Hunt P, Crowe PJ, Royle GT (1984) What do patients eat in hospital? *Hum Nutr App Nutr* **38A**:294–297.

Torrance C (1991) Pre-operative nutrition, fasting and the surgical patient. *Surg Nurse* **4(4)**:4–8.

Torrance C, Gobbi M (1994) Nutrition. In *Nursing Practice: Hospital and Home. The Adult*. Alexander MF, Fawcett JN, Runciman PC (eds). pp. 657–677. Churchill Livingstone, Edinburgh.

Chapter 7
Pain

Discomfort and pain are the most common reasons for seeking medical or nursing care. Pain represents one of the most common, but most misunderstood, problems in surgical nursing. Pain has been defined as 'an unpleasant, subjective sensory and emotional experience associated with actual or potential tissue damage, or described in terms of such damage (International Association for the Study of Pain, 1979). Another definition emphasizes that 'Pain does not occur in isolation but in a specific human being in psychosocial, economic and cultural contexts that influence the meaning, experience and verbal and non-verbal expression of pain' (National Institutes of Health, 1987). Pain is much more than a simple sensation caused by specific adverse stimuli: it is a complex phenomenon, with sensory, emotional and cognitive dimensions. Psychological and sociocultural factors affect the perception of pain and influence the way an individual experiences and responds to pain. Only the person in pain can know what it feels like and how much pain he is in. In assessing for pain, nurses should always be aware that no one can really know what being in pain is like for another person. Nurses also need to be aware of how much their own cultural beliefs may influence their perception of a patient's pain. Davitz et al. (1977) demonstrated that nurses from six different cultures assumed different degrees of suffering in the same patients. McCaffery (1972) states 'Pain is whatever the experiencing person says it is, existing whenever he says it does.' This should form our approach to pain control after surgery.

PHYSIOLOGY OF PAIN

The three types of nerve cells involved in the reception and transmission of pain are:

- Afferent or sensory neurons.
- Connector or interneurons.
- Efferent or motor neurons.

These nerve cells (each cell consisting of dendrites, a body, and an axon) have receptors in their endings that cause the pain impulse to be conducted to the spinal cord and the brain.

These receptors are highly specialized and initiate impulses in response to physical or chemical changes. Receptors that respond to painful stimuli are called nociceptors. Injury to the tissue stimulates the nociceptors to release chemicals including:

- Prostaglandins.
- Histamine.
- Bradykinin.
- Leukotrienes.
- Substance P.
- Proteolytic enzymes.

These chemicals sensitize nerve endings and transmit pain impulses to the brain. The peripheral nerve fibres that carry sensations to the brain are of three different sizes:

- A-alpha and A-beta fibres are large myelinated fibres. (Myelin is the lipo-protein surrounding the axons of some fibres.) These fibres carry sensations of touch and temperature.
- A-delta fibres are small, myelinated, and fast-transmitted fibres, and carry sharp 'pricking' sensations. These fibres allow us to judge the location and intensity of pain.
- C fibres are not covered with myelin. They are small and transmit slowly and are responsible for dull, diffuse, and persistent pain.

The immediate pain of an incision is mediated by A-delta fibres, but within a few seconds, the pain becomes more widespread due to C fibre activation. The pain impulse carried by the peripheral A-delta fibres travels quickly to the substantia gelatinosa of the dorsal horn of the spinal cord. Later slower-conducting C fibres may carry 'aching pain' impulses of longer duration (*Figure 7.1*). The sensory (afferent) impulse enters the dorsal horn of the spinal cord, forming chemical synapses using neurotransmitters (e.g. substance P). The pain impulse crosses over to the opposite side of the spinal cord and ascends to the brain via the

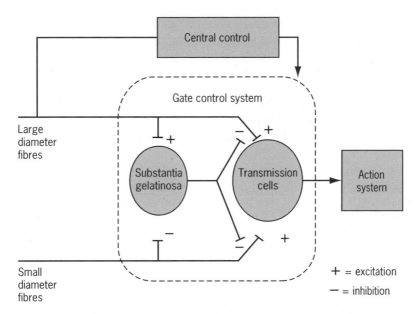

Figure 7.1   The gate control theory. (Reproduced from Melzack R, Wall PD (1988) *The Challenge of Pain*, 21st edn. Penguin Books, Harmondsworth.)

spinothalamic tract. The spinothalamic tract synapses in the thalamus and the impulse travels to the cerebral cortex where the painful stimuli are 'interpreted.'

When the pain transmission is relayed to the brain, the individual perceives the pain. Some pain impulses are passed directly to motor neurons via a reflex arc in the spinal cord. The motor neuron then emerges from the anterior horn of the cord to activate the relevant structure: for example, if a person touches a hot surface, the pain signal is converted into a motor impulse that stimulates the arm to draw away from the heat source.

Pain perception in the body may be modulated by substances called neuro-regulators. These may have an excitatory or inhibitory action. Substance P is an example of a neurotransmitter with an excitatory action. It results in the formation of an action potential, causing transmission of an impulse, and as a result the patient experiences pain. Serotonin is an example of a neurotransmitter with an inhibitory action. It reduces the effect of the pain impulse. Other neuroregulators act by modifying the activity of the nerve cells for example endogenous opioids, endorphins, and encephalins; these substances are called neuromodulators and have been described as the body's 'opioid-mediated analgesia system' (Fields and Basbaum, 1989). They reduce the impact of pain impulses.

The Gate Control Theory of Pain

Pain perception is a complex phenomenon and various theories have attempted to describe the interaction between the anatomical, physiological, and psychological factors influencing pain. The gate control theory proposed by Melzack and Wall (1965) combined physiological observations with information from clinical practice. The theory suggests that the transmission of the pain impulse can be modified or even blocked by some sort of gating mechanism located in the dorsal horn (see *Figure 7.1*). The gate acts to decrease or increase the flow of nerve impulses from the nociceptors to the brain. If the gate is closed, the pain impulse is blocked; if it is partially open some impulses get through; if it is fully open the complete pain is experienced. Two main elements may contribute to the gate:

- First, large diameter (A-beta) fibres involved in the sensation of touch may pass through the gating mechanism. When activated these fibres may compete with the pain-conducting A-delta fibres and so reduce transmission of the pain signal. For example, when an area around a source of 'pricking' pain is massaged, the intensity of the painful sensation tends to be reduced.
- Second, projections from higher areas, particularly the substantia gelatinosa, act on the gate to inhibit transmission of pain.

The gate control theory provides a basis for understanding why measures such as touch, massage, auditory and visual distraction, and transcutaneous electrical nerve stimulation (TENS) can reduce pain perception (Hargreaves and Lander, 1989). The original theory has undergone some modification. For example, there may be more than one gate, but it remains a useful theoretical basis for understanding pain. However, the anatomical location of the gate is not proven and some studies have failed to support the gate control theory.

Referred Pain

Referred pain is a painful sensation in a peripheral part of the body, for example the arm or skin, that is not the source of the pain stimulus. This sensation occurs when neurons from the same spinal segment innervate the source of the pain and the area where the pain is apparently experienced. The number of receptors is much greater in the peripheral areas than in the deeper structures. Examples of referred pain can be seen in conditions of the gall bladder when severe pain may be experienced in the right shoulder blade, and in disease of the ureter, when pain may be referred to the groin.

Phantom Pain

Phantom pain can be a frightening and disturbing pain for the patient who has had an amputation of a limb. The pain, which is sometimes intense, is perceived in the amputated structure. It happens when a nerve pathway that supplied the amputated limb is stimulated at some point along its path. The pain may be heightened because pressure, touch, and proprioceptive impulses from the amputated limb, which would normally suppress the pain impulses, are lacking.

POSTOPERATIVE PAIN

Pain assessment and management are critical skills for the surgical nurse. In elective surgery some degree of postoperative pain is normal and in acute situations the surgical patient is often admitted in pain. Unfortunately, many studies suggest that nurses' knowledge of postoperative pain management is inadequate. In 1991, the Royal College of Surgeons and Anaesthetists identified the need for better education of hospital staff in postoperative pain control:

■ Cohen (1980) reported that 75% of postoperative patients experienced marked or severe pain.
■ Seers (1987) found that the pain of 87% of postoperative patients was not adequately controlled.
■ Kuhns *et al.* (1990) reported relatively high postoperative pain scores up to six days after surgery.

Closs (1992) interviewed 100 patients who had had abdominal surgery about sleep disruption and pain over the first three postoperative nights. Only two patients reported pain-free nights; 25 patients reported no sleep problems, while 75 said their sleep had been disrupted by pain. Noise and pain were cited as the main causes of sleep disruption. Increased pain at night was reported by 49 patients, yet few analgesics were given at night. Clearly, postoperative pain remains a major problem.

Patients respond to pain in various ways and these can be categorized broadly into:

■ Behavioural responses.
■ Responses manifested in smooth muscle and glands (autonomic).

Behavioural responses to pain include:

■ Vocal responses (e.g. moaning, gasping).
■ Verbal statements.
■ Facial expression (e.g. grimacing, clenched teeth, wrinkled forehead).
■ Limited movement.
■ Adopting a guarding behaviour (protective rigidity), which will limit the patient's participation in postoperative mobilization and coughing and breathing exercises.

Responses manifested in smooth muscle and glands (Philips and Cousins, 1986) include:

■ Nausea.
■ Vomiting.
■ Gastric stasis.

- Decreased gut motility.
- Increased intestinal secretion.
- Impaired renal activity.

Postoperative pain can be an important factor influencing patients' perceptions of their progress and recovery. Seers (1987) reported that patients with pain in the first postoperative day felt tired, weak, and ill. Subsequently, the more pain the patients experienced, the lower they rated their recovery. Due to the subjective nature of pain, it is difficult to directly relate pain intensity to the level of physical or psychological postoperative complications. However, pain intensity has been directly linked to an increased incidence of collapse of some of the alveoli in the lung (atelectasis) in critically ill cardiovascular surgical patients (Puntillo and Weiss, 1994).

Pain Assessment

Although no one can really know what being in pain is like for another person, the surgical nurse needs to try to understand the patient's pain, and the use of a systematic approach to pain assessment and management is essential. It is also essential that nurses do not allow their own attitudes and biases to influence their assessments of patients' pain. Studies have shown that the cultural, religious, and ethnic background of both patient and nurse can influence the nurse's perception of the patient's pain. The patient's age and diagnosis also influence the nurse's perception of pain (Kitson, 1994). Verbal assessment of pain will prove subjective and open to different interpretation by different nurses. Physiological indicators such as pallor, sweating, restlessness, changes in pulse and blood pressure, and sleep disturbance can be assessed more objectively, but may vary for a variety of reasons other than pain. A systematic and objective approach to pain assessment and documentation is required to ensure adequate and consistent pain assessment. Various pain assessment tools are available; they include simple descriptive tools, detailed questionnaires, visual analogue scales, and numerical scales or pain thermometers (*Figure 7.2*). Such pain assessment tools can also be used to monitor the effectiveness of analgesia or other interventions.

Assessment should provide the following information:

- The time of onset and duration of pain.
- The site where pain is experienced.
- The severity of the pain.
- The precipitating factors influencing pain.
- The measures that relieve the pain.

Time of onset and duration of pain

The nurse should question the patient to determine the onset, duration, and time sequence of the pain: when the pain began, how long it lasted, and how frequently it occurs. An understanding of the time cycle of pain enables the nurse

(a)   **Simple descriptive**
 • Mild pain
 • No pain
 • Severe pain
 • Very severe pain

(b)   **Graphic verbal-rating scale**

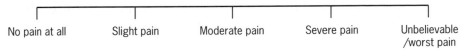

No pain at all   Slight pain   Moderate pain   Severe pain   Unbelievable
                                                                                        /worst pain

(c)   **Visual-analogue scale**

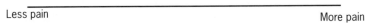

Less pain   More pain

(d)   **Numerical rating scale**

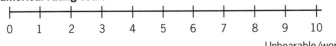

   0   1   2   3   4   5   6   7   8   9   10
                                                 Unbearable/worst pain
                                                 I can imagine

(e)   **Pain thermometer**

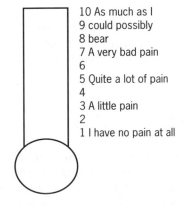

10 As much as I
9 could possibly
8 bear
7 A very bad pain
6
5 Quite a lot of pain
4
3 A little pain
2
1 I have no pain at all

(f)   **Pain relief measure–graphic rating scales**

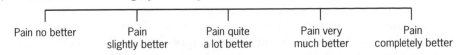

Pain no better   Pain   Pain quite   Pain very   Pain
                        slightly better   a lot better   much better   completely better

Figure 7.2   Pain assessment tools. (Reproduced with permission from Kitson (1994)).

to intervene at the appropriate time, for example to give analgesia before a change of dressing.

Site where pain is experienced

An assessment sheet with an outline of the body can be useful for the patient to indicate where the pain is felt. Sometimes the pain is referred from the original source to another part of the body as discussed earlier, so the nurse must have a sound knowledge of the nature of the patient's disease to be able to explain this to the patient.

Severity of the pain

A verbal descriptive scale can be used to assess the severity of pain. This scale consists of five descriptive terms placed along a line ranking from 'no pain' to 'unbearable pain'. Numbers from 1 to 10 can also be used on the scale instead of words. The visual analogue scale where the straight line of the scale has descriptive terms at each end, has proved to be a sensitive measure of pain severity because the patient can mark any point on the line rather than having to use a set word.

Precipitating factors associated with the pain

Once the nurse is aware of the factors that precipitate the pain, it is easier to perform the correct intervention; for example, if patients complain that coughing hurts their abdominal wound, the nurse can suggest that they support the area with a small pillow while coughing.

Measures to relieve pain

It is important to listen to patients and allow them to try their own methods of relieving their pain as long as they will not prove harmful. For example, changing position or sucking a peppermint may be the patient's remedy for a particular discomfort.

PHARMACOLOGICAL PAIN CONTROL

The use of analgesic drugs is the mainstay of immediate postoperative pain control. To achieve effective relief, pain control must be a high priority, and a planned and systematic activity. Seers (1987) noted that nurses and patients disagreed about the intensity of pain 77% of the time, and that nearly 35% of patients reported that they had not been able to have analgesia when they felt it was required. Cohen (1980) found that 87% of patients experienced pain breakthrough before their next dose of analgesia. Patients were uncertain about how and when to get their analgesia. Patients generally received less analgesia than prescribed (Cohen, 1980; Saxey, 1986). It appears that fear of addiction may be a major factor in nurses' reluctance to give sufficient analgesia. Later research suggests that nurses require more education about pain and pain control with analgesic drugs. Marks (1985) identified two important aspects of pharmaco-logical control of pain as:

- Provision of pain relief sufficient to allow mobilization, rest, and pain-free sleep, but avoiding drug side effects.
- Avoidance of breakthrough of pain between doses by sufficiently regular drug administration.

The key to effective pain control using analgesia is to give the correct dose fre-quently enough to prevent pain breakthrough. The time–response curve (*Figure 7.3*) demonstrates the relationship between the onset, peak, and duration of analgesic action and pain breakthrough. If doses are properly spaced (see *Figure 7.3a*) the drug concentration is maintained sufficiently to prevent pain break-through. However, if doses are administered less frequently (see *Figure 7.3b*), the drug concentration falls below the therapeutic level and pain is experienced.

Postoperative pain may be controlled using opiate or non-opiate analgesics (*Box 7.1*). The opioid analgesics are particularly suitable for treating moderate to severe pain of visceral origin. They are likely to be required in the immediate postoperative period after any but the most minor surgery. Opioid analgesics are associated with side effects including nausea, vomiting, constipation and drowsiness, and higher doses can cause respiratory depression and hypotension. They are often given by intramuscular injection, and an antiemetic (e.g. metoclo-pramide hydrochloride) may also be required. Patients receiving opioid anal-gesics require careful monitoring. The non-opioid analgesics and NSAIDS may relieve mild to moderate pain.

Patient-Controlled Analgesia (PCA)

PCA allows patients to give themselves their own analgesia by activating a syringe pump. It provides a flexible form of pain control, which is tailored by patients to meet their own needs. The problems of nurses' bias, inadequate pain assessment, and delays in administering drugs are avoided, and in addition, there are psychological advantages because the patient feels 'in control.' The patient presses a button to activate the pump and deliver an intravenous infusion of the analgesic. The research evidence suggests that PCA:

- Improves pain control (White, 1988).
- Reduces anxiety (Wheatley *et al.*, 1991).
- Allows earlier mobilization and therefore less risk of postoperative compli-cations (Lange *et al.*, 1988).
- Saves nursing time.

The pumps are set to prevent overuse; they are commonly set to allow 3–10 minutes between doses. Careful patient education is required for successful PCA, but if there are no problems with compliance or venous access, it is an effective form of pain control. Patients are able to titrate to maintain pain relief, but avoid

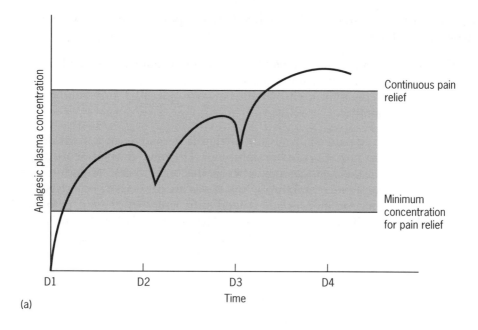

(a)

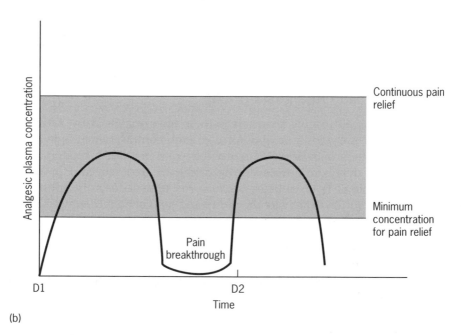

(b)

Figure 7.3 Time–response curves for analgesics. (a) Analgesic (D1–D4) given in sufficient dose at appropriate intervals. (b) Analgesic doses (D1, D2), overspaced.

> **Box 7.1** **Some common analgesics (*British National Formulary* (1996) No. 32, p. 189).**
>
> **Opioid Analgesics**
> - Diamorphine
> - Morphine sulphate, morphine hydrochloride
> - Pethidine hydrochloride
> - Buprenorphine hydrochloride
> - Codeine phosphate
> - Dihydrocodeine tartrate
> - Meptazinol
> - Nalbuphine hydrochloride
>
> **Non-opioid analgesics**
> - Aspirin (acetylsalicylic acid)
> - Paracetamol
> - Non-steroidal anti-inflammatory drugs (NSAIDs) (e.g. ibuprofen)
>
> **Compound analgesics**
> - Papaveretum (morphine hydrochloride, papaverine hydrochloride, and codeine hydrochloride)
> - Co-codamol (codeine phosphate and paracetamol)
> - Co-dydramol (dihydrocodeine and paracetamol)
> - Co-proxamol (dextropropoxyphene hydrochloride and paracetamol)

sedation (Check, 1982), and the overall consumption of opioid analgesics may be reduced. Patients receiving opioid analgesia by PCA still require careful monitoring to ensure that they are comfortable and satisfied with their pain relief.

NON-PHARMACOLOGICAL PAIN RELIEF

A variety of approaches including relaxation, distraction, massage, and breathing techniques can help alleviate postoperative pain. These may act on the physiological and psychological aspects of pain. TENS may activate the gating mechanism, impeding transmission of the pain impulse. Relaxation, music, and distraction techniques may act on both the higher centres involved in pain perception and the gating mechanism.

Relaxation

Relaxation is thought to diminish pain by reducing anxiety, which heightens pain perception. The use of appropriate music can help the patient to relax and simple deep breathing exercises enhance this effect.

Distraction

Focussing on something unrelated to the pain such as television, music, reading, or by talking has been found to be useful. Used correctly touch can also relieve anxiety and reassure the patient that someone cares and understands.

Complementary Therapies

There is a growing use of complementary therapies in nursing, and the role of complementary therapies in postoperative situations requires further research. Some health trusts have produced policies on the use of such therapies by nurses, and criteria for practice might include:

■ Consent by the patient.
■ Consultation with medical staff.
■ Authorization agreed between the nurse and nurse manager.
■ Documentation in the patient's notes.

Examples of complementary therapies that could be suitable for the post-operative patient include reflexology and aromatherapy. Reflexology is the ancient art of foot and hand massage. It is said to bring relief from stress while encouraging the body to heal itself. Aromatherapy is the use of essential oils that have been extracted from plants to treat problems such as dyspepsia, nausea, or flatulence, or they may be used as a deodorizing or relaxing agent. The oils are massaged into the skin in a lotion for absorption into the body or they may be absorbed via the lungs using an inhaler. It must be emphasized that correct implementation of these techniques requires certain training and expertise. Non-pharmacological methods may be used as a useful adjunct to analgesia in the immediate postoperative period.

COMMUNICATION AND PAIN RELIEF

Boore (1978) states that anxiety can produce a similar physiological response as acute pain, but although it is accepted that the degree of this response varies with different individuals. Most people will experience some anxiety about surgery, and hospitalization in itself may induce anxiety (Wilson-Barnett, 1976; Swindale, 1989). Hayward (1975), recognizing the link between anxiety and pain, found that preoperative information given in a manner that the patient could understand was beneficial to the patient. If patients wished to know what to expect after surgery, and they were correctly informed, decreased pain levels were recorded postoperatively and the patients tended to recover more quickly. The nurse should provide the information that is relevant to the patient, check that this information is clearly understood, and support patients' rights to make their own decisions (Kohnke, 1978). For example, as discussed in Chapter 12, the treatment for breast cancer entails a variety of procedures, and it is essential that the patient fully understands and complies with the particular treatment on which she is embarking.

In addition to explaining to patients about their operation or treatment, and listening carefully to their questions or comments, the nurse must ensure that the patient is prepared for the degree of pain they may experience postoperatively. The reason for this pain and how it will be relieved should be explained. The patient's attitude to pain control can be discussed at this time and whether they have any preference for a particular method of relief. If the patient has any particular fears about the anaesthetic the anaesthetist can be notified. It is useful if this sort of information is included in the patient information booklet or leaflet, but there should also be an opportunity for discussion. During this time communication should also include advice about deep breathing, coughing, leg movements, and any other information that will prevent painful postoperative complications.

Patients with abdominal wounds will usually move as little as possible so that pain is kept to a minimum. They will also avoid deep breathing and coughing because it is painful, and some patients fear that they will burst their wound if they cough or move. It is very important that patients are told that after suitable analgesia they should try to move around, deep breathe, bend and stretch their legs, and make rotating movements with their feet and ankles to avoid complications. which include respiratory infection, deep vein thrombosis, and potentially life-threatening pulmonary embolism.

ADDITIONAL SOURCES OF POSTOPERATIVE PAIN

A variety of factors can cause pain or make the patient feel uncomfortable or more aware of pain. Fear and distress can add to pain, and giving the patient a measure of autonomy or control can lessen these problems. Some of the many factors that contribute to discomfort and pain postoperatively include:

- Manual handling and turning the patient.
- Pressure sores.
- Abdominal distension caused by flatulence.

Manual Handling and Turning the Patient

Careful handling or turning of the patient is essential. The patient should be involved as much as possible in any turning or moving that is required. Postoperatively, patients may be reluctant to move and need to be nursed on good quality mattresses and encouraged to mobilize.

There are many aids to moving, including gliding or turning sheets to place under the patient, moving slings on which to slide the patient, and mechanical hoists. If the patient is able to pull himself up, an overhead handle or rope 'ladder' fixed to the foot of the bed can be used. At all times it is vital to explain to patients the reason a particular movement is necessary and how they can best help.

Pressure Sores

Pressure areas, especially the sacrum, heels, and elbows can easily become painful and the skin break down. A pressure-relieving mattress may be necessary, and it must be ensured that the sheet under the patient is wrinkle-free and clean.

Movement should be encouraged, and if the patient is to sit in a chair, the nurse must ensure that the seat is comfortable and supportive, and the patient must be given the opportunity to return to bed for rest periods.

Abdominal Flatulence

Postoperative flatulence is a common problem after abdominal surgery. Flatus is normally present in the stomach and intestines, but flatulence arises when it cannot pass. This results in abdominal distension and pain, which can be more troublesome to patients than the surgery they have undergone. Most patients who have had abdominal surgery have decreased bowel function for the first 2–3 days postoperatively due to:

- The anaesthetic agent.
- The cumulative effect of the surgical trauma and lack of bulk in the intestines.

When gas has accumulated in the intestines due to a lack of gastrointestinal (GI) motility a nasogastric tube can be used to maintain continuous suction for 48 hours. However, it is now generally accepted that the postoperative cessation of peristalsis acts as a mechanism to keep the GI tract at rest to allow healing (Vaughn and Nemcek, 1986). A careful assessment should be carried out as follows:

- Observe the patient for feelings of fullness and cramp-like pain in the abdomen.
- Auscultate the abdomen for bowel sounds.
- Palpate the abdomen for distension.
- Measure the patient's abdominal girth.

The following measures may help relieve abdominal distension:

- Change the patient's position frequently. If patients are able to, ask them to bend their knees onto their chests and rock backward and forward slowly five times each hour.
- Encourage patients to walk while gently massaging the abdomen.

- Avoid using drinking straws.
- Avoid carbonated fluids and iced liquids.

Other factors associated with treatment that may cause the surgical patient pain and discomfort include nasogastric tubes, wound drains, and intravenous infusions. It is important that patients' mouths are kept clean and moist, and that micturition and defaecation are not causing pain or embarrassment.

PAIN AND WOUND MANAGEMENT

Skin damage due to surgery or trauma inevitably causes a certain amount of pain or discomfort. It is the responsibility of the nurse to minimize this and to ensure the pain is not worsened by subsequent treatment. Thomas (1989) maintains that pain can be experienced while the dressing is in place or when an adherent dressing is removed. Correct assessment of the wound, and if necessary referral to the Tissue Viability Specialist Nurse, will enable the nurse to choose appropriate comfortable dressings for individual patients (see Chapter 9). Dealey (1991) describes some alginate and hydrocolloid types of dressings, which avoid localized dehydration of the wound area. Dehydration can stimulate nerve endings, resulting in pain. The patient can experience severe pain at the time of dressing changes. If a gauze or similar dressing has been used on the surface of the wound, it can become hard and adherent to the wound; if the dressing is then forcibly removed, it will cause pain and may damage the healing tissue. Soaking the dressing with sterile saline may allow it to be removed comfortably.

PAIN AFTER DAY SURGERY

Day surgery is becoming more common and the patient will usually leave hospital pain-free because of the local nerve block used during the operation. It is important that the nurse ensures that the patient has means of relieving any pain or discomfort once the effect of the nerve block has worn off. In a survey conducted by Firth (1991), 75% of the respondents expected to have pain after their operation, but 50% said they had not been informed of the possibility in clinic. Only 12% of people had prepared for relieving their pain when they got home by buying medication. Only 50% of patients said they were given any advice on how to deal with pain.

Ideally, patients should be assessed for fitness for day surgery in a preassessment clinic. At this time they should be provided with specific verbal and written instructions for both the pre- and postoperative periods. They should be told what to expect after surgery in terms of pain and discomfort and should be advised to obtain analgesia in preparation for their discharge. After operation and before discharge, patients should be advised in writing to consult their general practitioner if the analgesia proves inadequate. Spigelman (1991) describes postoperative care in relation to pain relief advocated for day surgery patients after repair of an inguinal hernia. Patients were supplied with oral analgesia and lactose for any consequent constipation to take at home and were visited by a community nurse in the evening after surgery. Of the 19 patients studied, only one complained of excessive postoperative pain.

CONCLUSION

The cause of pain in surgical patients is varied and sometimes complex. Control of this pain, particularly in the postoperative period requires adequate pre-operative preparation and skill on the part of the nurse in terms of both assessment and implementation of care. Effective evaluation is vital to ensure that the medication or treatment given is satisfactory for the patient. If the patient is not satisfied then the patient must be reassessed and further measures taken to ensure that the ultimate goal of patient comfort is attained as soon as possible

References

Boore J (1978) *A Prescription for Recovery* pp. 67–121. Royal College of Nursing, London.

British National Formulary (1996) No. 32. British Medical Association and Royal Pharmaceutical Society for Great Britain, London.

Check WA (1982) Results are better when patients control their own analgesia. *JAMA* **247**:945–947.

Closs JS (1992) Patients' night-time pain, analgesic provision and sleep after surgery. *Int J Nurs Stud* **29(4)**:381–392.

Cohen FL (1980) Post-surgical pain relief: patient's status and nurses' medication choices. **Pain** 9:265–274.

Davitz LL, Davitz JR, Highuchi Y (1977) Cross-cultural inferences of physical pain and psychological distress. *Nurs Times* **73**:521–523.

Dealey C (1991) Modern wound management products. *Nursing* **4(30)**:31–32.

Fields HL, Basbaum AL (1989) Endogenous pain control mechanisms. In *Textbook of Pain*, 2nd edition. Wall PD, Melzack R (eds). pp. 206–217. Churchill Livingstone, Edinburgh.

Firth F (1991) Pain after day surgery. *Nurs Times* **87(40)**:72–76.

Hargreaves A, Lander J (1989) Use of transcutaneous electrical nerve stimulation for post operative pain. *Nurs Res* **38(3)**:159–161.

Hayward J (1975) *Information: A Prescription Against Pain*, Series 2:5, pp. 113–121. Royal College of Nursing, London.

International Association for the Study of Pain (1979) Subcommittee on Taxonomy: Pain terms, a list with definitions and notes on usage. *Pain* **6**:249–252.

Kitson A (1994) Postoperative pain management: A literature review. *J Clin Nurs* **70**:440–442.

Kohnke MF (1978) The nurse's responsibility to the consumer. *Am J Nurs* **78(3)**: 440–442.

Kuhns S, Cook K, Collins M, Jones JM, Mucklow JC (1990) Perceptions of pain after surgery. *Br Med J* **300**:1687–1690.

Lange MP, Dahn MS, Jacobs LA (1988) Patient-controlled analgesia versus intermittent analgesia dosing. *Heart Lung* **17**:495–498.

Marks RL (1985) Terminal pain. *Surgery* **1(25)**:565–568.

McCaffery M (1972) *Nursing Management of the Patient in Pain*, Chap. 1, p. 8. Lippincott, Philadelphia.

Melzack R, Wall PD (1965) Pain mechanisms: a new theory. *Science* **150**:971–979.

National Institutes of Health Consensus Development Conference (1987) The integrated approach to the management of pain. *J Pain Symp Manag* **2(1)**:35–44.

Philips GD, Cousins MJ (1986) Neurological mechanisms of pain and the relationship of pain, anxiety and sleep. In *Acute Pain Management*. Cousins M, Philips G (eds). pp. 21–48. Churchill Livingstone, New York.

Puntillo K, Weiss SJ (1994) Pain: Its mediators and associated morbidity in critically ill cardiovascular surgical patients. *Nurs Res* **43(1)**:31–36.

Royal College of Surgeons and Anaesthetists (1991) *Report of the Working Party on Pain after Surgery, Commission on the Provision of Surgical Services* p. 4. Royal College of Surgeons, London.

Saxey S (1986) The nurse's response to postoperative pain. *Nursing* **3(10)**:377–381.

Seers K (1987) Perceptions of pain. *Nurs Times* **83(48)**:37–39.

Spigelman AD (1991) An initial experience of day surgery repair of inguinal hernias. *J One-Day Surg* **1(2)**:22–23.

Swindale JE (1989) The nurse's role in giving pre-operative information to reduce anxiety in patients admitted to hospital for elective minor surgery. *J Adv Nurs* **14(11)**:899–905.

Thomas S (1989) Pain and wound management. Community outlook. *Nurs Times* **85(28)**:11–15.

Vaughn JB, Nemcek MA (1986) Postoperative flatulence: causes and remedies. *Today's OR Nurse* **8(10)**:19–23.

Wheatley RG, Madej TH, Jackson IJB, Hunter D (1991) The first year's experience of an acute pain service. *Br J Anaesth* **67**:353–359.

White PF (1988) Use of patient-controlled analgesia for management of acute pain. *JAMA* **259**:243–247.

Wilson-Barnett (1976) Patients' emotional reactions to hospitalisation: an exploratory study. *J Adv Nurs* **1**:351–358.

Chapter 8
Infection Control

The hospital ward can be viewed as a pool of potential infection with nursing and medical staff providing a ready route for dissemination of micro-organisms within the surgical environment. The patient is exposed to increased numbers and varieties of infectious micro-organisms and illness. Invasive procedures and the effects of surgery increase susceptibility to infection. Infection control techniques are critical in preventing the spread of infection between patients and the surgical nurse and are central in controlling hospital-acquired infection (HAI). This chapter will briefly review the nature of infection, discuss the problem of nosocomial or HAI, and look at the role of the nurse in minimizing the spread of infectious organisms. Good infection control practices will help protect both patients and nurses from HAIs.

THE NATURE OF INFECTION

A pathogen is a micro-organism capable of producing disease, and infection is the invasion of the body by pathogens. However, most micro-organisms are not harmful. Commensal organisms such as the normal body flora do not invade or infect and can be beneficial: vitamin K is synthesized by bacteria in the small intestine. Extensive antibiotic therapy, for example before intestinal surgery, can destroy the intestinal flora and cause a temporary vitamin K deficiency. An opportunistic pathogen is a micro-organism that is normally present in the body that becomes pathogenic when host immunity or bacterial ecology is disrupted (e.g. thrush after antibiotic therapy). Colonization is the multiplication of micro-organisms in the body without causing disease while infection is the invasion and multiplication of a micro-organism with pathological effects. Pathogenicity is the capacity of micro-organisms to infect and cause disease and is determined by several factors including:

■ Virulence (the ability to cause disease).
■ Dose (the number of organisms).
■ Invasiveness (the ability to penetrate and spread through body tissues causing injury).
■ Host susceptibility or resistance (the host's ability to limit invasion or withstand the pathogenic effects of the organism).

A variety of micro-organisms can be pathogenic (*Table 8.1*) and pathogens may be resident or transient. Resident pathogens are normally present on the skin in stable numbers. They are the organisms the patient brings into hospital and are mainly found in the superficial layers of the skin. Resident pathogens are not easily removed by normal handwashing as 10–20% are found in deeper epidermal layers. Transient pathogens are acquired from contact and are usually loosely attached to the skin and can be removed by washing. Nursing and medical staff can easily transmit transient pathogens to patients.

Infections may be symptomatic, causing clinical signs and symptoms, asymptomatic, or subclinical, with no clear clinical signs or symptoms of injury or disease. Acute infections have a rapid onset with an immediate immune response and symptoms are usually severe, but generally of short course or duration. In contrast a chronic infection tends to have a slower onset, a more delayed immune response and milder symptoms, but is of longer duration. A latent infection occurs when the pathogen is present but dormant: symptoms may be intermittent and often flare up under stimuli such as stress. Herpes simplex (type 1) causing cold sores of the lips is a good example of a latent infection.

Table 8.1 Pathogenic micro-organisms.

Organism	Example	Infection or disease
Bacteria	*Escherichia coli*	Enteritis
Mycoplasma	*Mycoplasma pneumoniae*	Pneumonia, tracheobronchitis, pharyngitis
Rickettsiae	*Rickettsia typhi*	Epidemic typhus fever
Chlamydiae	*Chlamydia psittaci*	Psiittacosis
Viruses	Orthomyoviruses	Influenza
Fungi	*Candida albicans*	Thrush
Protozoa	*Plasmodium malariae*	Malaria
Helminths	*Enterobius vermicularis*	Threadworm

Infection can be localized causing focussed infection and injury as in an abscess or boil, or may be generalized or systemic, causing widespread infection and injury. A secondary infection occurs when infection by one pathogen encourages the invasion and multiplication of a second pathogen. A viral cold resulting in secondary catarrhal bacterial infection of the respiratory mucosa is a common example of secondary infection.

NOSOCOMIAL OR HOSPITAL-ACQUIRED INFECTION

The increased risk of acquiring an infection in hospital has been demonstrated by many studies. Meers *et al.* (1980) reported on one of the largest British studies, which surveyed 18,163 patients in 43 hospitals. It was found that 19.1% of hospital patients had an infection and 9.2% of the patients had acquired the infection in the hospital: urinary tract infection accounted for 30% of HAIs, wound infection 20%, and respiratory infection 19%. Taylor (1986) has estimated that 5–10% of surgical patients will develop an HAI, so on a 30-bed ward three patients are likely to have an HAI. Specific problems such as wound infection, the catheterized patient, and infection control and intravenous therapy are dealt with in Chapters 4, 5 and 9, respectively.

The cost of HAI to the health service is large. The DHSS/PHLS Hospital Infection Working Group (1988) estimated that HAI cost the NHS £ 111 million in 1986, while in the US costs have been estimated at $4 billion dollars a year (Miller *et al.*, 1989). Failure to prevent cross-infection can result in:

- Delayed recovery.
- Exposure of the patient to additional illness.
- Increased pain, anxiety, and stress affecting patients and their families.
- Extended hospitalization with human and financial costs.
- Serious morbidity and mortality in severe cases.

THE CHAIN OF INFECTION

The presence of a pathogen alone does not mean an infection will develop. The process of infection depends on a sequence of elements producing the chain of infection (*Figure 8.1*). There must be an infectious agent (see *Table 8.1*), and in surgery the pathogen is most often a bacterium or virus. *Table 8.2* lists some common infectious agents in the surgical setting. The pool or reservoir of pathogens may be a person, an animal, an insect, or an object in the environment. The body itself is the most problematic source of infection and human reservoirs may be symptomatic or asymptomatic carriers. Food, water, clothes, bedding, contaminated equipment, intravenous solutions, enteral feeds, and infusion apparatus can all act as reservoirs. Any environmental object, from the bed to a vase of flowers, can act as a refuge for micro-organisms if conditions are right.

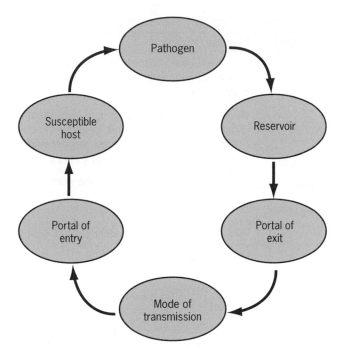

Figure 8.1 The chain of infection.

Although inanimate objects can harbour micro-organisms, patients and staff are probably the main reservoirs of infection in hospital.

The next step in the chain of infection is the release of pathogens from the reservoir via the portals of exit. If the human body is considered the major reservoir the main portals of exit are:

■ The respiratory tract.
■ The skin.
■ The alimentary tract.
■ The urogenital tract.
■ The blood.

All tissues of the body can harbour infectious organisms, but some sites are more commonly associated with releasing pathogens. The main portals of exit and associated micro-organisms are listed in *Table 8.3*.

The next stage in the chain of infection is transmission and there are several modes:

■ Direct contact.
■ Indirect contact.
■ Airborne.

Table 8.2 Some examples of surgically important pathogens.

Bacteria (gram-positive)	Disease/Infection
Staphylococci	Wound infection, abscess, carbuncle, osteomyelitis, endocarditis, septicaemia, pneumonia, toxic shock syndrome
Streptococci	Wound infection, cellulitis urinary tract infection, pneumonia, bacteraemia, septicaemia, neonatal infection (pneumonia, septicaemia, and meningitis), acute tonsillitis, abscess formation, endocarditis, dental caries
Clostridium perfringens	Wound infection (usually traumatic wounds)
Bacteria (gram-negative)	
Escherichia coli	Urinary tract infection, wound infection, septicaemia
Klebsiella	Urinary tract infection, wound infection, respiratory infection, septicaemia
Proteus	Urinary tract infection, chronic wound (pressure sore, leg ulcer)
Pseudomonas	Wound infection (particularly burns and chronic wounds), urinary tract infection, pulmonary infection
Viruses	
Herpes simplex	Risk of herpetic whitlow to health care workers
Human immunodeficiency virus (HIV)	Acquired immunodeficiency syndrome (AIDS), risk to health care workers from contaminated blood
Blood-borne hepatitis viruses	Risk to health care workers

- Vehicle-borne.
- Vector-borne.
- Blood-borne.

Direct contact is the most important mode of transmission of HAIs and is the transfer of pathogens, usually on the hands, between patients. Staff hands are the main source, but contact between patients is another route of transfer. Commensal organisms can become opportunistic pathogens. They may be spread from one patient to another or from their normal site to a more susceptible site, for example a surgical wound, where they are pathogenic. One man's commensals can be another man's pathogens. Endogenous infection can result when a patient's own microbes are transferred from one site to another site; they do not usually colonize. Exogenous or cross-infection occurs when patient or staff carriers spread infectious organisms to other patients. Many organisms can be transmitted by direct contact and it is probably the main source of endogenous

Table 8.3 Portals of exit with examples of micro-organisms and routes of transfer to hands.

Source	Micro-organism	Transfer to hands
Respiratory tract		
Nose	Staphylococci	Droplets, sneezing, handkerchiefs, touching nose
Mouth and throat	Staphylococci, streptococci	Coughing
Skin and hair	Staphylococci, streptococci	Shed into clothes and general environment, touching hair
Alimentary tract		
Lower gut	E. coli	Faeces, washing anogenital area
Urogenital tract		
Genitalia	Staphylococci	Shed into and from clothes
Surgical		
Blood	Hepatitis B	Invasive procedures, health care worker inoculation due to needlestick injury or uncovered skin break

and exogenous wound infections. It should be noted that research suggests that direct contact is also a major mode of transmission of respiratory infections such as colds. Gwaltney *et al.* (1978) showed that volunteers' hands became contaminated with rhinovirus after contact with subjects suffering from colds. People tend to touch their faces frequently and may transfer the viruses to their eyes and nose where they can then gain access to the respiratory mucosa and cause infection. It seems likely that hands rather than coughs and sneezes may spread diseases such as the common cold.

Indirect contact is the transfer of micro-organisms via fomites or inanimate objects. A fomite may be clothing, bedding, bedpan, or any other communal equipment that is not adequately cleaned between patients. For example, a recent report suggested that inadequately cleaned vaginal specula could be a source of cross-infection in general practice. Even transmission of respiratory infections may involve indirect contact. The viruses causing a cold can be deposited and survive on objects and surfaces. They are then picked up by the next person handling the contaminated object (Leclair *et al.*, 1987) and transferred from the hands to the respiratory membranes as described above.

Airborne transmission is infection by inhalation of droplets. Large droplets produced by coughing and sneezing can transmit bacteria and viruses and may be one method of transmission for streptococcal infection and the influenza viruses. Large droplets settle quickly and the main risk is during coughing and sneezing. However, much smaller droplets (aerosols) can transmit a range of bacteria and viruses. Small droplets can remain suspended in the air and be inhaled hours after production. *Mycobacterium tuberculosis*, the organism that causes tuberculosis, is an example of an organism transmitted by aerosol inhalation.

Contamination of water, food, enteral feeds, intravenous solutions, drugs, or blood products can cause vehicle-borne transmission. The use of proprietary, pre-prepared intravenous solutions and enteral feeds has reduced this problem, but occasional cases of contamination still occur. Hospital outbreaks of salmonella food poisoning are regularly reported. The infection of haemophiliac patients with HIV is a recent and tragic example of transmission by contaminated blood products.

Vector-borne infection via insects (e.g. mosquitoes transmitting malaria, ticks) is not a major problem in the UK, but can be an important route of transmission in other countries.

Portals of entry represent the next stage in the infection chain. The pathogen needs to gain entry to the host. The main portals of entry are essentially the same as the portals of exit and are:

- The respiratory tract (by inhalation).
- The skin (by penetration or inoculation).
- The alimentary tract (by ingestion).
- The urogenital tract (ascending infections).
- The blood (by inoculation).

The final deciding factor in the infectious process is the host. A variety of factors contribute to patient susceptibility to infection, including:

- Age.
- Immune status.
- Nutritional status.
- Exposure to trauma including surgery.
- Use of drugs and radiotherapy.
- Underlying diseases (e.g. diabetes mellitus, neoplasia).
- Use of invasive therapies.

The old and very young are particularly at risk from infection. The ageing process increases the incidence of neoplasia, infections, and autoimmune problems. The immune system is central to the body's ability to resist infection and depression of the immune system due to disease, poor nutrition, stress, drugs, or radiotherapy will increase susceptibility to infection. Common procedures or therapies such as urinary catheterization or inserting an intravenous cannula will bypass the body's normal defences and provide a ready access for microorganisms. Surgery itself is a source of stress: it may reduce immunity and the surgical wound may provide an additional portal of entry.

INFECTION CONTROL

The spread of infection in a surgical ward is summarized in *Figure 8.2*. Preventing cross-infection requires a general approach used for all patients, with additional precautions and care being taken when the patient has a known infection or is immunosuppressed. Measures to control HAIs aim to:

- Eliminate or reduce the reservoirs of infection.
- Minimize transfer of pathogens.
- Isolate known reservoirs.

This can translate roughly as either cleaning, general cross-infection control, and isolation or barrier nursing, or the environment, the staff, and the patient.

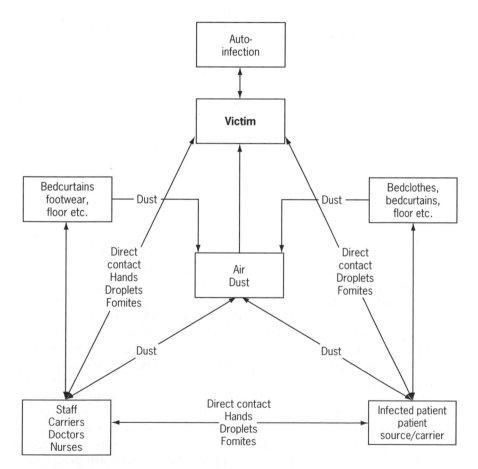

Figure 8.2 The spread of infection in a surgical ward.

The Patient

To help patients protect themselves from endogenous and exogenous infection the surgical nurse can attempt to reduce host risk factors and increase ability to resist infection. Important steps are:

- To encourage personal hygiene, especially handwashing. It is particularly important that the bedfast patient is offered handwashing facilities after using a urinal or bedpan. The patient's unwashed hands could touch and contaminate many articles in the ward with which other patients and staff might then be in contact. Good personal hygiene will not eliminate bacteria, but it should help reduce the problem of transient micro-organisms and reduce the problem of endogenous infection.
- To encourage good nutrition in the surgical patient as there is a clear link between nutritional status and immune function.
- To be aware of the disruptive effects of antibiotics, chemotherapy, and other treatments on bacterial ecology and immune function. The intestinal flora may be particularly affected and opportunistic infections can occur. It is essential that antibiotics are given on time to ensure that therapeutic levels are maintained. Antibiotic-resistant micro-organisms are a major problem and antibiotic therapy has to be appropriate and correctly administered.
- To encourage the patient not to interfere with lines, catheters, dressings, and drains. Both endogenous and exogenous transient micro-organisms on the patient's hands could be carried to these sites and lead to local or systemic infections.

Staff

Nurses are a major vehicle for transmitting pathogens and it is important that they take steps to protect themselves and the patient. Surgical nurses need to be aware of the impact of their own health on infection control. They need to keep all vaccinations and immunizations up to date. If they suspect that they have even a minor infection they should probably stay at home. The nurse's minor cold could become the postoperative patient's chest infection. Handwashing is essential, and in addition, particular care is required with any breaks in the skin. Even minor cuts and abrasions should be covered with a waterproof plaster. Doctors and nurses in contact with oral and genital secretions risk developing a finger infection (whitlow). The hands are a major instrument in nursing and a whitlow that might be a herpetic (herpes simplex) whitlow should not be treated as a minor infection. The surgical nurse should avoid patient contact until the whitlow is healed. The surgical nurse has to be aware of the ward infection control procedures and to use handwashing, gloves, and aprons appropriately. Handwashing and other specific aspects of infection control are dealt with in more detail below.

The Environment

In the past nurses were responsible for much of the general cleaning of a ward. Today this is carried out by domestic staff, but nurses are still responsible for ensuring that the general environment is safe and clean. The nurse must work with domestic staff and supervisors to ensure that the correct procedures for cleaning are carried out. In 1950 Lidwell and Lowbury showed that *Staphylococcus aureus* and β-haemolytic streptococci could survive in dust for long periods of time. Correct cleaning, mopping, or damp dusting is required to remove dirt and dust and reduce the numbers of micro-organisms. Incorrect cleaning procedures may simply result in a redistribution of the dirt (Ward, 1990). Cleaning is the removal of dirt or contamination, it is not a form of disinfection. Cleaning involves using a detergent or soap to degrease an object or area and then water to remove the dirt. Danforth *et al.* (1987) demonstrated that cleaning with a detergent was more efficient than using a disinfectant in reducing floor contamination. Cleaning equipment should be stored dry and it is essential that equipment designated for 'dirty' areas, such as the sluice, is not used in cleaner areas. Ideally mop heads require daily laundering.

Although maintaining a clean environment is important, it should be noted that hand contamination and not environmental contamination remains the main cause of HAIs. Bibby (1982) found that cleaning frequency and practices had little impact on infection rates, while Maki *et al.* (1982) concluded that micro-organisms in the hospital environment contributed little to the problem of nosocomial infection. It is, however, important to ensure immediate and effective cleaning if body fluids are spilled. Spillages of blood, urine, or other body fluids are usually dealt with by nursing staff. Staff should make appropriate use of gloves and aprons. Disposable cloths or paper wipes should be used to mop up the spillage, and an appropriate disinfectant used. Many hospitals now use chlorine-releasing granules to absorb and disinfect spills although these cannot be used in confined, poorly ventilated areas. Most hospitals now have set policies and procedures for dealing with spillage of blood and other body fluids and these should be followed. Proper handling and disposal of clinical and general wastes, careful bedmaking and handling of laundry, efficient terminal cleaning, and correct cleaning and disinfection or sterilization of medical and nursing equipment all contribute to maintaining a safe environment and are dealt with in more detail below.

HANDWASHING

Handwashing is probably the single most important factor in controlling HAI. Hands can pick up micro-organisms from many surfaces, including the nurse's own body, patients, clothing, laundry, taps, equipment, and furnishings: in fact almost any object in the ward environment. These transient pathogens are then spread to further surfaces and to patients unless removed by handwashing.

Gram-negative bacteria survive on skin better than most other strains. Klebsiella, a gram-negative enterobacterium that is frequently involved in pneumonia, and wound and urinary tract infections can survive during normal duties on nurses' hands for 150 minutes (Casewell and Philips, 1977). Effective handwashing by staff and patients will help reduce:

- Endogenous infection due to normal body flora being carried by the patient's (or nurse's hands) to another area of the body.
- Exogenous infection due to organisms being transmitted between patients on the nurse's hands.

Numerous studies have indicated that handwashing is inadequately carried out. Handwashing is often both incorrectly (Albert and Condie, 1981) and too infrequently performed (Broughall et al., 1984). Gould and Ream (1993) observed nurses' handwashing in two intensive care units have reported that 50% of all essential hand decontaminations were omitted. Fox (1974) identified that most nurses missed some part of the hand when washing, and that right-handed people tended to wash the left hand more thoroughly than the right (reversed for left handers). Taylor (1978a,b) demonstrated that the most frequently missed areas were between the fingers, the nails, and the thumb (*Figure 8.3*). Surveys of hand hygiene in intensive care units have reported that handwashing often

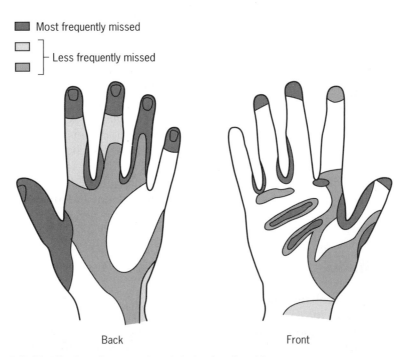

Most frequently missed

Less frequently missed

Back   Front

Figure 8.3 Distribution of areas missed during handwashing.

varied from recommended procedures (Conly *et al.*, 1989; Graham, 1990). Compliance with handwashing was especially poor before emptying urinary catheter bags, before mouth care, and before carrying out endotracheal suction. The duration of handwashing has been reported to range from a few seconds to several minutes. Quraishi *et al.* (1984) reported that handwashing in two intensive care units lasted an average of 8.6 seconds. Some authors have suggested that rings including wedding rings may increase the number of bacteria on the hands. It is probably best to avoid wearing rings, but if worn, they should be removed when washing the hands. Short, filed, and unvarnished fingernails are recommended, but nail brushes are not suitable for routine use as they may damage the skin.

Handwashing requires an easy-to-reach sink, preferably with elbow or foot-operated taps, warm running water, soap or soap substitute, and paper towels. The nurse should stand in front of the sink taking care not to let uniform or hands contact the sink surfaces. Elbow or foot-operated taps remove the need for contaminated hands to touch the taps, if the taps are hand operated a paper towel can be used when turning on the tap. The hands should be washed under running water with the water temperature as hot as is comfortable. Soap or a suitable substitute should be used and the hands washed with a vigorous action, rubbing the skin surfaces together for at least 10 seconds. Soap loosens any dirt and facilitates the removal of bacteria by the running water. Liquid soap dispensers are preferable to bar soap. Particular care is required to ensure that the areas that are often missed are washed (see *Figure 8.3*).

Care is required to avoid contaminating the uniform with water splashes. Hands and forearms should be kept lower than the elbows during washing so that water flows away from the least contaminated areas and organisms are washed down into the sink. If the hands are known to be contaminated or are visibly soiled washing should be extended to 1–3 minutes. After thorough lathering and rubbing, the hands must be well rinsed and then thoroughly dried using a paper towel. Towel waste is disposed of into a foot-operated waste bin.

Liquid soap or other detergents (medicated or non-medicated) and water can be used for routine washing and decontamination of the hands. Preparations that contain a disinfectant such as chlorhexidine gluconate may leave a residue on the skin that has a cumulative antibacterial effect. However Ayliffe *et al.* (1988) suggest that an effective washing technique is usually more important than the preparation used. Alcohol-based formulations can be used when the hands are not contaminated or visibly soiled. However, alcohol preparations must be used as recommended by the manufacturer and care is needed to ensure that all areas of the hands are treated. Generally 3–5 ml is recommended and the alcohol has to be applied to all skin surfaces before it drips off or evaporates. All soap or skin cleansers must be acceptable to the staff if the frequency of handwashing is to be maintained.

Taylor (1978a,b) also identified that nurses were uncertain of when as well as how to wash their hands. Handwashing is required:

- When starting work and at the end of a shift.
- Before and after patient care (between patients).
- Before and after handling or emptying urinary drainage (or wound drainage) bags.
- Before and after any invasive or aseptic procedure.
- Before handling food (including pouring drinks).
- Before handling intravenous equipment or other susceptible sites.
- Before any contact with high-risk (immunosuppressed) patients.
- After handling patients.
- After handling bedding, wastes, or other contaminated equipment.
- After visiting the toilet.
- After contact with any body fluid or excreta.
- After any contact with infected patients.

Sanderson and Weissler (1992) identified nursing activities that resulted in the recovery of coliform bacteria from the nurses' and patients' hands in an ortho-paedic hospital. Activities most frequently involved were touching patients' washing materials, touching patients' clothing, bedmaking, sluice room activi-ties, handling curtains, and handling clean or dirty linen. As a rule of thumb if the hands are visibly dirty or have been handling body fluids, wash well with soap and water. For apparently clean hands, the hands can be washed with a proprietary alcohol-based solution. If in any doubt, the hands should be washed, and if you cannot remember when you last washed your hands, they probably need washing. In the operating theatre a more rigorous technique of surgical handwashing is required.

GLOVES

Many types of disposable gloves are now available to the surgical nurse, and glove wearing has increased markedly over the last few years. Gloves are an essential protective measure for some activities, but cannot be viewed as replacing handwashing and careful attention to infection control. Gloves are used in addition to, not instead of, handwashing. Gloves are as easily contami-nated as the hands. If using gloves causes a false sense of security and replaces effective handwashing they may add to the problem of HAI. Handwashing is required before and after using gloves. Gloves are for single use only, they should be discarded after each patient and after contact with infected material during the care of an individual patient. Sterile and non-sterile gloves are available; both types are expensive and inappropriate use results in an unnecessary economic burden on the health services. Appropriate uses of sterile gloves are:

- Invasive procedures (e.g. insertion of urinary catheter, insertion of venous cannula)

- Invasive tracheal procedures or contact with tracheal secretions (e.g. endo-tracheal suction, tracheostomy care, removal of endotracheal or tracheostomy tube).
- Direct contact with wounds or open skin lesions (i.e. forceps are not used).
- Reverse barrier nursing (protective isolation).

Appropriate uses of non-sterile gloves are:

- Potential contact with blood (e.g. taking blood, capillary blood sampling).
- Potential contact with urine (e.g. meatal or catheter care, emptying urine bags, removing catheters).
- Potential contact with faeces (e.g. perineal hygiene, ostomy care).
- Handling soiled bedding or clothing (blood, urine, or faecal soiling).

Gloves can also be used if the nurse has a skin break or for any activity in which there is a risk of spilling or splashing blood or any body fluid on the hands. Gloves are not usually required for:

- Handling intravenous lines and equipment.
- Oral care (using toothbrush or forceps).
- Handling of nasogastric tubes, aspiration, and feeding.
- Skin contact and general hygiene (unless contaminated).
- Taping tubes, and handling dressings.
- Bedmaking, turning, lifting, and other general nursing activities (unless there is contamination or known infection).

UNIFORM AND APRONS

Nurses' uniforms are in almost continuous contact with the patients or bedding. Studies have identified micro-organisms, particularly *S. aureus*, on nurses' uniforms, and a Swedish study confirmed that uniforms can transmit organisms around the ward (Hambraeus, 1973). Ideally the uniform should be changed daily and laundered by the hospital. Home laundering may be insufficient to ensure adequate cleaning, especially if the uniform has been contaminated by body fluids. Plastic aprons can be used to reduce direct contact when making beds, dealing with body wastes, and other direct contact activities. Plastic aprons have two main functions:

- First, they can help reduce transmission of bacteria from the uniform.
- Second, they may reduce contamination of the uniform, and in particular protect from splashes.

Curran (1991) has suggested the simple guidelines listed below on the use of plastic aprons. Even when wearing a plastic apron contaminated articles should always be held away from the body. Aprons should be used for:

- Bedmaking, using a clean plastic apron and discarding after use. The beds of vulnerable patients should be made first. Discard the apron if visibly contaminated linen is handled.
- Total patient care, using a fresh apron for each patient.
- Toileting, using a fresh apron for each patient.
- Handling food or feeding, using a fresh apron, and discarding after the activity.
- Cleaning or other 'dirty' tasks, using a fresh apron and discarding it after the task.
- Aseptic techniques, using a fresh apron for each patient.

WASTE DISPOSAL

Careful disposal of general and clinical waste is an important aspect of infection control. Correct disposal will not only assist in infection control on the ward, but will help minimize the risk to portering staff and others handling the waste after it leaves the ward. Most hospitals use a standard colour-coded plastic bag system for waste disposal. It is important that the correct type of waste is placed in the right colour of bag. General or domestic waste, the equivalent to household waste, is placed in black bags and may be disposed of by incineration or dumping in a landfill site. Glass and aerosols are usually disposed of separately; broken glass must always be disposed of separately from general waste. Clinical waste for incineration is placed in yellow bags, except for sharps, which are discussed below. Clinical waste includes all human tissue, excreta, and body fluids, and all disposables contaminated by tissue or body fluids. Local policies should be consulted in relation to waste contaminated by cytotoxic or radioactive material. All waste bags should be securely sealed and regularly removed from the ward. Incorrect bagging of waste can be a major problem for portering and other staff handling the waste after it leaves the ward. Excreta and body fluids can be disposed of in the sluice or toilet, except in the case of some infectious conditions being treated by isolation. Care must be taken to prevent splashes and spills that will contaminate both the nurse and the environment.

Sharps

Although concern about HIV infection and AIDS has increased awareness of the risks associated with sharps injuries, they remain a major and probably under-reported problem (Torrance, 1993). A sharp can be any item contaminated with blood or body fluids that can puncture the skin. At least 20 different pathogens can be transmitted through sharps injuries (Collins and Kennedy, 1987). Lancets, stitch cutters, scalpel blades, and contaminated, broken glass can all cause sharps injuries, but needles remain the single largest cause. The largest numbers of needlestick injuries involve nurses, but all health care workers can be involved.

Incorrect disposal of sharps threatens ancillary workers, including domestic staff, porters, and laundry and incinerator staff. It should be noted that portering staff have the highest rate of sharps injuries per worker. The British Medical Association has produced the following simple rules to avoid sharps injuries:

- You used it – you bin it.
- Do not resheath needles.
- Discard needle and syringe as one unit.
- Dispose of sharps into a safe container immediately after use.
- Do not leave sharps lying around.
- Do not overfill sharps' container.
- Get immunized against hepatitis B.

Additional suggestions include:

- Use robust leak- and puncture-resistant sharps containers meeting the minimum British standard.
- Place the sharps container at the point of use to ensure immediate disposal.
- Seal the container when three-quarters full.
- Ensure staff transporting sharps bins use protective gauntlets.

Laundry

Dirty laundry represents a special type of hospital waste. Laundry can be classed as used, soiled, fouled, infected, and temperature-sensitive. Used laundry and laundry soiled with excreta or body fluids (except blood) are usually placed in white laundry bags. Blood-stained laundry or laundry from infectious patients should be double-bagged, the outer red laundry bag warns laundry staff of the need for special precautions. Personal garments, sheepskins, and other heat-sensitive laundry should be handled according to local policy. One of the main risks in handling laundry is the danger from objects bagged with the dirty laundry. Laundry staff have been injured by sharps in laundry bags, mainly scalpel blades and needles.

BEDS AND BEDMAKING

The bed is a central feature of the surgical patient's personal space in hospital. Even mobile patients are likely to spend a large part of their day on or by their beds. The bed and bedding will quickly become contaminated by the patient's resident organisms, and in addition may be contaminated by transient organisms. A number of studies have identified the mattress as a possible source of infection. Sherertz and Sullivan (1985) attributed an outbreak of infection on a burns unit to *Acinetobacter calcoaceticus* found inside mattresses, and *Pseudomonas aeruginosa* was identified in a damaged mattress in a Birmingham burns unit

(Lilly *et al.*, 1982). Loomes (1988) studied mattresses in an intensive care unit and found that 15 of 29 mattresses showed bacterial growth. An outbreak of methicillin-resistant *S. aureus* (MRSA) in a maternity unit resulted in 110 cases of cross-infection (wound infections, vaginal and urinary tract infections, breast abscesses and conjunctivitis) and ended only when all mattresses on the unit were destroyed (Ndawula and Brown, 1990). Conway (1990) studied 44 mattresses from an acute general unit and found that 36 showed some sign of damage, and seven produced bacterial growth of concern to the infection control team. Cleaning with soap and water is usually all that is required for undamaged mattresses, and the use of alcohol or some disinfectants may damage the waterproof covering. Mattresses should be allowed to dry completely to avoid the growth of mould. Loomes (1988) recommended that:

■ Mattresses should be examined at least every six months.
■ Stained mattresses should be discarded.
■ Mattresses should be cleaned according to the manufacturer's recommendations.

Adequate cleaning of bed, mattresses, and bedding is important. Hospital laundering is generally very effective. Duvets are becoming more popular for hospital use and Croton (1990) has emphasized the need for their use to be researched, particularly in relation to infection control. To reduce airborne bacteria and disturbance of dust, bedmaking should be carried out using a smooth unhurried bedmaking technique. If possible 'clean' beds should be made first. Aprons are required, and dirty linen should always be held away from the uniform and disposed of in the correct laundry bag. As in most situations, correct handwashing after bedmaking is the single most important infection control procedure.

STERILIZATION, DISINFECTION, AND CLEANING OF CLINICAL EQUIPMENT

Basic clinical equipment ranging from the bed to the stethoscope is a potential source of cross-infection. Studies have demonstrated pathogens on stethoscopes, auroscope earpieces, washing bowls, shaving brushes, baths, endoscopes, humidifiers, and surgical instruments. In fact any equipment may continue to harbour pathogens if improperly cleaned, disinfected, or sterilized. Murdoch (1990), for example, has shown that there is significant bacterial colonization of bath hoists, and noted that cleaning between patients was often perfunctory. Murdoch recommends that no major equipment should be bought without infection control advice. It is essential for the surgical nurse to be able to identify infection risk and the appropriate level of intervention required. It is not possible or appropriate to sterilize every piece of equipment used; cost alone would make it unrealistic. Three risk categories for sterilization and disinfection are suggested in *Box 8.1*. Single-use, sterile, disposable equipment has many advantages and is probably preferable whenever cost allows. Nurses should note that reusing single-use disposables will void the manufacturer's product liability and could make the nurse or employer liable.

Cleaning

Cleaning aims to remove organic contamination or dirt that may provide a growth medium for pathogens and protect them from chemical and physical disinfection. General cleaning is discussed above and is all that is required for furnishings and equipment not involved in direct skin contact. Often cleaning with hot water and detergent is all that is required for basic equipment such as beds, furnishings, bowls, and disposable bedpan holders. However, all such equipment must be stored dry. Effective bedpan washers, for example, use hot water of at least 80°C to clean the bedpan and will usually produce clean results. However, some viruses and spores are resistant to heat and autoclaving or chemical disinfection is then required. Guidance on cleaning this type of equipment should be included in infection control protocols as often the most prosaic equipment can be the source of cross-infection. Effective cleaning is also the first step in adequate disinfection and sterilization.

Disinfection

This is the removal or destruction of pathogenic organisms. Moist heat and chemical disinfection are the two main approaches used. Moist heat includes boiling in water, pasteurization, and the use of low pressure and temperature

Box 8.1	Risk categories for sterilization and disinfection (from Stucke, 1993).
High risk	Anything that penetrates the integument or comes into contact with a break in skin or mucous membranes (e.g. surgical instruments, cystoscopes, urinary or intravenous catheters). Usually requires sterilization
Intermediate risk	Anything in direct or indirect contact with skin and mucous membranes (e.g. respiratory equipment, endoscopes, bedpans). Usually requires a combination of cleaning and disinfection
Low risk	Equipment or material that does not have close patient contact (e.g. walls, sinks, beds). Cleaning is usually sufficient

steam. However, materials suitable for moist heat are also usually suitable for heat sterilization. Chemical disinfectants are used for equipment that is unsuitable for heat sterilization. In general chemical disinfectants should only be used if hot water and detergent cleaning is inadequate or a heat method such as autoclaving is inappropriate (Philpott-Howard and Casewell, 1994). *Table 8.4* lists some of the common cleaning and disinfecting procedures. Disinfectants are effective against most bacteria and viruses, but some bacteria, for example *Clostridium*, form spores that may be resistant to some disinfectants. All disinfectants must be used according to manufacturer's recommended concentrations. Common problems with disinfectants are:

- Inadequate cleaning. The presence of organic material increases the time for effective penetration and killing of pathogens.
- Concentration. Only the recommended strength should be used. If it is too weak or too strong it may be ineffective.
- Inadequate contact time.
- Inadequate contact with all surfaces. All of the contaminated area must be disinfected.
- Freshness. Most disinfectants need to be made up freshly every 24 hours.
- Inactivation and incompatibility. Many materials and chemicals can inactivate chemical disinfectants.
- Chemical hazard. All disinfectants must be stored, prepared, used, and discarded in line with Control of Substances Hazardous to Health (COSHH) regulations.

Sterilization

This is the destruction or removal of all organisms, including all viruses and bacterial spores. Sterilization may be achieved by heat or chemical methods, filtration, and irradiation. Irradiation, gas (ethylene oxide), and filtration tend to be used in the sterilization of commercial single-use equipment and solutions. Within the hospital, equipment may be sterilized by:

- Autoclaving (steam under pressure).
- Dry heat (one hour in the oven at $160°C$).
- Prolonged immersion in glutaraldehyde.

As with disinfection rigorous cleaning is necessary to remove dirt or organic material before sterilization.

NURSING THE PATIENT IN ISOLATION

Isolation or barrier nursing is sometimes necessary to prevent transmission of a virulent pathogen from an infected patient (source isolation or barrier nursing)

Table 8.4 Cleaning and disinfection of equipment.

Equipment	Method
Airways, non-disposable	Return to central sterilizing supply department
Auroscope speculum	Clean: alcohol wipe; contaminated: wash and disinfect
Baths	Clean before (unless certain it has been done) and after each use with non-abrasive, chlorine-based cleanser
Bath hoists	Rinse seat with hot water between uses; if contaminated clean according to manufacturer's recommendations
Bed, frames, cradles, backrests	Hot water and detergent clean between patients
Bowls, surgical	Return to central sterilizing supply department
Crockery, cutlery, feeding cups	Hot water (80°C), preferably in a dishwasher; allow to dry
Dressing trolleys and trays	Wipe with 70% alcohol and allow to dry between uses. Hot water and detergent if visible contamination
Electric razors	Wipe heads with alcohol; preferably use patient's own
Endoscopes	Clean and disinfect according to manufacturer's guidelines and hospital policy
Flower vases	Discard water down sluice; hot water and detergent clean; store dry and inverted. Avoid use in intensive care units or with immunocompromised patients
Faecal, or urine, or blood spillage	Disposable gloves and apron, and decontaminate with proprietary hypochlorite granules or hypochlorite solution according to hospital policy
Humidifiers and nebulizers	Use disposable units where possible. Totally replace fluid with sterile stock, never just top-up. Daily hot water and detergent wash
Lockers, furnishings, floors	Dusting, vacuuming, hot water and detergent cleaning
Mattresses	Impermeable covers. Wash with hot water and detergent or follow manufacturer's recommendations. Replace if stained or damaged
Oxygen masks and tubing	Use disposables. Change regularly and after every patient and if visibly contaminated
Pillows, foam troughs, cushions	Impermeable covers. Wash with hot water and detergent or follow manufacturer's recommendations. Replace if stained or damaged
Stethoscopes	Clean earpieces and diaphragm and bell with alcohol; use hot water and detergent if visibly contaminated
Suction equipment and bottles	Store bottles dry, ensure filters are changed regularly, change tubing daily and between patients
Thermometers	Cold water and detergent wash if dirty, alcohol wipe, store dry
Urinals and bedpans	Bedpan washer at 80°C, store dry
Urine measuring or emptying jugs	Central sterilizing supply department or bedpan washer at 80°C after each use, store dry
Washing bowls	Clean with hot water and detergent, store dry and inverted, do not stack. Patients should have their own bowl

or to protect an immunocompromised patient from exogenous infection (protective isolation or reverse barrier nursing).

Methicillin-resistant *S aureus* Infection (MRSA)

MRSA occurs throughout the world. It is an increasing problem in surgical units, burns units, and any area where patients are undergoing invasive procedures. Patients are often immunocompromised and are therefore vulnerable to infection, which in some cases can lead to fatalities (Waldvogel, 1986).

MRSA was first described in the 1960s; the number of cases decreased in the 1970s, but rose again in the 1980s, with a new strain of MRSA, which was also resistant to gentamicin and chloramphenicol (Casewell, 1986).

The spread of MRSA can be linked with poor infection control practices such as handwashing and overprescription of broad-spectrum antibiotics (Lambert, 1995; Kelly and Chivers, 1996). Handwashing techniques (using an antiseptic detergent) and the number of times hands are washed are important in preventing transmission of pathogens. An alcohol handrub can be used as an extra precaution. Infected patients must be isolated in a single room. Staff must wear gloves, and aprons and linen and waste must be disposed of correctly, as described earlier in this chapter (p. 152). Hands must be washed correctly before and after the use of gloves. Masks should be worn if sputum suction is necessary. MRSA can be effectively treated with intravenous vancomycin, but this antibiotic is toxic and must be used with caution. The situation can be frightening and confusing for patients who develop MRSA and their relatives. The necessity for isolation and all the precautions entailed in this care can distress them. It is important that the condition is clearly explained to them by the patient's nurse, and a patient information leaflet is useful.

Source Isolation or Barrier Nursing

On the general surgical ward it is often necessary to take extra precautions to isolate patients with a known infection. For some serious and notifiable diseases the patient may be transferred to an infectious diseases unit, but more often the problem has to be managed within the general ward setting. General cross-infection procedures and universal precautions are supplemented by additional protective measures. Isolation usually involves the use of a single side-room, but with careful attention can be carried out in the main ward. Affected patients can be nursed together in one area of the ward with their own designated staff if cross-infection has already occurred. All domestic and support staff involved must be made aware of the need for isolation and instructed in the appropriate precautions. Uninfected patients must be excluded from the isolation area. In general patients may require isolation if they have:

- Pyrexia of unknown origin.
- An undiagnosed rash.

■ Diarrhoea and vomiting of unknown cause.
■ A known infection requiring isolation.

They may also require isolation if they are known carriers of antibiotic-resistant strains, especially MRSA.

Philpott-Howard and Casewell (1994) suggest three categories of source isolation:

■ Standard isolation.
■ Excretion, secretion, and blood isolation.
■ Strict isolation.

Standard isolation is required to protect from transmission by direct contact (e.g. by hands, air, dust) and is needed, for example, for *S. pyogenes*-infected bedsores or wounds, infected dermatitis or eczema, impetigo, fleas, lice, and staphylococcal pneumonia.

Excretion, secretion, and blood isolation is protection from transmission of pathogens found in body fluids and excreta, for example protection from *Campylobacter*, *Clostridium difficile*, *Cholera*, diarrhoea of unknown origin, dysentery, staphylococcal enterocolitis, *Salmonella*, hepatitis A, non-A non-B hepatitis, resistant *Klebsiella*, syphilis, urinary tract infection due to gram-negative resistant bacilli, and wound infections due to resistant *S. pyogenes*.

Strict isolation is required for protection from highly infectious and transmissible pathogens that may infect both staff and patients. Strict isolation is mainly necessary for notifiable diseases, for example diphtheria, Ebola haemorrhagic fever, Lassa fever, and viral haemorrhagic fever.

General principles
A side-room with its own hand basin and if possible patient washing and toilet facilities should be used. An anteroom for changing into protective clothing is useful, but often not available. The room should be well ventilated to the outside, but the door needs to be kept closed and movement into and out of the room kept to the essential minimum. Ideally the room should have its own air supply and venting under negative pressure to prevent movement of air into the main ward. Notices stating the type of isolation and precautions required must be prominently displayed. Visitors should report to the nurses before entering the room and will require instruction in the correct procedures. Furnishings in the room should be kept to a minimum, and pillow and mattress covers must be impermeable. The room should be provided with all the necessary equipment, for example foot-operated bins (with yellow bags), laundry bags, domestic equipment, thermometers, and sphygmomanometers. Charts are usually kept outside the room and specific staff allocated to care for the patient. Daily cleaning is important: cleaning equipment must remain in the room and domestic staff must be instructed in correct procedures. In most cases disposable crockery and cutlery is not required provided a dishwasher with an adequate hot water cycle is used.

Visitors and staff must wash their hands on entry, before leaving the room, and after contact with the patient. Handwashing remains the single most important infection control measure. Protective clothing is required. Plastic aprons are preferable to cotton gowns and essential for activities involving patient contact. Aprons must be discarded after use within the room. Caps are not generally required, but may be used if there is likely to be contamination by splashing. Masks may be necessary protection with some infections, but must be of the close-fitting, filtering, surgical-type mask. Cheap paper disposables are probably a waste of money. Overshoes are also likely to be of little value, and due to the risk of hand contamination when putting them on or removing them may increase infection risk (Carter, 1990). Gloves are usually only required when handling body fluids or for other high-risk procedures. As in general infection control, gloves are not a substitute for effective handwashing and may engender a false sense of security.

Waste containment is an important aspect of source isolation. Clinical waste such as used dressings must be disposed of in yellow bags marked for incineration and a sharps box within the room is essential. Linen is treated as infected, and with some infections soiled or blood-stained linen may have to be incinerated. *En suite* toilet facilities are to be preferred, but if not available, then urine and faeces can usually be discarded and bedpans washed in the normal way. It is best to return the bedpan to the isolation cubicle for storage.

Psychological support
Patients who are nursed in isolation may be deprived of the normal social interactions offered by the ward environment. With appropriate understanding and attention to cross-infection control there is no real barrier to conversational and physical contact. Isolation patients do not need to be treated as outcasts. Eating and drinking is usually an enjoyable social activity. In isolation it may be solitary, but does not need to be cheerless or unstimulating. Radio, television, and newspapers can all help relieve the boredom of isolation, and contact with a limited number of nurses can offer an opportunity for establishing close nurse–patient relationships. The patient's visitors may feel inhibited or threatened by the isolation procedures, but the nurse can help them overcome their fears and encourage a more normal interaction with the patient by carefully explaining and emphasizing the key measures.

References

Albert RK, Condie F (1981) Handwashing patterns in medical intensive care units. *N Engl Med J* **304**:1465–1466.

Ayliffe GAJ, Babb JR, Davies JG, Lilly HA (1988) Hand disinfection: a comparison of various agents in laboratory and ward studies. *J Hosp Infec* **11**:226–243.

Bibby BA (1982) Mathematic modelling of patient risk. PhD thesis. Aston University.

Broughall JM, Marshman C, Jackson B, Bird P (1984) An automatic monitoring system for measuring handwashing frequency in hospital wards. *J Hosp Infect* **5**:447–453.

Carter R (1990) Ritual and risk. *Nurs Times* **86(13)**:63–64.

Casewell MW (1986) Epidemiology and control of the modern methicillin-resistant *Staphylococcus aureus*. *J Hosp Infect* **7** (Suppl. A):1–11.

Casewell M, Philips I (1977) Hands as route of transmission for *Klebsiella* species. *Br Med J* **2**:1315–1317.

Collins CH, Kennedy DA (1987) Microbiological hazards of occupational needlestick and 'sharps' injuries. *J Appl Bacteriol* **62**:385–402.

Conly JM, Hill S, Ross J, Lertzman J, Lowie TJ (1989) Handwashing practices in an intensive care unit: The effects of an educational program and its relationship to infection rates. *Am J Infect Control* **17(6)**:330–339.

Conway R (1990) Mattress conditions. *Nurs Times* **86(11)**:52.

Croton CM (1990) Duvets on trial. *Nurs Times* **86(26)**:63–67.

Curran E (1991) Protecting with plastic aprons. *Nurs Times* **87(38)**:64–68.

Danforth D, Nicolle LE, Hume K, Alfieri N, Sims H (1987) Nosocomial infections on nursing units with floors cleaned with a disinfectant compared with detergent. *J Hosp Infect* **10(3)**:229–235.

DHSS/PHLS Hospital Infection Working Group (1988) *Hospital Infection Control HC(88)33*, pp. 1–37. HMSO, London.

Fox MK (1974) How good are hand washing practices? *Am J Nurs* **74**:1676–1678.

Gould D, Ream E (1993) Assessing nurse's hand decontamination performance. *Nurs Times* **89(25)**:47–50.

Graham M (1990) Frequency and duration of handwashing in an intensive care unit. *Am J Infect Control* **18(2)**:77–80.

Gwaltney J, Moscalski PB, Hendley JO (1978) Hand to hand transmission of rhinovirus colds. *Ann Intern Med* **88**:463–467.

Hambraeus A (1973) Transfer of *Staphylococcus aureus* via nurses' uniform. *J Hygiene* **71**:799–814.

Kelly J, Chivers G (1996) Built in resistance. *Nurs Times* **92(2)**:50–54.

Lambert S (1995) Do staff follow guidelines for dealing with M.R.S.A.? *Nurs Times* **91(44)**:25–27.

Leclair JM, Freeman J, Sullivan BF, Crawley CM, Goldman DA (1987) Prevention of nosocomial syncitial virus infections through compliance with gown and glove precautions. *N Engl J Med* **317**:329–334.

Lidwell OM, Lowbury EJ (1950) The survival of bacteria in dust II. The effect of atmospheric humidity on survival of bacteria in dust. *J Hyg* **48**:21–27.

Lilly HA, Kidson A, Fujita K (1982) Investigation of hospital infection from a damaged mattress and the demonstration of its mechanisms. *Burns* **8(6)**:408–413.

Loomes S (1988) Is it safe to lie down in hospital? *Nurs Times* **84(49)**:63–65.

Maki DTG, Alvarado CJ, Hassemer CA, Zilz MA (1982) Relation of the inanimate environment to endemic nosocomial infection. *N Engl J Med* **307**:1562–1566.

Meers PD, Ayliffe GAJ, Emmerson AM (1980) Report of the National Survey on infections in hospital. *J Hosp Infect* **2**(Suppl.):29–34.

Miller PJ, Farr BM, Gwaltney Jr JM (1989) Economic benefits of an effective infection control programme: case study and proposal. *Rev Infect Dis* **11(2)**:284–288.

Murdoch S (1990) Hazards in hoists. *Nurs Times* **86(49)**:68–70.

Ndawula EM, Brown L (1990) Mattresses as reservoirs of epidemic MRSA. *Lancet* **337(8739)**:488.

Philpott-Howard J, Casewell M (1994) *Hospital Infection Control. Policies and Practical Procedures*, pp. 19–25. WB Saunders, London.

Quraishi ZA, McGuckin M, Blais FX (1984) Duration of handwashing in intensive care units: A descriptive study. *Am J Infect Con* **11**:83–87.

Sanderson PJ, Weissler S (1992) Recovery of coliforms from the hands of nurses and patients: activities leading to contamination. *J Hosp Infect* **21**:85–93.

Sherertz RJ, Sullivan M (1985) An outbreak of infections with *Acinetobacter calcoaceticus* in burns patients: Contamination of patients' mattresses. *J Infect Dis* **151(2)**:252–258.

Stucke VA (1993) *Microbiology For Nurses*, p. 121. Baillière Tindall, London.

Taylor L (1986) Hospital-acquired infections. *Self Health* **11**:8–9.

Taylor LJ (1978a) An evaluation of handwashing techniques. I. *Nurs Times* **74(2)**:54–55.

Taylor LJ (1978b) An evaluation of handwashing techniques. II. *Nurs Times* **74(3)**:108–110.

Torrance C (1993) Sharps injuries. *Surg Nurse* **6(1)**:5–9.

Waldvogel FA (1986) Treatment of infection due to methicillin-resistant *Staphylococcus aureus*. *J Hosp Infect* **7(Suppl. A)**:37–46.

Ward K (1990) All that glisters. . . . *Nurs Times* **86(24)**:32–34.

Chapter 9
Wounds and Wound Care

Any type of surgery results in some damage or destruction of tissue. The surface wound, the obvious break in the continuity of the skin, is only one manifestation of surgical trauma. All the tissues cut or manipulated during an operation will have suffered some degree of injury and inflammation and will need to heal. The importance of treating patients rather than wounds has been emphasized for patients with chronic problem wounds (Torrance, 1987), but it is just as important for the surgical nurse to be aware of this when treating apparently simple surgical incisions. In this chapter, tissue responses to injury, healing of wounds and tissues, wound assessment, management, and closure, and wound drainage will be considered. One system for classifying surgical wounds is given in *Box 9.1*.

TISSUE RESPONSES TO INJURY

Cell injury or death can be due to a range of mechanisms (*Box 9.2*). In surgical wounds mechanical trauma and hypoxia are important causes of death and injury. All wounds will cause some blood loss, and the haemostatic response may add to the local hypoxia. The severity of damage experienced by cells at the site of injury will depend on the extent of the trauma, the duration and degree of hypoxia, and the type of cells present. Neurones in the brain are irreversibly damaged by more than a few minutes of anoxia, while epithelial or fat cells may

---

Box 9.1 Wound classification (adapted from Smeltzer and Bare, 1992).

Mechanism of injury
- Incised wound (e.g. surgical incision)
- Contused wound (e.g. blunt injury, blow)
- Lacerated wound (e.g. ragged edges made by broken glass)
- Punctured wound (e.g. stab wound)

Degree of contamination
- Clean wound: uninfected surgical incision
- Clean-contaminated wound: surgical wound in which gastrointestinal, respiratory, urinary or genital tracts have been breached
- Contaminated wound: open wound, wound known to have been contaminated
- Dirty or infected wound: wound in areas known to be contaminated by infecting organisms before surgery

---

Box 9.2 Causes of cell injury.

Mechanical
- Cutting, crushing, and other mechanical injuries disrupt the cell membrane
- If damage is extensive or irreversible the cell dies

Chemical
- Chemicals act like poisons, disrupting cell metabolism
- If the damage is irreversible the cell dies

Heat
- Extremes of heat coagulate cytoplasmic organelles, disrupting cell metabolism

Radiation
- Acts on cellular deoxyribonucleic acid (DNA) and disrupts cell regulation and replication

Micro-organisms
- Bacteria, viruses, and other organisms may directly attack cells or release toxins, which act like chemical poisons

Inflammation and immune responses
- Inflammatory and immune responses can become misdirected and destroy body cells

Hypoxia
- All cells require oxygen to maintain cell metabolism and integrity; lack of oxygen and a build-up of metabolites will eventually cause cell lysis

recover after hours of hypoxia. The severity of injury and so the extent of healing required depend on the type of trauma and the nature of the cells affected. The potential tissue responses to injury are summarized in *Figure 9.1*. As this figure shows, full healing or regeneration is only possible for certain cell types. Most injury results in some scar formation and loss of normal structure, and a consequent reduction in function.

THE PHYSIOLOGY OF WOUND HEALING

The general process of wound healing is described in this section, while healing of specific tissues is discussed in the next section. Wound healing is a complex continuous process (*Figure 9.2*), but for clarity of description can be conveniently separated into four overlapping and interdependent main stages (Torrance, 1985):

- The acute inflammatory phase (days 0–3).
- The destructive phase (days 1–6).
- The proliferative phase (days 3–24).
- The maturational phase (days 24–365).

In reality these stages represent a continuous overlapping process in which the exact timing and sequence of events varies depending on a variety of factors such as site, extent, and nature of the injury; general condition and medical treatment of the patient; and local wound management. In addition to these phases the processes of wound contraction and epithelialization will also be considered.

The Acute Inflammatory Phase (*Figure 9.3*)

The first response to injury is activation of haemostatic mechanisms to limit blood loss from damaged blood vessels. Platelet activation, coagulation, and complement activation are the key processes. Vasoactive substances released by the damaged cells cause a short period of vasoconstriction of small blood vessels at the site of injury. Coagulation is initiated by platelet activation. Trauma disrupts the endothelial lining of blood vessels and platelets adhere to the exposed subendothelium and degranulate, releasing a range of chemical mediators including adenosine diphosphate (ADP) and serotonin. The chemical mediators encourage further platelet adhesion and aggregation and mediate the conversion of fibrinogen to fibrin. Blood cells and other blood components are trapped in this growing clot and the fibrin stabilizes the clot, plugging the injured blood vessel. Platelets and other cells involved in wound healing also release cytokines or growth factors (i.e. essential signalling and regulating chemical or 'local hormones'), which are thought to have a major role in controlling the healing process (*Box 9.3*).

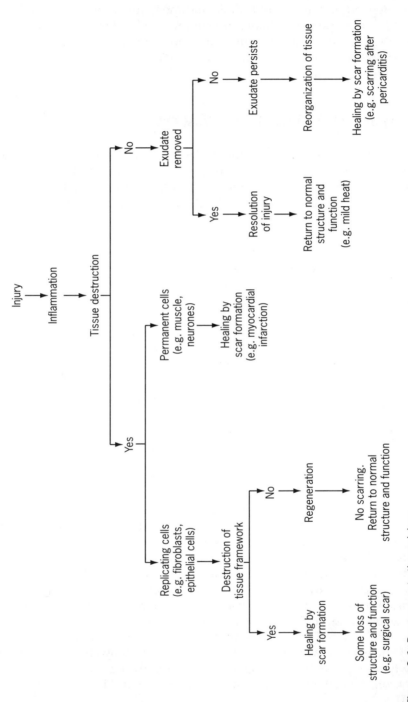

Figure 9.1 Responses to tissue injury.

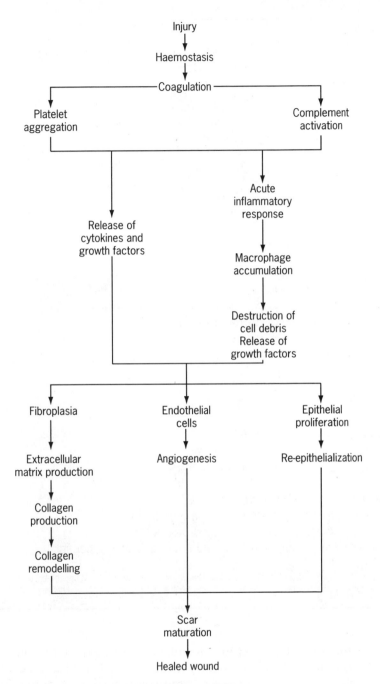

Figure 9.2 Wound healing (adapted from Whitby, 1995).

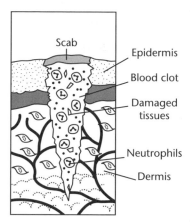

Figure 9.3 The acute inflammatory phase of wound healing.

Box 9.3 Growth factors and their effects in wound healing.

Platelet-derived growth factor (PDGF)
- Fibroblast chemotaxis and proliferation
- Granulocytes and monocyte chemotaxis

Epidermal growth factor (EGF)
- Fibroblast, epidermal, and endothelial cell proliferation

Fibroblast growth factor (FGF)
- Fibroblast and endothelial cell proliferation
- Stimulates new blood vessel formation in the wound

Transforming growth factor beta (TGFβ)
- Proliferation of fibroblasts and some other cells
- Inhibits proliferation of epithelial and other cells
- Stimulates the production of wound collagen and fibronectin

(Note: The role of growth factors has been demonstrated in culture and their value is under investigation. In the future they may be used therapeutically to accelerate rather than simply facilitate wound healing.)

Vasoconstriction is followed by vasodilation and increased capillary permeability. This is initiated by inflammatory mediators such as histamine released by damaged cells, coagulation processes, and complement activation. The capillaries become abnormally permeable, allowing plasma, plasma proteins, and other blood components to leak out into the damaged tissues. The exudate formed by this leakage is rich in fibrin, which together with other blood elements and blood cells lost into the injury, forms a clot that plugs the defect and provides a limited degree of protection. As the clot dries out it forms a hard scab over the wound. The fibrin clot also provides a framework for later stages of healing. Leukocyte migration into the injury is initiated in this stage. In the first 24 hours granulocytes, mainly neutrophils, are the main white cells found in the wound, followed later by a range of other white cell types. The inflammatory responses of this first phase are essential and set the stage for the next phases of the healing process. However, if tissue loss is extensive or if the wound is infected or contaminated by foreign material, inflammation can be prolonged and this can disrupt healing resulting in excessive granulation, chronic inflammation, and a problem wound. Gentle handling of the wound and rigorous asepsis are important in promoting haemostasis and limiting inflammation.

The Destructive Phase *(Figure 9.4)*

The main feature of this phase is removal of dead tissue and any micro-organisms contaminating the wound. Neutrophils, monocytes, and macrophages infiltrate and proliferate within the wound. Neutrophils dominate in the first 24 hours, but macrophages proliferate to become the dominant cell type. Wound macrophages are derived from two sources:

- Proliferation of local tissue macrophages.
- Differentiation of circulating monocytes attracted into the wound into macrophages.

The macrophages remove tissue debris bacteria by phagocytosis and releasing proteolytic enzymes. Macrophages are the key cells for this phase of wound debridement. They are the major phagocytic cells, but they also release a range of regulating chemicals or 'local hormones', which stimulate endothelial cell and

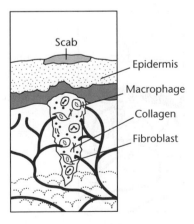

Figure 9.4 The destructive phase of wound healing.

fibroblast proliferation, production of extracellular matrix (ECM), and smooth muscle replication (Whitby, 1995). Experiments in which macrophage activity is disrupted by antibodies have resulted in decreased fibroblast migration, decreased fibroblast proliferation, reduced collagen production, and delayed wound healing. Disruption of neutrophil activity does not impede healing.

The Proliferative Phase (*Figure 9.5*)

In this phase there is a marked increase in metabolic activity within the wound as it enters a period of intense proliferation and production. The two main players in this phase are endothelial cells and fibroblasts, and the two main processes, angiogenesis and fibroplasia.

Angiogenesis is the formation of new blood vessels in the wound. Endothelial cells migrate into the wound and proliferate, forming a delicate network of capillary loops or buds. These capillary loops grow into the spaces created by macrophages during the destructive phase.

Fibroplasia involves the proliferation of fibroblasts and production of ECM. Fibroblasts migrate into the wound following behind the capillary loops and begin to multiply. There is evidence that fibroblasts can use some of the serum glycoproteins of the wound clot to produce new tissue. Initially ECM production results in the formation of new ground substance, but from about day four, collagen production begins to dominate. At first wound collagen is produced randomly, but as the proliferative phase continues it is reorganized and cross-linked to increase the tensile strength of the wound. The high level of cellular activity that marks this phase requires an abundant supply of oxygen and nutrients. Vitamins and minerals (notably vitamin C and iron) are essential for collagen synthesis.

The capillary buds and supporting connective tissue give the base of the wound a red, bumpy, or granular appearance (i.e. granulation tissue). Early in

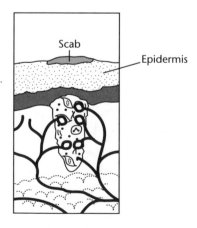

Figure 9.5 The proliferative phase of wound healing.

the proliferative phase the supporting connective tissue is loosely arranged and contains little collagen; new granulation tissue is very fragile and the wound requires gentle handling and cleaning. As the proliferative phase matures, the initial hyperactivity dies down and the number of capillaries and fibroblasts in the wound decreases. A month after injury the wound still lacks strength and will have only 35–50% of the tensile strength of the original tissue (*Figure 9.6*).

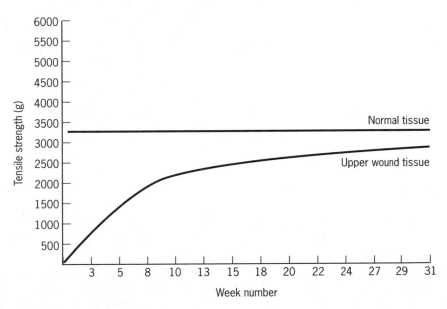

Figure 9.6 Wound tensile strength with time.

The Maturational Phase (*Figure 9.7*)

This phase is characterized by a continued increase in the collagen content of the wound. By the end of the proliferative phase the tissue defect appears closed, but fibroblast activity continues. Wound collagen is constantly being remodelled to increase the strength of the wound tissue, and the maturational phase can continue for weeks, months, or up to a year. The number of blood vessels and fibroblasts in the scar continues to decrease towards more normal levels, and the scar loses its red angry appearance, becoming paler, flatter, and softer. However, it should be noted that scar collagen has a different microstructure from normal collagen and the scar will never recover the full tensile strength of the original tissue (see *Figure 9.6*). Scars usually have a thinner epithelial covering than the surrounding tissue.

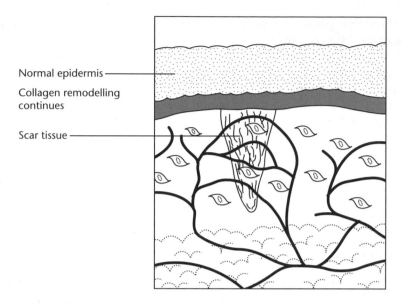

Normal epidermis

Collagen remodelling
continues

Scar tissue

Figure 9.7 The maturational phase of wound healing.

Wound Contraction

When first cut, the edges of a full thickness wound retract, increasing the area of the wound by 10–15%. In simple wounds contraction may be observed after 3–4 days. This contraction involves both the dermal and epidermal elements and the edges of the wound begin to move inwards. Wound contraction is caused by specialized fibroblasts, the myofibroblasts. In small uncomplicated wounds, wound contraction makes a major contribution to healing and improves the functional quality of the repair. The contribution of wound contraction is less significant if there is a large area of tissue loss or if the wound is in an area where the skin and subcutaneous tissue are more tightly bound to underlying structures.

Epithelialization

Epithelialization is the process of epithelial cell proliferation and migration. Within a few hours of injury, epithelial cells begin to migrate into the wound and proliferation begins within 1–2 days. Epithelial cells can only migrate across moist viable tissue. Normal scab formation results in dehydration of the wound surface with further loss of tissue increasing the depth of the wound. Epithelial cells have to migrate under the scab or eschar. Optimal epidermal healing occurs across a moist wound surface and epithelialization is about three times faster under an occlusive dressing that keeps the wound surface moist than under a scab. The edges of the wound represent the main source of new epithelial cells, but in shallow dermal wounds remnants of epithelial structures such as hair follicles also act as focal points for proliferation and migration. These epidermal remnants will be destroyed if the wound surface dries out to form a scab. As the epithelial cells migrate they lose their ability to divide. The tongues of migrating epithelial cells are only loosely adherent to the wound surface and are easily damaged by poor handling or inappropriate wound treatments.

HEALING BY FIRST AND SECOND INTENTION

Healing of surgical wounds has traditionally been described as ocurring by first, second, and third intention. These terms describe the form of healing rather than the physiological processes. Healing by first intention or primary union (*Figure 9.8a*) occurs in sharp, clean surgical wounds where there has been little tissue loss and the wound margins are sutured with careful apposition. In wounds healed by first intention the skin is sutured to close the wound and granulation tissue forms under the skin. Scar formation is usually minimal.

Healing by second intention or granulation occurs when there is more tissue loss and the wound edges cannot be closely apposed (*Figure 9.8b*). Healing is concentrated in the base of the wound and the defect fills slowly. Infection or prolonged inflammation results in healing by granulation rather than first intention. Healing by second intention is slow and can produce a poor cosmetic appearance or functional result. Closure with skin grafts or flaps may be a better alternative in these cases.

Healing by third intention or secondary closure results when an established granulating wound is sutured together. This may be necessary if a suture line has broken down or dead tissue has been excised from a wound and the two bleeding surfaces are sutured together.

HEALING IN SPECIFIC TISSUES

All types of tissues and organs are cut during surgery and these may heal at different rates and in slightly different ways. The healing of surface skin wounds has been described above, healing of other tissues such as fascia, muscle, bone, organs and nervous tissue is briefly considered here.

Connective Tissues

The deep fascia is a thin, dense, fibrous connective tissue that encloses and separates muscles. Bone and other structures have their own form of fascia. Fascia heals by a process of fibroplasia, and small tears can be repaired by simple suturing. Larger defects may require treatment by fascia transplantation. Bone heals by the process of callus formation, and fracture healing is analogous to the processes of skin healing. Cartilage heals by chrondrocyte proliferation and increased production of proteoglycans with only limited collagen production

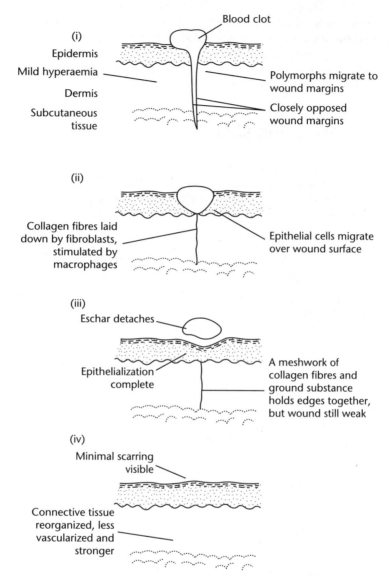

Figure 9.8 (a) Healing by first intention.

and poor filling of cartilage defects. Tendon repair is also slow, because tendons have a poor blood supply and because the number of tendon fibroblasts is low compared with the tendon mass. Healing is by fibrous scar formation.

Muscle

Both skeletal and smooth muscle have limited ability to regenerate. Muscle fibre processes can interdigitate and fill small defects, but any connective tissue

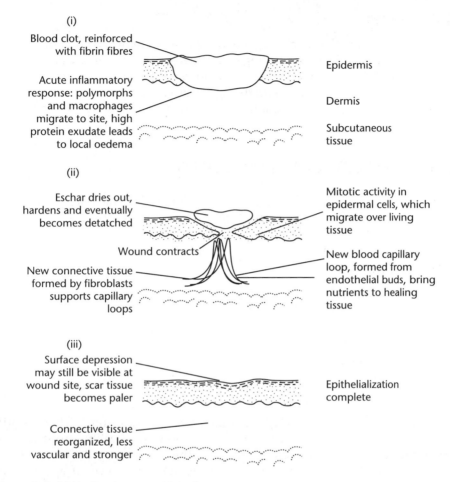

(i)

Blood clot, reinforced with fibrin fibres

Epidermis

Acute inflammatory response: polymorphs and macrophages migrate to site, high protein exudate leads to local oedema

Dermis

Subcutaneous tissue

(ii)

Eschar dries out, hardens and eventually becomes detatched

Mitotic activity in epidermal cells, which migrate over living tissue

Wound contracts

New connective tissue formed by fibroblasts supports capillary loops

New blood capillary loop, formed from endothelial buds, bring nutrients to healing tissue

(iii)

Surface depression may still be visible at wound site, scar tissue becomes paler

Epithelialization complete

Connective tissue reorganized, less vascular and stronger

Figure 9.8 (b) Healing by second intention.

between the damaged muscle ends will impede this process. Excision of damaged tissue and close apposition of the muscle ends maximizes the chances of regeneration with minimal scarring. If the tissue loss is moderate or extensive, healing is mainly by scar formation.

Nervous tissue

Support cells of nervous tissue can regenerate, but neurones lack mitotic activity and cannot replicate. Damaged central nervous system neurones have limited repair processes. Dead neurones cannot be replaced. Healing will be by glial (support cell) proliferation and formation of a glial scar. Peripheral nerves can regenerate damaged axons provided the damage does not include the cell body. Regeneration of axons is slow and the restoration of function is uncertain.

Other Tissues

Most epithelial lining tissues can regenerate with a full return to normal structure and function provided the underlying connective tissue and muscle are intact. In the kidney the tubular epithelium can recover, but complete nephrons cannot be replaced. The liver is exceptional for its regenerative capacity and can restore lost tissue even after extensive resection. Haemorrhage is a major problem in liver trauma.

FACTORS AFFECTING WOUND HEALING

Wound healing is influenced by both systemic and local factors that may delay or disrupt wound healing. Understanding and managing these factors is an important part of the surgical nurse's art.

Systemic Factors

Systemic factors include:

- Age.
- Nutritional status.
- Medical condition.
- Drugs and treatments.

Age

Age is often identified as an important factor in wound healing. There is little direct evidence that normal ageing necessarily slows the healing process. It has been suggested that wound complications in the elderly may have more to do with cardiovascular and respiratory problems than the effects of ageing itself (Hunt *et al.*, 1978).

Nutritional status

The metabolic demands of healing processes are high and nutritional deficiencies can seriously disrupt healing (Chapter 6). Tissue replacement increases the need for protein, and collagen production is particularly disrupted by protein deficiency. Animal studies indicate that a high protein diet can improve healing. Vitamins are also critical in wound healing. Experimental studies clearly show that vitamin C deficiency disrupts collagen synthesis, and vitamin A may also be of particular importance. Of the minerals, iron, zinc, and copper seem to be particularly relevant to healing. Copper and ferrous iron are critical for collagen metabolism, but serious deficiency states are not commonly identified. Zinc is involved in many metabolic processes and there is evidence that correcting zinc deficiency can improve healing. There is no evidence that mineral supplements will improve healing in cases where there is no deficiency. It is clear that feeding the patient feeds the wound, and nutritional support is an important element of wound care. Pinchcofsky-Devin (1994) emphasizes that early nutritional assessment and intervention are necessary to provide the protein, energy, vitamin, and mineral nutrients required to promote healing. Wound healing follows trauma and the nutritional aspects of trauma are reviewed in Chapter 6.

Medical condition

Treatment of concurrent illness, particularly respiratory and cardiovascular disease, will have a beneficial effect on wound healing. The high metabolic demands of healing mean that treating any condition that reduces oxygen and nutrient availability at the site of healing is critical. A blood transfusion for an anaemic patient may be more effective in promoting wound healing than any local wound treatment. Diabetics have a decreased resistance to infection due to decreased phagocytic ability and diminished neutrophil chemotaxis and may have problems with wound healing due to wound infection (Porth, 1990). Systemic infection may also have adverse effects on wound healing. Uraemia or liver failure is also likely to disrupt healing.

Drugs and treatments

A variety of drugs and treatments can adversely influence healing processes, but glucocorticosteroid and anti-inflammatory drugs are of particular importance. The administration of adrenocorticotrophic hormone (ACTH), cortisone, and other glucocorticosteroids may delay healing by decreasing capillary permeability during the early stages of inflammation. Glucocorticosteroids also tend to reduce the phagocytic properties of leukocytes and inhibit fibroblastic proliferation and function. However, there is little evidence that glucocorticosteroids will significantly delay surgical wound healing by first intention in practice, although healing by granulation in open wounds may be delayed.

Chemotherapy agents may also disrupt healing, and the local effects of radiotherapy may reduce vascularity and inhibit granulation and wound contraction. Rigby (1992) and Siana *et al.* (1992) have suggested that catecholamines liberated in the presence of nicotine accelerate the formation of chalones, which inhibit epithelialization.

Local Factors

Local factors are also important in influencing the course of wound healing. Important local factors include:

- Wound infection.
- Foreign bodies.
- Type of wound.
- Poor blood supply.
- Movement.
- Wound dehydration.
- Wound temperature.

Wound infection

Infection is one of the most important local factors disrupting wound healing. Infection delays healing, and a local wound infection can progress to a serious systemic infection. The problem of wound infection is addressed in more detail later in this chapter (p. 182).

Type of wound

The nature, extent, and position of the wound are important. A gaping wound tends to heal more slowly than one easily closed by suturing; a wound with large tissue loss obviously tends to take longer to heal than a small wound. The presence of adhesions may prevent adequate apposition of wound edges and wound contraction. Rigby (1992) uses the example of adherence of wound edges to the underlying tibia thus delaying healing of a wound in this area. Wounds in some locations may be easily contaminated or subject to excessive movement.

Foreign bodies

The presence of any foreign material within the wound will delay healing. Foreign bodies may be splinters of glass or wood, clothing fragments, or other material introduced during traumatic wounding, but surgical debris, bone fragments, and sutures can be equally problematic. Sutures should be removed promptly; a suture, like any foreign body, may prolong the inflammatory responses, causing a localized problem within the healing wound such as abscess formation. Dead tissue or slough can act as a foreign body and can also harbour bacteria, thus early removal of devitalized tissue can be an important factor in the treatment of problem wounds.

Poor blood supply

Wound healing is a demanding event metabolically and a poor blood supply will delay healing. Wounds in areas with an abundant blood supply heal much more rapidly than those in areas with a poor blood supply. A skin wound on the anterior thigh, for example, will heal more rapidly than a similar wound over the anterior aspect of the tibia. Wounds in areas affected by peripheral vascular disease also heal slowly. A pressure sore of the heel provides a good example of a slow-healing wound due to ischaemia because of poor blood supply and the local effects of pressure.

Movement

The healing wound is fragile and easily damaged by excessive movement of the wound margins. Newly formed granulation tissue has little collagen supporting it and the tongues of epithelial cells spreading across a wound surface are only lightly adherent to underlying dermis. Disruption of these tissues by movement will act like a fresh injury, prolonging inflammation and impeding healing. It may be necessary to splint or otherwise immobilize wounds in areas such as joints where movement is likely to be a problem. Overfrequent dressing changes will also disrupt these new tissues.

Wound dehydration

As discussed previously (p. 174) scab formation occurs when the wound surface dries out. This seals the wound, but the dehydration causes a loss of tissue, increasing the depth of the wound and slowing healing, particularly epithelialization. There is now sufficient evidence to support moist wound healing as a more effective approach to treatment for most wounds. Some dressings such as dry gauze dressings may encourage wound dehydration.

Wound temperature

The active metabolic and proliferative processes involved in wound healing are very sensitive to local temperature changes. A fall in temperature of only 2°C is sufficient to decrease the rate of mitosis and reduce leukocyte activity to zero (Barton and Barton, 1981; Johnson, 1988). Exposure of wet wounds can markedly reduce surface temperature, and mitosis can take several hours to recover (Turner and Stevens, 1982). Lengthy dressing changes should be avoided where possible. Dressings should not be removed until the nurse is ready to apply the new dressing, and the dressing used should be capable of maintaining thermal insulation.

HEALING OF ABDOMINAL WOUNDS AND THE GASTROINTESTINAL TRACT

Foster and Williams (1994) emphasized that the aim of an abdominal wall repair is to achieve a strength equal to that of the area preoperatively. The repair should be pain free and not look unsightly. Failed healing can lead to an incisional hernia, wound dehiscence, and possibly a 'burst abdomen'. The older, obese, anaemic patient with a malignant bowel obstruction has a considerable risk of experiencing a wound healing problem. When there is a previous incision in the abdominal wall it is often difficult to gain access through the same area as this may interrupt the blood supply and cause subsequent necrosis of the skin bridge between the two incisions. It may also weaken the abdominal wall. It takes about 120 days for the abdominal wound to attain its maximum strength. Initially, the wound relies entirely on the strength of the non-absorbable nylon sutures. Any discharge of clear fluid from the wound site should be reported immediately as this may herald a 'burst abdomen' where the abdominal contents slide out onto the exterior abdominal wall. If this happens, the intestines must be covered with warm saline packs and the patient returned to theatre for resuturing as quickly as possible.

Healing within the gastrointestinal tract depends on the fine balance between synthesis and lysis of collagen. Foster and Williams (1994) states that the tensile strength of the anastomosis is low in the first 3–4 days. There is then a rapid gain in tensile strength, which coincides with collagen synthesis. If the fine balance between synthesis and lysis of collagen is disrupted, the anastomosis can be affected. Excessive lysis, for example, may produce a fistula, while excessive synthesis may cause stenosis of the wound site. Wounds in the abdomen and gastrointestinal tract are clean-contaminated, and possibly contaminated if there has been a spillage of intestinal contents.

WOUND ASSESSMENT

An understanding of the process and stages of wound healing is essential for effective wound assessment and treatment. Wounds may require different treatments and dressings depending on the stage of healing and the importance of specific local factors. Dealey (1991) states that the appearance of the wound gives a clear indication of the stage of healing of the wound. However, it may be important to clean the wound before assessment as many of the dressings used form a gel on the wound surface. Wound assessment allows the nurse to identify problems and priorities for wound treatment.

Necrotic wounds may present as a hard black scab or as a thick black, brown, or grey slough. There is often an increase in the amount of exudate, which may have an offensive odour. Removal of necrotic tissue or slough is the priority with these wounds, and treatment will be directed towards debridement. An infected wound may be identified by redness around the wound, localized heat, cellulitis, swelling in the tissues, offensive exudate, and pain in the area. Treatment of an infected wound will concentrate on combating infection and allowing drainage. The patient needs to be monitored for signs of systemic infection, and a wound swab should be taken to identify the bacteria involved so that appropriate systemic antibiotics can be prescribed. Granulating wounds are very delicate, and if the new cells and capillary loops are damaged then the wound will bleed. Epithelialization occurs once a cavity is filled with granulation tissue, treatment is then directed towards protecting the wound and facilitating the natural healing processes. Wounds may be more extensive than they appear, with undermining of the skin margins, and they may also contain concealed pockets or sinuses.

When assessing a wound the surgical nurse should note:

- The position of the wound.
- The shape of the wound.
- The area and depth of the wound.
- The colour of the wound and wound margins.
- The presence and amount of exudate.
- The presence of slough or eschar.
- Wound odour.
- Any pain.

An accurate record is needed of all aspects of the wound and the patient's general condition. Factors that should be considered in systematic wound assessment tools are listed in *Box 9.4.*

Box 9.4 Wound assessment (adapted from Kozier *et al.*, 1995).

Appearance
- Colour of the wound
- Colour of the skin at the wound margin
- Approximation of wound edges
- Any changes in colour

Size
- Length, width, area
- Depth
- Increase or decrease in either of these dimensions

Drainage
- Colour
- Consistency
- Odour
- Volume and degree of saturation of dressings
- Location (e.g. from a specific area of the wound or a sinus)

Swelling
- Induration at wound margins or within the wound (sterile gloves can be worn to palpate the wound edges for tension in the tissues)

Pain
- Persistent severe pain or sudden onset of pain may indicate infection or internal bleeding

Wound drains
- Monitor placement and security of drains
- Monitor patency of the drains
- Check that suction or vacuum apparatus is functioning
- Note the amount and character of the drainage

WOUND COMPLICATIONS

The incidence of wound complications varies, but the general rate is about 5%. Wound infection is the major complication of surgical wounds, but oedema, haematoma or seroma formation, secondary haemorrhage, wound failure or breakdown, fistula formation, inplantation cysts, contracture and adhesions, and abnormal healing or scarring are other problems. Factors that alter the complex processes of wound healing may result in abnormal patterns of healing.

Wound Infection

Wound infection occurs in 2–4% of clean surgical wounds and in emergency surgery of the gastrointestinal or urinary tracts may occur in as many as 50–60% of cases (Hochberg and Murray, 1991). Infection confined to the wound that is not making the patient ill can be classed as minor. If the infection is spreading, causing a systemic response, or delaying discharge, it should be considered as major. A primary wound infection arises from organisms within the wound; a secondary wound infection occurs if the wound is contaminated by blood-borne bacteria or by organisms from the environment.

Many wound infections are endogenous and due to opportunistic infection by enteric or other commensal organisms. However, cross-infection is a serious problem, particularly with the increase in resistant strains such as methicillin-resistant *Staphylococcus aureus* (MRSA). Safe preoperative preparation, scrupulous surgical technique to avoid contamination, and attention to aseptic techniques in the postoperative period, particularly handwashing by staff and patients, all help reduce the incidence of wound infection. *Box 9.5* summarizes the nursing measures that can be used to help reduce the risk of wound infection. For wounds classed as clean-contaminated wounds, contaminated, or known to be infected, appropriate antibiotic prophylaxis and treatment will be considered. Wound swabs can be taken to identify infecting organisms and determine appropriate antibiotic therapy. Wound infection may be indicated by the signs of inflammation (i.e. local heat and redness, swelling and induration, pain, increasing exudate, odour, or pus). Systemic signs of infection may also be apparent, and any unexplained pyrexia in a postoperative patient suggests that the wound should be reassessed for infection.

Drainage is the main approach to treating an infected wound. Any necrotic tissue should be removed and the wound allowed to drain freely. Absorbent dressings or wound irrigation may be used to treat infected wounds. The choice of dressing will depend on the volume of exudate, the presence of slough or necrotic tissue, and problems with wound odour.

Wound infection has several adverse effects. In the short term it delays healing and is likely to prolong hospitalization. It increases the risk of cross-infection and the patient may need to be isolated. In susceptible patients wound infection can progress into a serious systemic infection, even septicaemia, bacteraemia, and death. More long-term effects may derive from the quality of healing. Infected surgical wounds heal by secondary rather than primary intention. The resulting scar will be larger than otherwise and may have adverse effects on body image, sexuality, and self-esteem. In some cases scarring can cause serious alterations of lifestyle.

Haematoma and Seroma

A haematoma is a collection of blood, while a seroma is a collection of serous fluid (not blood or pus) within a wound. A degree of oedema and haematoma

---

Box 9.5 Measures to reduce wound infection.

Preoperative
- Reduce preoperative hospitalization
- Reinforce patient handwashing and personal hygiene
- Treat concurrent infections
- Avoid shaving operative site (if required use depilatory cream or clippers and shave immediately before surgery)
- Clean operative site
- Use antibiotic prophylaxis when appropriate
- Isolate patients with wound infection

Operative
- Safe and correct preparation of operative site
- Pay careful attention to aseptic techniques, gowning, gloving, and draping
- Remove powder from sterile gloves
- Constantly monitor sterile field
- Use scrupulous surgical techniques, and meticulous haemostasis
- Avoid prophylactic use of drains

Postoperative
- Reinforce patient handwashing and personal hygiene
- Reinforce staff handwashing and infection control procedures
- Minimize wound disturbance
- Ensure aseptic handling of wound
- Ensure adequate nutrition
- Treat concurrent infections
- Isolate patients with wound infection

---

can be expected in a wound, but the excess fluid is usually reabsorbed or removed in the wound drainage. A haematoma generally results from poor haemostasis and the risk is greatest in patients receiving anticoagulant therapy or with a coagulation disorder. A seroma is often associated with procedures that involve extensive disruption of lymphatic vessels, for example a mastectomy with axillary clearance. The fluid stasis of a haematoma or a seroma provides an excellent environment for bacterial growth; the swelling also increases local pain and prevents good approximation of wound edges. Haematoma or seroma formation may need treatment involving reopening the wound, ligation of any bleeding points, evacuation of the fluid collection, and possibly insertion of a wound drain. Secondary haemorrhage is bleeding from the wound several days after surgery. It is most commonly seen in open wounds, for example after tonsillectomy or tooth extraction.

Wound Failure

In wound failure there is a total or partial disruption of the wound layers, resulting in wound dehiscence in the early stages or an incisional hernia if it occurs later in the healing process. Wound dehiscence can occur at any site, but is probably most common with abdominal incisions. Obesity, heavy coughing, vomiting, or retching, or the development of ascites will increase the strain on an abdominal wound and predispose to wound failure (Hochberg and Murray, 1991). Wound dehiscence is more likely in malnourished patients, patients receiving glucocorticosteroids, and patients with systemic infections, or conditions such as uraemia, liver failure, and diabetes mellitus. With abdominal wound dehiscence there is a risk of evisceration or burst abdomen when the abdominal contents escape through the wound. About one in five cases of burst abdomen result in death. In a normally healing incision it is often possible to identify a ridge or hardened thickening lying about 5 mm from each edge of the incision at about day 5–7. Lack of this feature may be used to identify a wound at risk of dehiscence; leakage of serosanguinous fluid is another strong indicator. However, dehiscence may occur spontaneously during an episode of coughing or vomiting. An incisional hernia may develop weeks to months after surgery. It can be difficult to repair, recurrence is common, and there is a risk of strangulation or obstruction of the bowel segment protruding through the hernia.

Fistulas and Implantation Cysts

Fistulas or tracts can form between internal organs and the skin surface or between two organs, for example the bladder and vagina. Fluid leakage from fistulas can cause extensive skin excoriation and present a major nursing problem.

An implantation cyst forms when epidermal cells are trapped within the healing wound and proliferate to form an epidermal cyst.

Contracture and Adhesions

Adhesions are often a late complication of healing and result from fibrous scarring forming bridges between internal organs. Adhesions can cause problems ranging from discomfort to complete loss of function. Further surgery may be needed to release the adhesions. Contracture occurs when scar tissue contracts producing deformity and loss of function. It is a particular problem across joints or with structures such as the urethra and oesophagus where it can cause strictures.

Abnormal Healing

Infection, foreign bodies, or chronic inflammation may cause an overproduction of connective tissue, resulting in a larger more obvious scar than would have occurred if healing had progressed normally. In some individuals these scars do not resolve, but enlarge, forming hypertrophic and keloid scars. Hypertrophic and keloid scars are most frequently seen after burns in children, but can occur after even minor injury. Keloid scars can develop to become much larger than the original wound. The cause of hypertrophic and keloid scar formation is uncertain, but it has been suggested that genetic factors and infection are contributing factors. Keloid scars are more common after burns, in the head and neck region, in the young, and in patients with dark-coloured skin. Formation of excessive granulation tissue can also be a problem. The excess granulation tissue may protrude into the wound, preventing apposition of the wound edges.

WOUND MANAGEMENT

Nursing care can contribute to wound healing by facilitating the patient's own healing process and by minimizing the impact of local factors that might impede wound healing. Patient-centred approaches are as important as wound-focused care in aiding healing (Torrance, 1987). Wound healing is likely to be improved by promoting nutrition, comfort, rest, sleep, and psychological well-being. There is evidence of increased tissue repair during sleep (Torrance, 1990). Adam and Oswald (1984) have suggested that hypnotic drugs may facilitate tissue restoration by providing uninterrupted sleep. Local wound care is, however, important, and it is essential that any dressings or treatments applied to the wound assist rather than impede the healing processes. Topical applications or a wound dressing applied to an open wound should be prescribed with the same care and scientific rationale as any drug. Wound cleansing, debridement, and dressing are discussed below.

Wound Cleansing

A clean surgical incision removed from any source of contamination such as a stoma requires little intervention. Any dressing put on the wound in theatre can be removed within 48–72 hours and if necessary, the wound sprayed with a plastic dressing spray. Chrintz et al. (1989) advocated early removal of the theatre dressing for ease of inspection. Patients may feel more comfortable without a dressing. Such wounds are sealed and heal well, and Cutting (1990) points out that there is little need to clean them any further. With these wounds less care is often better care. However, wounds often do need cleansing. Such wounds are those with:

- Profuse exudate causing discomfort or hygiene problems.
- Foreign body contamination. Irrigation is often the best method of removing particulate foreign material.
- Gross contamination. Surgical cleansing or debridement may be required.

A simple approach can be adopted. If nothing can be seen in the wound for removal and there are no local or systemic indications of infection, cleansing is not necessary. A clean granulating wound base is unlikely to benefit from swabbing with a saline-soaked gauze. If cleansing is required, the approach will depend on the nature of the contaminant to be removed. Removal of loose material or exudate or the reduction of bacterial contamination is probably best achieved by simple irrigation, and tepid normal saline solution can be used. Mechanical pressure such as swabbing may be needed to loosen and remove more adherent contaminants; slough and necrotic tissue can often be removed using forceps and scissors. Extensive slough or necrosis is likely to require full surgical debridement or lengthy treatment with dressings such as the hydrogels, which facilitate natural debriding processes (phagocytic activity).

A variety of detergent and antiseptic solutions have been advocated for wound cleansing. These solutions will not create a sterile wound environment and may be harmful. Deas *et al.* (1986) have demonstrated that common cleansing agents (chlorhexidine, chlorhexidine with cetrimide, chloramine-T, hydrogen peroxide, and povidone–iodine) have toxic effects on fibroblasts in culture. Brennan and Leaper (1985) have suggested that the toxic effects of the hypochlorite solutions (e.g. Eusol) preclude their clinical use.

Wound Dressings

Clean, incised and sutured wounds usually heal uneventfully by first intention and require minimal care. They should be left undisturbed for the first 48–72 hours and then observed. Wounds healing by secondary intention (granulation) present a more diverse problem. Bale (1993) states that a dressing should be selected depending on the requirements. Selection should be based on:

■ An holistic assessment of the individual.
■ A sound knowledge of the range of products.
■ Assessment of the stage of healing and state of the wound.
■ Identified priorities for local intervention (treatment and dressings).
■ Review and evaluation of previous treatment.

The range of wound treatments and dressings is large and constantly changing. Some of the main types of dressing are presented in *Box 9.6*, but the reader is advised to consult an annually updated source for a full listing of dressings and their use.

Patient Care

The surgical nurse has a central role in caring for a patient with a wound. The nurse will regularly observe the wound, monitor wound drainage, carry out wound cleansing, change dressings, and remove sutures. However, wound care extends beyond the wound itself. For example, observation of vital signs may identify pyrexia due to a wound infection. A patient's reaction to a wound is

Box 9.6 Wound dressings and treatments (categories are adapted from Thomas, 1994; the dressings listed are examples only).

Cleansing or debriding agents
- Polysaccharide bead dressings (e.g. Debrisan beads, paste, and pads, Iodosorb beads and ointment)
- Hydrogel dressing (e.g. Intrasite gel)

Low exudate wounds (superficial)
- Hydrocolloid dressings (e.g. Granuflex Extra Thin)
- Hydrogel dressings (e.g. Spenco 2nd Skin, Geliperm, Vigilon)
- Polyurethane foam dressing (e.g. Lyofoam)
- Semipermeable adhesive film dressings (e.g. Opsite, Opsite Flexigrid, Tegaderm, Bioclusive)

Low to moderate exudate wounds (superficial or full thickness)
- Alginate dressings (e.g. Kaltoclude, Kaltostat, Sorbsan, Sorbsan SA, Tegagel)
- Collagen–alginate dressings (e.g. Fibracol)
- Hydrocolloid dressings (e.g. Biofilm, Comfeel, Granuflex, Granuflex Extra Thin, Tegasorb)
- Polyurethane foam dressing (e.g. Allevyn, Lyofoam, Tielle)

Moderate to high exudate wounds (superficial or full thickness)
- Alginate dressings (e.g. Kaltostat, Sorbsan, Sorbsan Plus, Tegagel)
- Collagen–alginate dressings (e.g. Fibracol)
- Polyurethane foam dressing (e.g. Allevyn, Tielle)

Cavity wounds
- Alginate dressings (e.g. Sorbsan packing, Kaltostat cavity dressing)
- Hydrocolloid dressings (e.g. Comfeel paste, Granuflex paste)
- Hydrogel dressing (e.g. Intrasite gel)
- Polyurethane foam dressing (e.g. Allevyn cavity wound dressing)
- Silicone foam dressing (e.g. Silastic foam)

Sinuses
- Alginate dressings (e.g. Sorbsan ribbon)
- Hydrogel dressing (e.g. Intrasite gel)

Infected wounds
- Medicated dressings (e.g. Bactigras, Inadine, Metrotop, Serotulle, Sofra-Tulle)
- Polysaccharide bead dressings (e.g. Iodosorb beads)
- Semipermeable adhesive film dressings (e.g. Tegaderm Plus)

Wound odour control
- Activated charcoal dressings (e.g. Actisorb Plus, Lyofoam C)
- Medicated dressings (e.g. Metrotop)

variable and a small wound that will be shrugged off by one patient may be of major concern to another. Prominent wounds, facial wounds, and wounds that might be thought to reduce physical or sexual attractiveness can all cause alterations in body image and self-esteem. Some patients may be interested in their wounds and eager to look at them and take part in wound care. Others will be reluctant to view their wounds and will prefer the nurse to carry out wound care and 'cover it up' as quickly as possible. A careful assessment of the individual and the meaning or impact of the wound is important. Anxiety or fear of the wound may be reduced if the site, extent, and appearance of the wound has been discussed with the patient before surgery. Certainly the patient will need to be reassured that the angry-looking raised early wound will usually resolve and fade to a thin pale line. If the wound is likely to be intrusive, for example after mastectomy, genital surgery, or facial surgery it may help if the patient can talk to a specialist nurse or counsellor from an appropriate support organization.

Patients' involvement in their own wound care can be helpful. They will need information both in the preoperative and postoperative period about the role of personal hygiene and handwashing in reducing wound infection. They will want to know when and how they can wash, bathe, or shower, how to manage drains and drainage bottles, how much wound pain they will experience, whether dressing changes, and drain or suture removal will hurt, whether lifting or carrying will open up the incision, when they can dispense with the dressing and resume a normal life. The surgical nurse will need to be prepared to answer these questions with regard to the type, size, and position of the wound, method of wound closure, and the patient's occupation and lifestyle.

Effective management of wound pain, particularly at dressing changes, will assist in relieving anxiety and help the patient adjust to the wound. Graffam (1979) suggested that nurses should assess the patient's pain before dressing procedures and plan pain-relieving strategies with the patient. Hollinworth (1995) recommends the use of a simple visual analogue scale in combination with an assessment chart incorporating pain and wound assessment. An analgesic prescribed for general pain relief can be given before dressing changes, or analgesia such as nitrous oxide and oxygen (Entonox) may be prescribed specifically for use at dressing changes. Nitrous oxide and oxygen provides rapid, safe, patient-administered pain relief with no measurable adverse effects (Baskett and Bennett, 1971). Patient participation during dressing changes should be encouraged, and where suitable, patients can be taught appropriate relaxation and distraction techniques to control their pain. All information obtained during assessment of the patient's pain and the interventions used that effectively relieve the problem must be clearly documented.

WOUND DRAINAGE

Surgical drains are used to aid the removal of fluids such as exudate, blood, pus, and other body fluids that can collect in cavities or dead spaces within a wound

(Torrance, 1993). Fluid accumulation and stasis predispose to infection and drainage reduces this risk and allows closer tissue apposition. Drainage may be passive (draining by gravity or capillary action) or active (using a suction or vacuum system) (*Figure 9.9*). Dougherty and Simmons (1992) have suggested three main categories of wound drainage:

■ Therapeutic drainage.
■ Prophylactic drainage.
■ Decompressive drainage.

Therapeutic drainage has three objectives:

■ The removal of bacteria, dead tissue, pus, and other infected material.
■ The removal of excess inflammatory mediators, phagocytic enzymes, and other elements of the inflammatory response found in wound exudate.

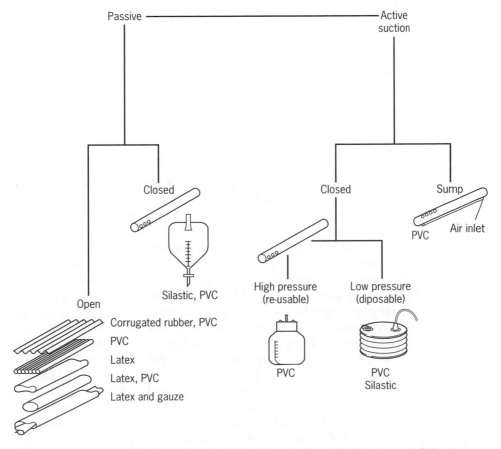

Figure 9.9 Wound drains. (Reproduced with kind permission of *British Journal of Nursing*, Mark Allen Publishing Ltd.)

Removal of these excess elements will reduce further tissue damage and aid healing (Dougherty and Simmons, 1992).

■ Reduce dead space and the risk of abscess formation or recurrence.

Techniques for therapeutic drainage include needle aspiration, catheter aspiration, incision and drainage, incision and curettage, and complete surgical excision.

Prophylactic drainage is intended to prevent infection, but this practice has been largely replaced by the use of antibiotics. A surgical drain can act like a foreign body, providing a surface for bacterial adhesion and a tract for ascending infection, so there is little justification for the routine use of prophylactic drainage and the practice has generally been abandoned.

Decompressive drainage is used to prevent fluid accumulation in, or leakage from, the wound. The drain removes serous fluid and blood from the wound, thus reducing the possibility of seroma or haematoma formation; the drain also serves to obliterate dead spaces. Decompressive drainage is used to prevent leakage of fluid such as urine, bile, intestinal, and pancreatic fluids.

It should, however, be noted that the use of drains is often controversial as wound drains can cause complications (see below). In a trial of suction drainage after thyroid surgery the 'no-drain' group suffered no more complications than the 'with drain' group (Wihlborg et al., 1988). Conversely a trial of suction drainage of the axilla found that it did help reduce the problem of seroma (Cameron et al., 1988).

Types of Drains

Drains come in a range of materials and types from a simple gauze wick to more complex closed-circuit systems. There are capillary, simple tubular, multitubular, corrugated, suction, or sump drains. Drains may be made out of red rubber, silicone rubber, latex, and polyvinyl chloride (PVC). Drains can be made with open blunt ends or rounded ends with single or multiple drainage holes. They may drain into a dressing, into a collecting bag, or into a drainage bottle.

Passive drainage may be open into a dressing or collecting bag placed over the wound, or closed into a collecting bag or bottle connected directly to the drain. Open passive drainage is usually used with a simple tubular or rubber wick type of drain; closed systems are used with tubular or catheter-style drains. For passive drainage the drain is inserted at an upward angle and is usually secured to the patient's skin by a single suture. Gravity or capillary action draws fluid into the dressing or collecting bag. In open passive drainage, exudate is collected into a dressing or drainage bag by a gauze wick or pack, a simple sheet drain (such as corrugated rubber or plastic cut to the right size), or a tube drain. The suture must be cut before the drain is removed. Skin irritation or erosion can occur if wound fluid has prolonged contact with the skin.

Active drainage depends on vacuum or suction for drainage. Vacuum or suction can be achieved by using a continuous action pump, but modern systems often use pre-evacuated drainage bottles, compressible bulbs, or concertina evacuators (air is expelled by squeezing the bulb or concertina before attaching it to the drain). Vacuum systems can be used with a range of drains, but the drains used in suction systems tend to be more rigid. The bore of the drain and number and placement of drainage holes will depend on the expected type of drainage. Narrow-bore tubes are more easily blocked, but a larger tube will cause more tissue erosion.

Complications of Surgical Drainage

Surgical drains should not be viewed as innocuous (Hochberg and Murray, 1991); they are associated with a variety of risks, and these may be increased if the wrong type of drain is used or the drain is inappropriately managed (Torrance, 1993). The complications are summarized in *Box 9.7*, and generally can be classed as:

Box 9.7 Complications of surgical drainage (Dougherty and Simmons, 1992).

Foreign body effects
- Inflammation
- Bacterial adherence
- Ascending infection
- Haemorrhage
- Fistula formation
- Perforation
- Obstruction
- Impaired healing

Mechanical effects and problems
- Tissue ingrowth
- Herniation of visceral tissue through drain tract
- Movement or misplacement
- Breakage or accidental removal
- Kinking or obstruction
- Wrong type of drain or drainage

Physiological impairment and disruption
- Pain
- Fluid and electrolyte loss
- Decompression effects (e.g. in brain or lung)
- Pneumothorax

- Those associated with the drain as a foreign body.
- Mechanical effects and problems.
- Physiological impairment and disruption.

Nursing Management of Drains

There is a variety of reasons for using wound drains, and the range of drains and drainage systems is large. Before planning nursing care of the patient with a drain it is essential to establish:

- The type of drain.
- The internal location of the drain (where is it draining?).
- The exit point.
- How it is secured.
- Whether it is passive or active drainage.
- The drainage system.
- The patency or level of suction in active drainage.

Observation and careful handling are central to managing wound drains. The colour, amount, nature, and viscosity of the drainage fluid is recorded. Excessive drainage, changes in the type of fluid observed (particularly fresh bleeding), or cessation of drainage should be recorded and reported. Drains, drainage bags, and bottles have to be well secured to prevent accidental removal and provide easy observation for kinking or obstruction of the tubing. The drain site should be observed for signs of inflammation or damage from leaking exudate. An aseptic approach is essential when handling drains or components of a drainage system. Closed systems are best left undisturbed, but a vacuum evacuator should be checked to ensure an adequate vacuum. If there is a large volume of exudate bottles should be changed, the drain may need to be clipped shut, and a fresh sterile bottle attached using aseptic techniques. Passive drains may require regular shortening as the wound cavity heals from the base up. The retaining stitch is removed and 1–2 cm of drain withdrawn. A sterile safety pin is used to prevent the drain slipping back into the wound. Drains can be tricky to handle with forceps and using sterile gloves may be more convenient for the nurse and easier on the patient.

Drains are one of the more visible signs of surgery and can be of major concern to the patient. The surgical nurse needs to help the patient understand why the drain is there and to explain how it will be managed. Patients will need practical assistance in learning how to cope with the drain, to ensure it remains patent, effective, and aseptic, and to ensure that their mobility is not unnecessarily restricted. Patients will want to know how long the drain will be in place and how it will be removed. The length of time the drain is left in the wound will depend on the purpose of the drain and the volume of drainage. When a drain is to be removed it is important to explain the procedure fully and ensure adequate pain relief (oral, injected, or inhaled analgesia may be required). Drains are removed using an aseptic technique. Usually the vacuum is released to reduce trauma to the tissues as the drain is pulled out. The retaining suture is cut and the drain is smoothly and firmly pulled out. Difficulty in withdrawing the drain or excessive pain may indicate adhesion and medical advice should be sought. Care is essential when handling drains, drainage bottles, and drainage fluid. As with any body fluid wound exudate represents a biological hazard and carries the risk of transmitting a variety of diseases. Wound drains are disposed of as clinical waste. The final volume of drainage is recorded before it is discarded. The drain site will require a sterile dressing and should be observed for leakage or bleeding. The patient is advised to report any persistent pain at the drain site.

WOUND CLOSURE AND SUTURES

Selecting appropriate sutures and needles is important in minimizing tissue trauma while ensuring adequate apposition and support for the tissues. Sutures hold together or close internal structures, hold the wound layers together, and close the skin. Sutures for internal use are often made of an absorbable material such as catgut. The rate of absorption depends on the material used: plain catgut is absorbed in about ten days; chromic catgut (catgut treated with chromium salts) in about 20 days (Hochberg and Murray, 1991). Skin sutures are made of a variety of nonabsorbable materials such as nylon, cotton, and silk. *Box 9.8* lists some common suture materials and their properties. Wounds can also be closed by surgical staples, tapes, and adhesives.

Suturing Methods (*Figure 9.10*)

It is essential that the surgical nurse knows the suturing method used and how this will affect suture removal. The primary suture line is made up of the

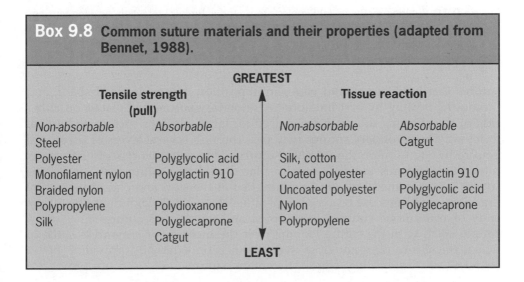

Box 9.8 Common suture materials and their properties (adapted from Bennet, 1988).

Tensile strength (pull)		GREATEST	Tissue reaction	
Non-absorbable	*Absorbable*		*Non-absorbable*	*Absorbable*
Steel				Catgut
Polyester	Polyglycolic acid		Silk, cotton	
Monofilament nylon	Polyglactin 910		Coated polyester	Polyglactin 910
Braided nylon			Uncoated polyester	Polyglycolic acid
Polypropylene	Polydioxanone		Nylon	Polyglecaprone
Silk	Polyglecaprone		Polypropylene	
	Catgut	LEAST		

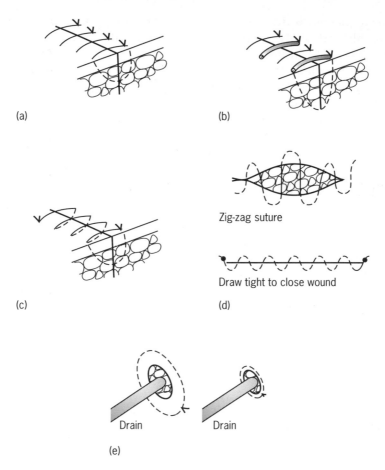

(a)

(b)

Zig-zag suture

Draw tight to close wound

(c)

(d)

Drain   Drain

(e)

Figure 9.10 Suturing methods. (a) Simple, interrupted suture; (b) retention, or deep tension, sutures – used to reinforce primary sutures line, may be inserted deep into fascia or muscle; (c) continuous suture; (d) subcuticular suture; (e) purse string suture, stitches run parallel to circular wound – often used to stitch wound drains in place.

sutures that hold the wound edges in apposition, removing dead space, and promoting healing by first intention. A secondary suture line placed on either side of the primary sutures may be used for large incisions such as abdominal incisions. The secondary sutures may pass through several layers of tissue and help reduce tension on the primary sutures, decreasing the risk of dehiscence. Interrupted sutures are individually placed and tied sutures. A continuous suture line is formed by a single suture tied at the start and end of the suture line. Some surgeons use beads or clips rather than simple knotting to tie off the ends of continuous sutures. Interrupted and continuous sutures may use a simple stitch with the suture looping over the incision, or a mattress stitch in which the suture does not cross over the incision externally, providing better eversion of the healing edges. Retention sutures are used to provide a secondary interrupted suture line at some distance from the primary sutures. Retention sutures support all the wound layers; strong nonabsorbable sutures such as steel, heavy silk, or nylon are used and the suture is tied with some tension. To prevent the suture cutting into the skin the exposed section of the suture is placed in a small piece of plastic tubing. A subcuticular suture is a continuous suture placed under the epidermis of the skin with only the ends exposed. A purse-string suture is a single continuous suture placed around a circular opening or structure.

Surgical staples are now widely used for both internal and external closure. Harris and Graham (1992) list five types of stapling devices:

- Linear stapling devices.
- Linear cutters.
- Intraluminal stapling devices.
- Skin closure devices.
- Mechanical ligators.

Surgical stapling is advancing rapidly, and absorbable staples are becoming available. The use of staples for skin closure produces excellent cosmetic results, but staple removal requires a special removal device designed for that specific type of staple.

Adhesive skin tapes are also used to close wounds. They have the advantage of holding wound edges together without the need to puncture the skin surface and are particularly useful for minor wounds in casualty and with children. They can also be left in place for much longer than sutures or staples. Skin tapes can also be used after suture removal to give some additional support. Tapes may be simple strips or in butterfly forms, which can be applied with a little more tension. However, tape may not produce effective eversion of the wound edges and can easily become loose if moistened by blood or exudate. Skin tapes can be particularly valuable when combined with subcuticular sutures.

Surgical adhesives such as autologous fibrin glue, fibrin seal adhesive, and cyanoacrilate are being used and developed (Hochberg and Murray, 1991) for internal closure. Autologous fibrin glue has been used with some success to hold skin grafts in place instead of suturing and pressure dressings (Saltz *et al.*, 1989).

Removal of Sutures and Staples

The timing of removal of skin sutures or staples varies depending on the type and the wound. Fine sutures used in facial surgery may be removed within three days, but most sutures are removed within 7–10 days of surgery. Retention sutures, however, may be left for 14–21 days. Removal is an aseptic technique. Sutures are removed using a curved suture-removing blade or a pair of suture scissors. Staples are removed with a special disposable instrument that squeezes the centre of the clip to remove it from the skin. All the sutures may be removed at one session or it may be requested that only alternate sutures are removed. The procedure is explained to the patient. Suture and staple removal may be uncomfortable, but is not generally regarded as painful or requiring analgesia.

Simple interrupted sutures are removed by gripping the suture and raising it slightly so it can be cut as close to the skin as possible directly under the knot (*Figure 9.11a*). The suture is cut, gripped under the knot, pulled out in one piece, and inspected carefully to ensure that the entire suture has been removed. If the suture is not cut close to the skin, the exposed suture will be drawn through the

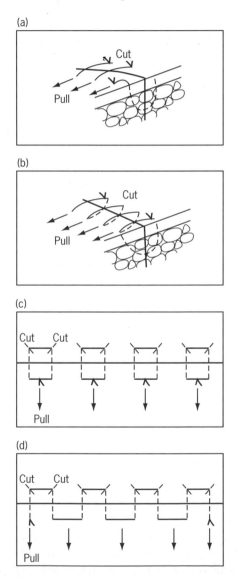

Figure 9.11 Suture removal. (a) Simple interrupted sutures. (b) Simple continuous suture. (c) Mattress interrupted suture. (d) Mattress continuous suture.

suture tract with the risk of wound contamination. Suture material left in the skin can act as a foreign body and cause infection. Alternate sutures are removed and then if there is no sign of the incision separating, the remaining sutures can be removed. If the wound tends to split open where the sutures have been removed the remaining sutures should be retained for 48 hours, and the wound inspected again. Slight wound dehiscence can be treated by applying a sterile 'butterfly' tape to hold the wound edges together and promote healing. (Kozier *et al.*, 1995). Simple continuous sutures are removed in a similar way, taking great care not to leave any part of the suture in the skin (*Figure 9.11b*). Mattress stitches require two cuts opposite the knot to remove the visible part of the suture (*Figure 9.11c,d*). A subcuticular suture is removed by cutting under the knot or bead at one end and pulling the suture out at the opposite end.

References

Adam K, Oswald I (1984) Sleep helps healing. *Br Med J* **289**:1400–1401.

Bale S (1993) Intervention in wound management. *Surg Nurse* **6(3)**:17–20.

Barton A, Barton M (1981) *The Management and Prevention of Pressure Sores*, p. 40. Faber and Faber, London.

Baskett PJF, Bennett JA (1971) Pain relief in hospital: the more widespread use of nitrous oxide. *Br Med J* **2**:509–511.

Bennet RG (1988) Selection of wound closure materials. *J Am Acad Dermatol* **18**:619.

Brennan SS, Leaper DJ (1985) The effects of antiseptics on the healing wound: a study using the rabbit ear chamber. *Br J Surg* **72**:708–782.

Cameron AEP, Ebbs SR, Wylie F, Baum M (1988) Suction drainage of axilla: a prospective randomized trial. *Br J Surg* **75**:1211.

Chrintz H, Vibits H, Cordtz TO, Harreby JS, Waaddegaard P, Larsen SO (1989) Need for surgical wound dressing. *Br J Surg* **76**:204–205.

Cutting K (1990) Wound cleansing. *Surg Nurse* **3(3)**:4–6.

Dealey C (1991) Assessment of wounds. *Nursing* **4(27)**:23–24.

Deas J, Billings P, Brennan S, Silver I, Leaper D (1986) The toxicity of commonly used antiseptics on fibroblasts in tissue culture. *Phlebology* **1**:205–209.

Dougherty SH, Simmons RL (1992) The biology and practice of surgical drainage. Part 1. *Curr Probl Surg* **29**:561–623.

Foster ME, Williams P (1994) Wound healing – a surgical perspective. *J Wound Care* **3(3)**:135–138.

Graffam S (1979) Nurse response to patients in pain: an analysis and imperative for action. *Nurse Leadership* **2(3)**:23–25.

Harris DR, Graham TR (1992) Surgical stapling devices. *Surgery* **10** (Sutures suppl.):1–8.

Hochberg J, Murray GF (1991) Principles of operative surgery: antisepsis, techniques, sutures and drains. In *Textbook of Surgery*, 14th edition. Sabiston DC (ed.) pp. 210–220. WB Saunders, Philadelphia.

Hollinworth H (1995) Nurses' assessment and management of pain at wound dressing changes. *J Wound Care* **2(2)**:77–83.

Hunt TK, Conolly WB, Aronson SB, Goldstein P (1978) Anaerobic metabolism and wound healing. A hypothesis for the initiation and cessation of collagen synthesis in wounds. *Am J Surg* **135**:328.

Johnson A (1988) Criteria for ideal wound dressings. *Prof Nurse* **3(6)**:191–193.

Kozier B, Erb G, Blais K, Wilkinson J (1995) *Fundamentals of Nursing*, 5th edition, pp. 1380–1382. Addison-Wesley, Reading, MA.

Pinchcofsky-Devin RD (1994) Nutrition and wound healing. *J Wound Care* **3(5)**:231–234.

Porth C (1990) *Pathophysiology. Concepts of Altered Health States*. 3rd edition, p. 175. JB Lippincott, Philadelphia.

Rigby H (1992a) Tissue healing, Part 1. *Surgery* **10(11)**:261–264.

Rigby H (1992b) Tissue healing, Part 2. *Surgery* **10(12)**:286–288.

Saltz R, Dimick A, Harris C, Grotting JC, Psillakis J, Vasconez LO (1989) Application of autologous fibrin glue in burn wounds. *J Burn Care Rehabil* **10**:504–507.

Siana JE, Frankild S, Gottrup F (1992) The effect of smoking on tissue function. *J Wound Care* **1(2)**:37–39.

Smeltzer SC, Bare BG (1992) Wound classification. In *Textbook of Medical–Surgical Nursing*. Smeltzer SC, Bare BG (eds), 7th edition, p. 450. JB Lippincott, Philadelphia.

Thomas S (1994) *A Handbook of Surgical Dressings*. The Surgical Materials Testing Laboratory, Bridgend.

Torrance C (1985) The physiology of wound healing. Wound Care in Accident and Emergency Supplement. *Nursing* **2(42)**(Suppl.):1–3.

Torrance C (1987) Chronic wounds patient care versus wound care. *Care Science and Practice* **5(1)**:10–13.

Torrance C (1990) Sleep and wound healing. *Surg Nurse* **3(2)**:12–14.

Torrance C (1993) Introduction to surgical drainage. *Surg Nurse* **6(2)**:19–23.

Turner TD, Stevens P (1982) Which dressing and why? *J Wound Care* No. 11, *Nurs Times* **78(29)**:41–44.

Whitby DJ (1995) The biology of wound healing. *Surgery* **13(2)**:25–28.

Wihlborg O, Bergijung L, Martensson H (1988) To drain or not to drain in thyroid surgery. *Arch Surg* **123**:40–41.

Chapter 10
Day Surgery

CONTENTS

- ❏ The Day Surgery Unit
- ❏ Patient Selection
- ❏ Day Surgery Procedures
- ❏ Nursing Management

Day surgery is becoming an increasingly popular option for short surgical procedures on relatively fit patients. Jarrett (1995) reported that from 1992 to 1993 day cases made up 21.7% of elective surgery in the UK. The corresponding figure for the USA was 53.8%, and 25% for the Australian state of New South Wales. The Royal College of Surgeons (1992a) has stated that 'day surgery is now considered the best option for 50% of all patients undergoing elective surgical procedures, though the proportion will vary between specialities.' The advantages for the patient are:

- Short stay and reduced disruption to the patient.
- Shorter waiting time for 'minor' surgery.
- Little risk of cancellation.
- Decreased risk of cross-infection.

The advantages to the health system are mainly economic and include:

- Increased efficiency and use of resources.
- Little risk of cancellation, so more efficient scheduling.
- Reduced staffing needs.
- Reduced waiting lists.
- Shorter stay in hospital.
- Release of inpatient beds.
- Increased patient satisfaction.

Day surgery cannot, however, be viewed as a cheap alternative in terms of facilities and staff training. It has to be effectively organized and requires efficient administration, and to gain full patient and economic advantages from this approach, appropriate selection of patients and surgical procedures (Reilly,

1991). Not every patient or every short procedure will be suitable as a day case. The main disadvantage for patients is the need for another adult to be available to escort them home and help care for them in the first 24–48 hours after surgery. For the staff, the main problem may be the need for experienced staff and reduced opportunities for junior staff to gain 'hands on experience' (Jarrett, 1995).

THE DAY SURGERY UNIT

The day case unit is usually attached to a general hospital with full back-up services. It should have a reception area, dedicated rooms or cubicles, and its own anaesthetic room, theatre, and recovery room, or be situated near the main theatre suite. Ideally it is located on the ground floor with its own entrance. Equipment and facilities in the patient care areas and operating theatre must be of the same standard as that required for general surgery. The unit will need to be equipped with oxygen, suction, and emergency equipment such as a crash trolley. Day patients need to be observed in the recovery room until it is safe to return them to the day unit for postoperative care.

PATIENT SELECTION

Appropriate patient selection is the key to successful day surgery (Reilly, 1991; Jarrett, 1995). A detailed medical history should be available and a full physical examination is required. The anaesthetic assessment and preoperative screening will be the same as for conventional surgery. Ogg (1976) developed a simple questionnaire that can be used to check essential details of the patient's medical and drug history (*Box 10.1*). The American Society of Anaesthesiologists (ASA) classification system can be used to assess preoperative health status and suitability for anaesthesia and day surgery. The ASA (1963) classification is:

- Class I:　normal, healthy patient.
- Class II:　patient with mild to moderate systemic disease associated with the surgical condition or caused by any other disease.
- Class III: severe systemic disease or disturbance of any origin.
- Class IV: severe systemic life-threatening disorders.
- Class V:　moribund patient unlikely to survive for more than 24 hours.

Only patients in ASA classes I and II are likely to be suitable for day surgery. *Box 10.2* lists some common problems that usually preclude day surgery. The elderly are suitable candidates for day surgery provided the same criteria for preoperative screening as applied to hospitalized patients are also applied, for example chest X-ray, ECG, and biochemical and haematological tests (Reilly, 1991). It is important to ensure when admitting patients for day surgery that they

Box 10.1 Preoperative assessment questionnaire (Ogg, 1976).

1. Have you or your family had any problems connected with anaesthesia or operations?   Yes   No

2. Are you allergic or sensitive to anything?   Yes   No

3. Have you suffered any recent illness from which you do not feel fully recovered (colds, cough, etc.)   Yes   No

4. Have you ever suffered from heart disease, high blood pressure, chest disease, bronchitis, asthma, a bleeding tendency, jaundice, rheumatic fever, tuberculosis?

   Yes   No

If yes please specify..

5. Are you having, or have you had in the past year, any form of medicine, tablets, injections, inhalers, etc. including tranquillizers, sedatives, antibiotics, cortisone or steroids, and drugs for epilepsy, high blood pressure, diabetes, thyroid disease, asthma, and bronchitis?   Yes   No

If yes please specify..

6. Do you have any crowned teeth, wear dentures, wear contact lenses?

7. Any woman patient who is, or thinks she is pregnant must let the anaesthetist know.

8. Is there anything else you feel the anaesthetist should know?.......................

   ....

9. When did you last have anything to eat or drink?...

   (Applicable only if form is completed on day of appointment)

have an escort home and a family member or friend to look after them for the first 24–48 hours postoperatively. Inadequate social support or problems with access to a telephone, toilet, and bathroom can also be contraindications for day surgery. The patient should live within 20 miles of the day surgery unit (Murphy, 1994).

Murphy (1994) describes a pre-surgery assessment clinic that is an integral part of the day surgery unit. Patients are referred to the assessment clinic after an outpatient surgical assessment. The patient is interviewed by the assessment clinic nurse to establish suitability for day surgery, using agreed protocols and guidelines. Murphy lists the functions of the pre-surgery assessment clinic as:

■ To assess suitability for day surgery (using clinic guidelines and ASA classification)

> ## Box 10.2 Contraindications to day surgery (adapted from Reilly, 1991).
>
> **General**
> - Unfit (not ASA class I or II)
> - Obese (body mass index greater than 35)
> - Operation longer than one hour
> - No escort or no competent adult available for first 24–48 hours
> - Psychologically unsuitable or day surgery unacceptable to the patient
> - Previous problems with anaesthetics (e.g. vomiting, intubation problems, poor venous access)
> - Drug therapy that might complicate anaesthesia or analgesia (e.g. monoamine oxidase inhibitors, pethidine)
>
> **Cardiovascular and haematological**
> - Hypertension, family history of malignant hypertension
> - Angina
> - Cardiac failure
> - Recent myocardial infarction (within last six months)
> - Anaemia
> - Anticoagulant therapy
> - Coagulation disorders
>
> **Respiratory**
> - Acute respiratory infection
> - Asthma
> - Chronic obstructive airways disease
>
> **Endocrine**
> - Diabetes mellitus
> - Glucocorticosteroid therapy
>
> **Musculoskeletal**
> - Kyphoscoliosis
> - Arthritis of jaw or neck
> - Neuromuscular disorder

- To carry out preoperative investigations and screen results (full blood count, urea and electrolytes, electrocardiography, chest radiography).
- To carry out preoperative preparation with written and verbal information and advice.
- To provide date for surgery or admission to waiting list.
- To refer to inpatient services if appropriate.

■ To refer to general practitioner (for treatment of conditions such as anaemia or hypertension that currently precludes day surgery).
■ To assess vital signs, and record height and weight.
■ To promote health and wellbeing.

Murphy (1994) observed that the non-attendance rate on the day of surgery was much higher for patients who had not experienced the pre-surgery assessment clinic.

DAY SURGERY PROCEDURES

A wide range of procedures from many surgical specialities can be performed as day cases (*Box 10.3*). The Royal College of Surgeon's (1992b) guidelines suggest that a procedure suitable for day surgery will last about 30 minutes, with a maximum time limit of 60 minutes. As with minimal access surgery there is a positive link between duration of operation and postoperative complications. Linked with this is the need for experienced medical and nursing staff. Viewing day surgery as minor is not justified. Inexperienced surgeons or anaesthetists can take significantly longer to perform 'routine' procedures. Suitably qualified operating room, recovery, and day unit nurses are equally essential. The NHS Management Executive (1991) stated that 'The nursing skills required for work in day surgery units differed from those required on an inpatient basis.' Hodge (1994), commenting on nurse education for day surgery noted that 'nurses in this speciality need to be expert communicators and carers and must be able to develop a rapport with their patients in a short period of time.' The availability of suitably qualified and experienced staff will be critical in deciding if a particular procedure can be carried out safely as day surgery.

NURSING MANAGEMENT

Preoperative preparation will start before the patient presents for surgery. The patient will usually have been assessed as an outpatient and should have received a detailed explanation of the procedure and the requirements of day surgery. Before admission the patient should be sent clear, written instructions detailing:

■ The surgical procedure.
■ Preoperative fasting time.
■ Time of arrival at the day unit.
■ Assistance in the first 24 hours postoperatively.
■ Arrival and discharge travel arrangements.
■ Avoidance of driving and operating machinery.
■ Analgesia and drug requirements.

Box 10.3 Procedures suitable for day surgery (adapted from Reilly, 1991 and Hodge, 1994).

General surgery
- Hernia repair (inguinal, femoral, umbilical, para-umbilical, epigastric)
- Varicose veins (ligation and stripping)
- Anal stretch or anal fissure
- Excision of cysts, sebaceous cysts, skin tags, benign tumours
- Excision of breast lumps
- Removal of naevus, mole, papilloma
- Removal of lipoma
- Pilonidal sinus

Orthopaedic surgery
- Carpal tunnel release
- Dupuytren's contracture surgery
- Injection of glucocorticosteroids
- Ingrown toenails
- Excision of exostosis
- Interphalangeal fusion of toes
- Arthroscopic menisectomy
- Removal of plates, pins, wires, and screws
- Trigger finger release
- Arthroscopy
- Amputation of a digit
- Removal of neuroma
- Excision of bursa
- Tenotomy
- Ganglionectomy

Urological surgery
- Circumcision
- Hydrocoele surgery
- Vasectomy or vasectomy reversal
- Urethral dilatation
- Testicular biopsy
- Division of penile adhesions
- Cystoscopy
- Excision of epididymal cyst
- Renal biopsy
- Varicocoele surgery
- Penile wart diathermy
- Urodynamic studies

Paediatric surgery
- Circumcision

- Hydrocoele surgery
- Orchidopexy
- Inguinal herniotomy
- Umbilical hernia repair

Gynaecological surgery
- Dilatation and curettage
- Laparoscopy
- Colposcopy
- Cautery or laser treatment of cervix
- Excision of Bartholin's cyst
- Termination of pregnancy
- Laparoscopic sterilization
- Cervical polypectomy
- Removal of vulval warts or cysts

Ear, nose, and throat surgery
- Myringotomy
- Direct laryngoscopy or pharyngoscopy
- Submucosal resection
- Antral washout
- Insertion of grommets
- Reduction of nasal fracture
- Submucosal diathermy of turbinates
- Removal of foreign bodies

Dental surgery
- Dental clearance
- Extraction of wisdom teeth
- Other routine extractions requiring general anaesthesia

Plastic surgery
- Correction of bat ears
- Breast augmentation
- Nipple and areola reconstruction
- Z-plasties
- Blepharoplasty
- Insertion of tissue expanders
- Excision of skin lesions
- Urethral meatotomy and dilatation

Ophthalmic surgery
- Cataract surgery
- Correction of squint

On arrival in the unit the patient is admitted and a nursing assessment made, concentrating on preoperative risk factors, the patient's understanding of the operative procedure, organization of discharge arrangements, and postoperative care. As the patients are relatively healthy, nursing should be able to focus on preoperative anxiety, knowledge deficits, and planning postoperative care. The nurse will need to ensure that informed consent has been completed before carrying out the usual preoperative preparation and checks. Day surgery may be performed under local or general anaesthesia. The choice of anaesthesia should reflect the need for rapid reversal of the anaesthetic and the expectation of same day discharge.

On return to the unit the patient will require observation, rest, and then preparation for discharge. Observation is essential, as 2–4% of day patients are likely to require overnight admission (Reilly, 1991). *Table 10.1* lists some simple indications for delayed discharge or overnight admission. Appropriate pain relief in the immediate postoperative period is essential, and in addition the patient and carer will need guidance on pain control after discharge. Oral analgesia, paracetamol, codeine, ibuprofen or other non-steroidal anti-inflammatory drugs (NSAIDs) are usually recommended. Printed instructions of postoperative needs and a list of 'dos and don'ts,' will help, but it is also essential that the nurse discusses these with the patient and carer. Such printed instructions cannot cover every eventuality and patients will usually have additional anxieties, questions, and problems that need to be discussed. It is particularly important that the patient is alerted to any postoperative symptoms or signs that require medical advice. They need to be told when to contact the unit or their general practitioner if there are postoperative problems.

The skills required for nursing in a day surgery unit are not the same as for inpatient care. The nurse has little time to assess the patient and establish a rapport: Hodge (1994) estimated an average of only four hours. The key skills identified by Hodge for the day surgery nurse are:

■ Assessment for safe patient selection.

Table 10.1 Indications for overnight admission (adapted from Reilly, 1991).

Problem	Action
No escort home or overnight carer	Admit
Bleeding	Delay discharge, reassess, admit if not resolved
Pain relief not effective	Delay discharge, reassess, admit if not resolved
Nausea or vomiting	Give antiemetic, reassess, admit if not resolved
Unable to tolerate oral fluids	Delay discharge, reassess, admit if not resolved
Not able to walk without staggering	Delay discharge, reassess, admit if not resolved
Unable to dress	Delay discharge, reassess, admit if not resolved

- Anaesthesiology.
- Theatre technique and management.
- Postoperative recovery.
- Surgical nursing care.
- Information provision and education.
- Supporting patients and carers.
- Liaison with primary care team.

References

American Society of Anesthesiologists (1963) New classification of physical status. *Anesthesiology* **24**:111–112.

Hodge D (1994) Introduction to day surgery. *Surg Nurse* **7(2)**:12–16.

Jarrett PEM (1995) Day case surgery. *Surgery* **13(1)**:5–7.

Murphy SJ (1994) Preoperative assessment for day surgery. *Surg Nurse* **7(3)**:6–9.

NHS Management Executive (1991) Day Surgery, Making it Happen, p. 31. HMSO, London.

Ogg TW (1976) Assessment of preoperative cases. *Br Med J* **1**:82–83.

Reilly CS (1991) Day case surgery. *Surgery* **98**:2332–2335.

Royal College of Surgeons for England (1992a) *Commission on the Provision of Surgical Services. Guidelines for Day Case Surgery*, p. 2. Revised edition. Royal College of Surgeons, London.

Royal College of Surgeons for England (1992b) *Commission on the Provision of Surgical Services. Guidelines for Day Case Surgery*, p. 8. Revised edition. Royal College of Surgeons, London.

Chapter 11

Minimal Access Surgery

Minimal access surgery (MAS) aims to achieve the same outcome as an open surgical operation, but reduce the trauma of access while maintaining the view of the area of the body under treatment (Cushieri, 1993b). Although Troidle (1990) noted that urologists, gynaecologists, and other surgical specialists had used endoscopes for years to assist diagnosis. In 1990 Dubois *et al.* reported that thirty-six patients had undergone coelioscopic cholecystectomy with few complications. The value of MAS now appears to be gaining recognition. With the rapid pace of development in the fields of medical imaging, fibreoptics, and computer-aided instrumentation, it is likely that MAS procedures will eventually replace many open surgical procedures. MAS is not confined to minor surgery. Major surgery such as coronary artery grafting procedures are performed by a minimal access technique. Although the visible effects of the operation on the patient are minimal, the surgery should still be considered major and full provision made for postoperative recovery, observation, and care. This chapter discusses the perceived benefits of MAS and examples of where it can be used. The perioperative care from the time patients are admitted until their discharge will be considered, including factors related to the anaesthetic. Possible complications of MAS are explored, and the chapter concludes with a short review of the use of lasers in MAS.

Some of the procedures currently carried out using minimal access approaches are listed in *Box 11.1*.

The approach may be:

■ Laparoscopic.
■ Endoluminal.
■ Perivisceral.
■ Intra-articular.

Box 11.1 Examples of MAS procedures.

General Surgery
- Laparoscopic cholecystectomy
- Laparoscopic cholangiogram
- Laparoscopic exploration of the common bile duct
- Laparoscopic appendicectomy
- Laparoscopic herniorrhaphy
- Laparoscopic colectomy

Gynaecology
- Laparoscopic treatment of hypermenorrhoea
- Laparoscopic-assisted vaginal hysterectomy
- Laparoscopic myomectomy
- Laparoscopic bladder repair

Urinary tract surgery
- Laparoscopic percutaneous nephrolithotomy
- Laparoscopic insertion or removal of stents
- Laparoscopic ureteroscopy
- Laparoscopic nephrectomy
- Laparoscopic prostatectomy

Vascular surgery
- Atherectomy
- Balloon angioplasty
- Laser angioplasty

Orthopaedic surgery
- Arthroscopy (e.g. knee, shoulder)
- Synovectomy

MAS is usually performed because it is thought to be 'patient-friendly' surgery (Troidle, 1993), with more advantages and fewer risks than the conventional approaches. Some of the benefits of MAS include:

- Accelerated recovery.
- Decreased postoperative pain.
- Reduction in the size of the operation scar.
- No risk of incisional hernia.
- Less trauma inflicted on the body.
- Less stress exerted on the body.
- Shorter stay in hospital.
- Earlier return to full activity.

MAS reduces the visible signs of surgery and shortens the time spent as an inpatient during postoperative recovery. This results in some major changes in the delivery of perioperative nursing care. The time available for both pre-operative preparation, postoperative care, and discharge planning are likely to be markedly reduced. Achieving adequate levels of patient preparation and understanding may involve more innovative techniques in preoperative assessment, preparation, and information delivery.

PERIOPERATIVE CARE

The nurse's role is to provide quality patient care appropriate to the needs of the individual patient. Actual and potential problems are identified, goals set in conjunction with the patient, and nursing care planned and implemented. The results of this care can then be evaluated. In common with conventional surgery, MAS imposes a physical and mental stress on patients. Nursing research has repeatedly demonstrated that these stresses can be reduced by giving preoperative information correctly and allowing the patient time to ask questions.

Admission

The patient should be welcomed and shown around the ward. Ideally this should be carried out by the nurse who will be responsible for planning the patient's care during the hospital stay. As the stay is likely to be short, the admitting nurse must attempt to develop a friendly relationship with patients quickly, so that they will feel at ease to ask questions. A full nursing history must be obtained with an emphasis on discharge planning, as it is important to ensure that the patient has someone to care for them when they first go home. The use of a preassessment clinic is very helpful for obtaining and providing valuable information related to pre- and postoperative care in a quiet and less busy environment

Informed Consent

It is the responsibility of the medical staff to explain the nature of the operation to the patient and to obtain the patient's written consent. The patient needs to be made aware that there may be complications during a laparoscopic procedure, and that as a result the surgeon may have to revert to a more conventional surgical approach. The surgical nurse must be prepared to answer patients' questions about their forthcoming operations. A preoperative visit by the theatre nurse who will be present at the patient's operation can be very helpful, particularly if the nurse is also available to greet the patient on arrival to theatre. MAS is a relatively new concept, and with newer procedures, patients may need more explanation and reassurance. The criteria for informed consent presented in Chapter 2 are particularly important if the minimal access route is being presented as a better alternative to a conventional procedure.

Preparation for Theatre

The patient is fasted for the required time and mouthwashes can be offered to promote oral comfort. The patient is encouraged to take a shower, and if necessary a depilatory cream or clippers are used to remove hair. Temperature, pulse, respiratory rate, and blood pressure are recorded to provide a baseline for future recordings. Urine is tested for abnormalities such as glucose. The patient will be wearing an identity band and theatre gown. All jewellery is removed to safe keeping, except for the patient's wedding ring, which can be covered with tape. Dentures, spectacles, wigs, and prosthetic devices can be worn into the anaesthetic room if the patient wishes. These valuable items must then be kept safely until they are required by the patient.

Antiembolism stockings are particularly important as MAS is technically more demanding than open surgery (Cushieri, 1993a) and so may prolong the time the patient is on the theatre table. Premedication is given. The accompanying nurse may need to reassure the patient that if a general anaesthetic is used, sleep will be maintained throughout the operation. If a local anaesthetic is used the patient should be reassured that pain should not be experienced, but if discomfort is felt, the accompanying nurse should be informed. The patient may find it reassuring to be accompanied to the theatre by the admitting nurse. All the patient's notes, results of any investigations, and radiographs should be available.

In the Operating Theatre

To ensure that the patient's condition remains stable, electrocardiograph (ECG) electrodes and a blood pressure cuff are applied. The diathermy plate is positioned and the patient is carefully checked to avoid contact with metal that could result in diathermy burns. The patient is positioned safely and securely, ensuring that the arms and legs are not overextended or joints damaged. As with all surgery, checks are made before, during, and after the operation to account for all swabs and cutting instruments used during the procedure. After the operation special care is needed to ensure that all drains are secured and that the patient continues to be positioned safely and comfortably. Staff in the recovery area need to be fully informed of the details of the operation and any complications that may have arisen.

Postoperative Care

The major cause of pain following laparoscopic surgery results from the presence of trapped carbon dioxide (CO_2) under the diaphragm causing pain in the shoulders. This pain can be relieved by heat pads, analgesia via patient controlled analgesia (PCA) and gentle passive exercise. It is important that PCA is explained to patients in the preoperative period so that they are fully aware of how it is used. Patients should also be aware that they may be attached to an intravenous infusion and have a wound drain after the operation. A nasogastric tube is sometimes present after surgery and this will prevent discomfort from abdominal distension and nausea. If nausea persists, it can be relieved by anti-emetic drugs administered by injection, suppositories, or skin patches (Gosling and Mason, 1994). The potential problems of postoperative haemorrhage and infection must be considered as after conventional surgery.

Discharge

Arrangements are made for patients to be taken home when they are fit for discharge. The community nurse must be contacted to perform a home visit two or three days after discharge. Patients should be told that the stitches are usually removed in seven days and they should be given an outpatient appointment for a check-up in four weeks. They should be advised to avoid heavy lifting and strenuous exercise for one week. They may resume normal activities as soon as they feel able, and return to work when they are comfortable.

COMPLICATIONS SPECIFIC TO MINIMAL ACCESS SURGERY

Complications related specifically to MAS are associated with the following procedures:

- Introduction of the operating media.
- Insertion and manipulation of the endoscopic instruments.
- Insertion of Verres needles, trocar, and cannulas.
- Creation of pneumoperitoneum in abdominal surgery.

Introduction of the Operating Media

In order to perform MAS, it is necessary to introduce a transparent operative medium to allow the surgeon to be able to see the operation site within the relevant body space. It is often necessary to expand actual or potential body spaces with this medium by instilling it at greater pressure than atmospheric pressure. Substances used include liquids (e.g. saline, glycine) and gas (e.g. CO_2).

Saline is used in arthroscopic surgery, which is usually performed using a tourniquet, so diathermy is not required. Saline is a good conductor of electricity and would be unsuitable in surgery requiring diathermy.

Glycine is used in bladder and uterine surgery. It is near-isotonic and a poor conductor of electricity, so diathermy may be used. However, if large amounts of glycine are absorbed into the tissues and blood, fluid overload, hyponatraemia, and hypokalaemia can occur. The patient may then become breathless (as a result of pulmonary oedema), tachycardic, and hypotensive. This is referred to as the transurethral resection syndrome as glycine is used in transurethral resection of the prostate gland.

CO_2 is used to insufflate the abdomen in general, gynaecological, and urological surgery. There is a danger of rapid CO_2 absorption leading to increased arterial CO_2 pressure, resulting in acidosis and cardiac arrhythmias. An embolus can occur if CO_2 enters the circulation. It may then travel through the circulation and pass to the right side of the heart, interfering with venous return and ultimately reducing cardiac output. If this occurs, it is vital that CO_2 excretion is increased either by hyperventilation or by aspirating CO_2 via a central venous pressure line. Insufflation of CO_2 must be discontinued immediately.

Insertion of Endoscopic Instruments

This can traumatize organs or tissues if the equipment is not handled skilfully.

Insertion of Verres Needles, Trocars, and Cannulas

These instruments are used to allow visualization of the operation site and to allow the introduction of the operative medium. If these instruments are not handled with skill, they can puncture blood vessels, resulting in haemorrhage or peritonitis.

Creation of a Pneumoperitoneum

When a pneumoperitoneum is created, the diaphragm is displaced by the increased abdominal pressure, reducing the functional capacity of the lungs. This effect can be particularly severe when the patient is placed head down to allow access to the lower abdomen. It is important to maintain the intra-abdominal pressure at less than 15 mm Hg, and this can be achieved with positive pressure ventilation.

LAPAROSCOPIC CHOLECYSTECTOMY – AN EXAMPLE OF MINIMAL ACCESS SURGERY

Although the exterior wounds are minimal in laparoscopic cholecystectomy compared with conventional cholecystectomy, the tissue trauma is similar internally and the loss of tactile feedback will alter how tissues are handled. The preparation of the patient is as previously described and the operation requires a general anaesthetic. In theatre an intravenous infusion is started and a nasogastric tube is passed to decompress the patient's stomach during the operation. The patient is placed in the lithotomy position with the legs supported and abducted, but not raised. A Foley catheter is inserted for continuous bladder drainage during the operation to prevent injury to the urinary bladder. A diathermy plate is attached to the patient, and after draping, the patient is placed in Trendelenburg's position. A Verres needle is introduced through a subumbilical incision to create a pneumoperitoneum using CO_2. Insufflation of the peritoneal cavity is maintained at 12–14 mm Hg throughout the operation. The Verres needle is removed, the small subumbilical incision slightly enlarged, and a 10 mm laparoscope is introduced.

The camera is attached to the telescope of the laparoscope, the patient is placed in a reverse Trendelenburg's position with a left lateral tilt to allow better visualization of the gall bladder and cystic duct. A 12 mm Surgiport is introduced into the patient's left hypochondrium, and two cannulas are inserted into the patient's right hypochondrium. Forceps are introduced through these cannulas to grasp the gall bladder. Other instruments are introduced though the Surgiport to dissect the gall bladder and divide the cystic duct and cystic artery. The gall bladder is dissected from the liver by the use of diathermy and cautery; it is decompressed by suction and the stones are removed. Haemostasis is ensured and as much CO_2 as possible is removed before the cannulas are withdrawn. Skin staples are used to close the small abdominal incisions, and the urinary catheter and nasogastric tube are removed.

Postoperatively, the patient requires PCA for the first 12 hours, but is then helped to ambulate and requires oral analgesia only (McKay, 1992).

LASERS AND MINIMAL ACCESS SURGERY

Lasers are particularly useful in MAS for two main reasons:

■ They are the safest high-power energy source that can be transmitted through long deflectable ultra-thin channels.
■ Laser tissue effects are absolutely controllable and tissue selective.

As surgeons increase their use of minimal invasive techniques in a wide range of specialities using small endoscopic diameters, lasers will become essential for every theatre (Slatkine and Mead, 1994). Lasers are expensive and great care is needed when using them, requiring protocols and equipment for the use of operating staff. Electrosurgical equipment for incisions and coagulation is widely accepted in operating rooms, but it does not provide the same control of thermal damage to tissue as lasers. This is because electrical current, and therefore thermal damage, tends to follow the path of least resistance (e.g. along blood vessels) rather than going through tissue. Optical lasers, however, provide highly controlled tissue effects in relation to:

■ Incision.
■ Coagulation.
■ Single-layer surface ablation.

THE IMPACT OF MINIMAL ACCESS SURGERY ON NURSING

As White and Carthew (1995) point out, the treatment of surgical patients is changing due to the development of techniques related to MAS. It is important that hospital- and community-based nurses develop specific skills and adopt new roles to meet the needs of patients who are undergoing these new techniques. The ability to make an efficient nursing and medical assessment of a patient in a limited time is one of the skills the nurse and doctor must develop. One important assessment is whether the patient is suitable for MAS. This is one of the functions that can be carried out in preassessment clinics that are now being developed in many centres. Patients and their relatives may be anxious about new procedures and may need repeated explanation and reassurance about the nature of the technique, particularly if laser treatment is being used. As a result of MAS, community nurses care for patients at an earlier stage of their recovery than they would if the patient had undergone conventional surgery. It is important that nurses, patients, and relatives acknowledge that patients have had organ and tissue removal, even though the external wound is minimal. Patients may be reluctant to admit that they do not feel well if they have no external wounds to justify their claim. This can result in patients going back to work too soon, resulting in tiredness and depression. Nurses must use all their skills in communication to help patients and their relatives and friends understand the nature of the developing techniques of MAS.

References

Cushieri A (1993a) Ergonomics of minimal access surgery. *Surgery* **11(10)**:526–528.

Cushieri A (1993b) Foreword and Introduction. *Minimal Access Surgery. Implications for the NHS*. London, Department of Health.

Dubois F, Icard P, Berthelot G, Levard H (1990) Coelioscopic cholecystectomy: preliminary report of 36 cases. *Ann Surg* **211(1)**:60–62.

Gosling M, Mason J (1994) Perioperative care. In *Minimal Access Surgery for Nurses and Technicians*. Hall FA (ed.). pp. 49–61. Oxford: Radcliffe Medical Press Ltd.

McKay M (1992) Laparoscopic cholecystectomy: theatre implications. *Br J Theatre Nurs* **1(10)**:24–26.

Slatkine M, Mead D (1994) Lasers. In *Minimal Access Surgery for Nurses and Technicians*. Hall FA (ed.). pp. 194–213. Oxford: Radcliffe Medical Press Ltd.

Troidle H (1990) The general surgeon and the trauma surgeon – binding the wounds. *Theoret Surg* **5**:64–74.

Troidle H (1993) The philosophy of patient-friendly surgery. In *Minimal Access Medicine and Surgery. Principles and Techniques*. Rosin D (ed.). Oxford: Radcliffe Medical Press. pp. 10–21.

White J, Carthew L (1995) The hazards of minimal access surgery. *Surg Nurse* **8(3)**:9–12.

Section Two

Nursing Care and Management

CONTENTS

Chapter 12

Breast Surgery

Any diagnosis of breast disease can have a major psychological impact on a woman. In many societies the breasts have strong associations with femininity and sexuality as well as their role in lactation and motherhood. In addition, cancer is a common fear when a breast lump or discharge is found. This chapter deals with the anatomical structure and physiology of the breast in relation to patients with breast conditions. The conditions discussed range from benign lesions such as fat necrosis and mastitis to the more serious conditions relating to breast malignancy. The pre- and postoperative nursing care is discussed with regard to the physical and psychological problems that may arise.

ANATOMY AND PHYSIOLOGY

The breasts or mammary glands (*Figure 12.1*) are found on the anterior chest wall, on either side of the sternum between the third to seventh ribs. The breasts are supported by the pectoral muscles and ligaments (Cooper's ligaments). These ligaments extend from the skin to the underlying deep fascia, and some types of carcinoma can pull on them causing dimpling of the skin. Cooper's ligaments stretch with age, causing the breasts to droop. The adult breast contains three main types of tissue:

- Glandular epithelium.
- Fibrous stoma.
- Fatty tissue.

The amount of fibrous and fatty tissue in the breast varies with age. In young women the epithelial and fibrous tissues predominate, in older women there is

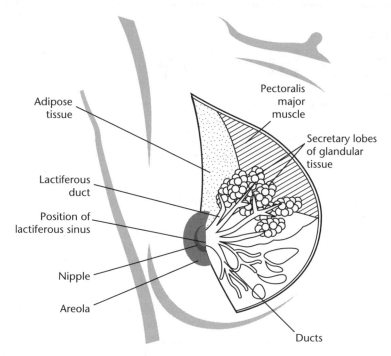

Figure 12.1 The breast or mammary gland.

more fatty tissue. As the presence of fatty tissue helps to define a lesion, mammography is of particular value in older women and should be offered to all women from 50 years of age on an annual basis (Novitskie Pool and Judkins, 1990). The breast is surmounted by a pigmented area of firmer tissue, the areola, which surrounds the nipple. There is a great deal of individual variation in size and shape of the breasts and the size and pigmentation of areolae and nipples.

The functional tissue of the breast is essentially a type of modified sweat gland. Each breast contains 19–25 lobes radiating out from the nipple and separated by intralobular regions of fibrous stroma (*Figure 12.1*). The lobes are drained by the lactiferous ducts. Each lactiferous duct widens in the region below the areola to form a lactiferous sinus. The sinuses act as a milk reservoir and open through short ducts onto the surface of the nipple. Cancerous cells arising from tumours in the lactiferous sinuses can traverse the short duct separating the sinus from the surface to invade the epithelium of the nipple. This results in Paget's disease of the nipple, which is described below. The lobes in turn form lobules, which are composed of the tubular alveolar ducts. The terminal structures are the globular alveoli or acini. The alveoli are lined by a secretory epithelium, which produces the milk. Underlying the epithelium is a layer of myoepithelial cells, which contract to help eject the milk.

The breast is an active vascular organ supplied by the internal and external mammary arteries medially and branches of the axillary artery laterally. Venous return is via the internal mammary veins and the axillary veins. Innervation is from branches of the fourth to sixth thoracic nerves. The nipple region is particularly sensitive. Stimulation of the nipple may cause it to become erect, and during lactation initiates the milk let-down reflex. The lymphatic drainage of the breast is particularly important in relation to spread of malignancy. Lymphatic vessels follow the pathway of the blood vessels, draining into the central axillary, scapular, subclavicular, internal mammary, and interpectoral groups of lymph nodes (*Figure 12.2*).

The development and physiological functions of the breast are under hormonal control. The onset of puberty marks the start of breast maturation. The adolescent breast consists mainly of fibrous stroma with a scanty, poorly developed system of scattered ducts lined by an epithelium. As puberty progresses the glandular system develops with branching and elongation of the ductile system and the formation of distinct lobular units. At the same time the stromal components multiply and there is deposition of fatty tissue.

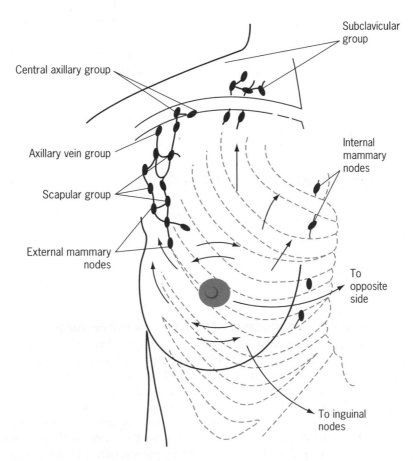

Figure 12.2 Lymphatic drainage of the breast.

Breast development is under complex hormonal control. Oestrogens and progesterone have a central role, but many other hormones including adrenal, thyroid, and pituitary hormones are important. The adult breast responds to hormonal cycles. There is a cyclic hypertrophy of glandular epithelium and stromal components during the menstrual cycle. Fluid accumulation and oedema of the intralobular tissues can lead to feelings of fullness, engorgement, and pain during the late luteal phase of the cycle. Pregnancy causes a further maturation and development of the glandular tissues. Additional lobular units will form and the amount of stroma is reduced. The menopause results in an involution of the glandular system and the lobular units largely disappear; the quantity of stroma and connective tissues decrease and the functional tissue is largely replaced by fat.

The breast is usually viewed as a female characteristic, but the male also has rudimentary breasts. Gynaecomastia (hypertrophy of the breast tissue) is the most commonly seen breast problem in men. This can occur in puberty and in older men (senescent hypertrophy), frequently as a side effect of medications. Breast cancer can also occur in the male, but is rare, probably less than 1% of the female incidence. The reported figures for incidence of female breast cancer in 1983 was 24,410 (DHSS, 1987). Delayed recognition of the condition combined with the sparseness of male breast tissue may result in presentation with a very advanced tumour. However, problems of the male breast in relation to surgical treatment are comparatively rare and the male breast will not be further considered in this chapter. The female breast and conditions requiring surgical treatment are the central topic.

INITIAL PRESENTATION OF BREAST DISEASE

Breast disease is often diagnosed when a woman presents with one or more of three common problems:

- A lump in the breast.
- Nipple discharge.
- Pain.

Ellis and Calne (1993a) state that 95% of breast lumps will be due to carcinoma of the breast, a cyst, fibroadenoma, or a localized area of fibroadenosis. Less common causes are listed in *Box 12.1*. Nipple discharge and breast pain can indicate a range of infectious and neoplastic breast conditions. However, a nipple discharge is common even in nonlactating women and does not usually indicate a breast carcinoma. *Box 12.2* lists different types of discharge and possible implications.

Breast pain is a common reason for seeking medical advice. Most breast pain is probably related to fluctuating changes due to the hormonal cycle such as engorgement, discomfort, and pain occurring premenstrually. Irregular menstrual cycles may be associated with irregular patterns of breast pain. However,

Box 12.1 Possible causes of breast lumps (adapted from Browse, 1978).

Common causes associated with the breast
- Breast abscess
- Fibroadenosis
- Cystic hyperplasia
- Fat necrosis
- Cysts of the glands of Montgomery
- Carcinoma

Less common causes associated with the breast
- Sarcoma
- Mondor's disease (spontaneous thrombophlebitis of the superficial veins of the breast and anterior chest wall)

Box 12.2 Types of discharges from the nipple and their causes (adapted from Ellis and Calne, 1993).

Bloodstained discharge
- Duct papilloma
- Intraduct papilloma
- Paget's disease

Yellow, brown or green discharge
- Fibroadenosis

Purulent discharge
- Abscess

Serous discharge
- May be an early sign of pregnancy

Milky discharge
- Following lactation

Note whether the discharge is bilateral or unilateral. Bilateral nipple discharge rarely indicates underlying carcinoma.

breast pain can indicate carcinoma of the breast, a breast abscess, or fibro-adenosis. Pain associated with fibroadenosis is often most noticeable just before the period. Breast pain may also be a sign of Tietze's disease, which is a condition characterized by a nonsuppurative swelling of the second, third or fourth costal cartilages.

DISORDERS OF THE BREAST AND NIPPLE

The three main groups of breast disease that might require surgical treatment are:

- Inflammations, trauma, and infections (e.g. mastitis).
- Non-neoplastic hyperplasia (e.g. fibroadenoma).
- Neoplastic hyperplasia (benign and malignant tumours).

Benign Conditions

Fat necrosis of the breast
This condition often occurs in fatty pendulous breasts. It may follow an injury to the breast, but frequently there is no obvious history of trauma. The condition presents as a lump that initially consists of fat-laden macrophages and other inflammatory cells. The axillary lymph nodes may be enlarged. The lesion may regress, but calcification and distortion of surrounding tissue give an appearance similar to that of a carcinoma on mammography. Treatment is usually excision with biopsy to exclude malignancy. The biopsy reveals a pale fibrous mass (Ellis and Calne, 1993b). The central region may be filled with fluid from necrotizing fat cells or more chalky consolidation. As this condition may initially present with features similar to carcinoma the patient may be very anxious until the biopsy results are known.

Acute mastitis and abscess
Acute non-infectious inflammation of the breast or mastitis can occur during periods of hormonal change, for example mastitis of the newborn, mastitis of pregnancy, and during lactation. However, the most common cause of acute mastitis and breast abscess is bacterial infection during lactation. Mastitis usually presents in the 1–2 months after delivery. Breast abscess is less common in nonlactating women and is rarely seen in postmenopausal women. Bacteria (commonly staphylococci) gain entry from cracked nipples or via the milk ducts. An ascending cellulitis develops from the nipple, and the breast becomes progressively more reddened, hard, and painful. Antibiotic treatment of the cellulitis within the first 24 hours may resolve the situation, but if the mastitis has persisted for more than one or two days there is a strong likelihood of abscess formation (Ellis and Calne, 1993c). Abscesses are often multiloculated, so needle aspiration is unlikely to prove effective. The abscess may be managed

conservatively until a single, drainable mass has formed. Cold poultices may help comfort the patient, and it may be necessary to suppress lactation. Drainage of the abscess and excision of the surrounding capsule is required. Recurrent abscesses may require a wider excision that includes the diseased subareolar ducts.

Fibrocystic diseases

Fibrocystic disease or fibroadenosis is the most common of the benign conditions affecting the breast and some degree of fibrocystic changes may be present in most women. There is an increase in fibrous stroma usually accompanied by cystic dilation of terminal ductules and acini. Breast cysts can range from microcysts to cysts containing 20–30 mL of fluid. Adenosis, an increase in the formation of new ductules or acini, may occur, along with simple fibrocystic changes. Fibrocystic disease may result in lumps or areas of calcification requiring biopsy to exclude carcinoma. Fibroadenosis is often bilateral and may be cyclic.

Fibroadenoma

A fibroadenoma is a firm encapsulated benign breast tumour containing both epithelial and stromal tissues. The mobile mass will not be attached to the skin. Fibroadenoma is the most common breast tumour in women under 30 years of age. Treatment is by excision with histological assessment to confirm the diagnosis and exclude carcinoma.

Duct papilloma

Papillomas (polyps of the ductal epithelium) may be solitary or multiple. They are often located in one of the 15–20 subareola ducts and the patient may report bleeding from the nipple. Treatment is by excision and histological examination to exclude carcinoma.

NURSING MANAGEMENT IN BENIGN BREAST CONDITIONS

Any women requiring even minor surgery or biopsy of the breast is likely to worry about possible cancer and will require careful explanation and support from the nurse. It is important that the nurse listens carefully to any fears the patient may have about her breast cyst or benign tumour and reassures her accordingly. Information may have to be presented and discussed several times. Benign disorders account for the majority of breast disease, but fear of cancer is likely to be one of the patient's major concerns.

After a minor breast procedure such as removal of a cyst, recovery is usually rapid and the case may be dealt with as day surgery or perhaps an overnight admission. Wound care and pain control are particular features, and the vascularity of the breast may predispose to extensive bruising. Wound drainage is often required, but drains are usually removed the next day. In the case of a cyst the nurse can reassure the patient that the lesion is not cancerous. However, if a lump has been removed the nurse must avoid false reassurances until definitive histology reports exclude carcinoma.

The breast may be painful for several days and over-the-counter analgesics such as paracetamol may be sufficient for pain control at home. However, if the patient has extensive bruising and oedema, a more powerful analgesic may be required. A well-fitting bra will help support the breast, promoting comfort and reducing the tension of the healing wound. Before discharge the nurse should assess the patient's knowledge of breast health and discuss issues such as regular breast screening, mammography, and self-examination. The nurse should explain to the patient that she should examine her breasts each month after her menstrual cycle, as lumps may become more pronounced before menstruation. Some women have reported a reduction in premenstrual oedema and breast pain by reducing salt intake and avoiding coffee. Gamolenic acid in evening primrose oil has been reported to provide symptomatic relief of cyclic breast pain. Some reports also suggest that pyridoxine (vitamin B_6) may help relieve premenstrual syndrome, but the evidence is not convincing and an overdose can be toxic.

BREAST CANCER

Breast cancer is the most common malignant tumour in women in developed countries, accounting for about 20% of all female cancers. The UK has the highest mortality rate from breast cancer in the European Community (Gaze, 1991). It is estimated that one in 12 women in the UK will develop breast cancer at some time in their lives (Hollingworth, 1992) and, as the report to the *Breast Cancer Services* (1995) points out, the disease kills 30–50% of its victims. Breast cancer can affect women of any age, but is not common under the age of 30 years. The cause of the disease is not yet known, but several major and minor risk factors have been identified (*Box 12.3*).

Prevention and Screening

As research has been unable to identify causative factors there is no clear preventive strategy currently available. Treatments have developed over the years, but the overall mortality from the disease has not been significantly decreased. However, it is important to diagnose the condition as early as possible. Treatment is more effective if instigated at an early stage. Therefore screening programmes for early detection of breast cancer are probably the best way currently available to reduce the number of deaths from breast cancer. The three components of good breast health advocated by Novitskie Pool and Judkins, (1990) are:

- Annual physical examination by a doctor.
- Mammography.
- Monthly breast self-examination.

> **Box 12.3** Risk factors for breast cancer (adapted from Inglehart, 1991).
>
> **Major risk factors**
> - Female sex
> - Age (less than 2% of patients are under 30 years of age)
> - Family history (there is a 2–3 times higher risk if mother, sister or daughter is affected by breast cancer; this risk is even higher if the cancer was premenopausal or bilateral)
> - Previous breast cancer
> - Atypical benign epithelial hyperplasia
>
> **Minor risk factors**
> - Early menarche
> - Late menopause
> - Obesity

Breast screening by mammography

This is the most important element of an early detection programme. Studies suggest such programmes can reduce breast cancer deaths in the 50-plus age group by 30% (Shapiro *et al.*, 1982; Tabar *et al.*, 1985). Mammography can detect breast lumps before they are palpable by clinical or self-examination. In the UK all women between 50 and 65 years of age are offered mammography every three years. The American Cancer Society guidelines recommend that women between the ages of 40–49 years should have mammography every 1–2 years and annual mammography after the age of 50 years. Ellis and Calne (1993) report that early data from screening programmes reveal one suspicious mammogram in 1000 and of these selected cases 50% are likely to be malignant. Some women avoid mammography because they fear pain and radiation. It is important that nurses emphasize that with experienced technologists and modern equipment the procedure can be carried out using low-dose radiation and with minimal discomfort. Although uncomfortable compression of the breast is necessary for a satisfactory mammogram, it may be possible to schedule the procedure following menstruation when the breasts are less tender.

Clinical and self-examination of the breast

This is less effective in early detection of breast cancer as micrometastases are often present by the time a small lump can be detected by palpation. However, annual examination by the general practitioner and monthly self-examination of the breast may contribute to early detection of other problems of the breast. It may also help detect some cancers while they are still small enough to allow for a wider range of surgical options.

Types of Breast Cancer

According to Haagensen (1986) breast cancer is a generic term because there are at least 15 histological subtypes of the disease. The World Health Organization (WHO) classification of breast cancers recognizes five main groups of malignant tumours with numerous subdivisions (*Box 12.4*). Infiltrating ductal carcinoma represents more than 50% of histological diagnoses.

Breast cancer is a local disease capable of rapid systemic spread. In the early stages it affects the ducts, but once the lesion attains the size of 5 mm, there is an increasing risk of the growth invading the lymphatic nodes and the systemic

---

Box 12.4 The World Health Organization classification of malignant breast tumours (adapted from Inglehart, 1993).

Noninvasive epithelial tumours
- Intraductal carcinoma
- Lobular carcinoma *in situ*

Invasive epithelial tumours
- Invasive ductal carcinoma
- Invasive ductal carcinoma with a predominant intraductal component
- Invasive lobular carcinoma
- Mucinous carcinoma
- Medullary carcinoma
- Papillary carcinoma
- Tubular carcinoma
- Adenoid cystic carcinoma
- Secretory carcinoma
- Apocrine carcinoma
- Carcinoma with metaplasia
- Others

Paget's disease of the nipple

Mixed connective tissue and epithelial tumours
- Fibroadenoma
- Phyllodes tumour
- Carcinosarcoma

Miscellaneous tumours
- Soft tissue tumours
- Skin tumours
- Tumours of haemopoietic and lymphoid tissue

circulation. The tumour usually starts in the upper outer quadrant of the breast, but as it grows it becomes attached to the chest wall or overlying skin. Without treatment the tumour will invade surrounding tissues and the lymph glands of the axilla. Metastases may spread to the lungs, bones, and liver. The patient may present with a painless mobile lump in the upper outer quadrant of the breast. Later the lump becomes fixed and irregular in shape and appears to be adhering to the chest wall. Some women will complain of burning or aching of the affected breast and nodules may appear in the axilla. There may be nipple retraction, and because the tumour infiltrates the fibrous divisions of the breast, the lymphatic drainage becomes blocked, causing oedema of the overlying skin between the hair follicles and sweat glands, giving the skin of the breast the appearance of orange peel called 'peau d'orange.' If the condition remains untreated, the breast tissues ulcerate and the patient's general health rapidly deteriorates. It is vital that breast cancer is detected early as the success of treatment is directly related to the stage of the cancer at diagnosis.

TNM Classification

A variety of systems have been used for staging breast cancer, but the TNM (T, tumour; N, status of regional lymph nodes; M, distant metastases) devised by the International Union Against Cancer (1986) is the most widely adopted. The classification as applied to primary breast cancer is shown in *Box 12.5*.

Using the TNM system breast cancer can be classified both clinically and pathologically into stages:

- Stage I: T_1 N_0 M_0
- Stage IIa: T_0 N_1 M_0 or T_2 N_0 M_0
- Stage IIb: T_2 N_1 M_0
- Stage IIIa: T_3 N_1 M_0 or $T_{1,2,3}$ N_2 M_0
- Stage IIIb: T_4 any N M_0
- Stage IV: any T   any N M_1

Investigations of Breast Tumours

The following procedures may be carried out to exclude malignancy or to determine the extent of the disease process:

- Clinical examination of the breast.
- Mammography.
- Ultrasound to distinguish solid from cystic lesions.
- Fine-needle aspiration to obtain fluid for cytology and to drain a cyst.
- Biopsy.

In fine-needle aspiration cytology of the breast, a syringe with a fine-bore needle is inserted into the breast mass and suction is applied. The contents are

---

Box 12.5 **TNM classification of breast cancer (International Union Against Cancer, 1986).**

Primary tumour – T
- T_x, primary tumour cannot be assessed
- T_0, no evidence of primary tumour
- TIS, carcinoma *in situ* (e.g. intraductal or lobular carcinoma *in situ*)
- T_1, tumour ≤ 2 cm in greatest dimension.
- T_2, tumour > 2 cm, but ≤ 5 cm in greatest dimension
- T_3, tumour > 5 cm in greatest dimension
- T_4, tumour of any size with direct extension to chest wall or skin

Regional lymph nodes – N
- N_x, regional lymph nodes cannot be assessed
- N_0, no regional lymph node metastases
- N_1, metastases in four or less ipsilateral axillary nodes (none greater than 3 cm diameter)
- N_2, metastases in four or more ipsilateral axillary nodes, and/or any larger than 3 cm, or in any ipsilateral internal mammary lymph node

Distant metastases – M
- M_x, distant metastasis cannot be assessed
- M_0, no evidence of distant metastases
- M_1, distant metastases present

---

withdrawn, placed on a slide, and sent to the laboratory for examination. Cytology results will be graded C0–C5. C0 represents an insufficient specimen, C1 and C2 benign cells, C3 and C4 suspicious of carcinoma, and C5 carcinoma. It is important to remember that a benign result may simply indicate that the needle missed the target. If there are other signs of a cancerous lesion, a biopsy is recommended. Three types of biopsy are commonly used.

- In Trucut biopsy a core of tissue is removed with a large-bore needle. This is usually performed using a local anaesthetic.
- In excision biopsy the suspicious lump is entirely excised. The patient is given a general anaesthetic and is usually in hospital for 24 hours.
- In localization biopsy, which may be used when a lesion has been illustrated on mammography but there is no palpable mass, a wire is inserted into the abnormal area under X-ray control. This ensures that the surgeon removes the right area.

It is important that the nurse understands these procedures and can explain them accurately to the patient. Although breast biopsy is a relatively minor surgical procedure, it is not without complications. Haematoma formation, wound sepsis, and pain are not unknown, and the cosmetic results vary. In a study of breast biopsy it was found that 24 of 39 woman reported significant pain lasting an average of 27 days postoperatively (Hirst and Whitehead, 1984). Two patients said that the biopsy had disfigured their breasts to such an extent that they would wait as long as possible before reporting further breast symptoms. Also due to the anxiety associated with breast cancer the patient may require extensive support from the nurse.

Management of Breast Cancer

Treatment of breast cancer will depend mainly on the stage at diagnosis. With early diagnosis surgical treatment offers a chance of cure. In later stages surgery will need to be more radical and the chances of cure are reduced. Radiotherapy or chemotherapy or both may be used in addition to surgical removal. Once diagnosis has confirmed the cancer, the patient is advised of the preferred choice of treatment. Fentiman (1991) points out that mastectomy is not always the appropriate treatment. It is very important at this stage particularly that the patient's questions are answered fully and honestly and that time is given for decisions to be made. The patient may wish her partner and family to be involved in the discussion and opportunity should be provided for this. Surgical procedures include:

- Lumpectomy (removal of the tumour plus a small rim of normal tissue).
- Wide local excision (removal of the tumour and all abnormal tissue plus a 1–2 cm ring of normal tissue).
- Quadrantectomy (resection of the tumour, all tissue of that portion or quadrant of the breast, and overlying skin).
- Simple mastectomy (removal of all breast tissue, skin, and nipple, but underlying muscles are left intact).
- Radical (Halsted) mastectomy (breast, underlying pectoralis muscles, and axillary lymph nodes are all removed; not commonly used today).
- Extended radical mastectomy (internal mammary nodes are also resected; additional benefits over a radical mastectomy are not proven).
- Modified radical (Patey) mastectomy (all breast tissue, overlying skin and nipple removed, pectoralis major muscle left intact, pectoralis minor muscle removed along with axillary lymph nodes).

The most appropriate form of surgery for stage I or II breast cancer remains controversial. Clinical trials have not demonstrated that any particular procedure is clearly superior. Current practice tends to favour a more conservative approach to surgery. A small tumour with no lymph node involvement can be treated by lumpectomy followed by radiotherapy of the remaining breast tissue and axillary nodes. This conserves the breast and tends to produce better cosmetic results. There is evidence that less radical (breast conservation) surgery combined with radiotherapy is just as effective as radical mastectomy (Veronesi *et al.*, 1990). Patients with large tumours are usually advised to have a mastectomy together with clearance of the axillary lymph nodes. For those women who do not wish to have a breast removed, chemotherapy or radiotherapy may shrink the tumour sufficiently to avoid mastectomy. Hollingworth (1992) points out that some women feel happier if the breast is removed as it should follow that the cancer is removed. However, it has been shown that mastectomy is not always a cure and a proportion of patients develop secondary cancer. Lymph node involvement suggests that micrometastatic spread is likely and additonal treatment may be required. The Early Breast Cancer Trialists' Collaborative Group (1992) research shows that improved survival rates are being obtained with adjuvant therapy (i.e. radiotherapy, chemotherapy, or hormonal therapy).

Adjuvant therapy

Radiotherapy, chemotherapy, and hormonal therapy may be used as the main treatments for later stage cancers that are untreatable by surgery or with widespread metastases. However, they also have an important role as adjuvants to surgery. They are particularly useful after partial or conservation procedures to reduce the risk of recurrence in the remaining breast tissue.

Radiotherapy

Radiotherapy may be administered by external irradiation or by the use of iridium wire implants. Postoperative external irradiation will be given several times a week over 5–6 weeks. Preserved breast tissue and axillary nodes may be irradiated. The main problems associated with the radiotherapy are redness and soreness of the skin over the treated area. The women may also experience a general fatigue as the treatment progresses.

Chemotherapy

Systemic chemotherapy may be indicated if there are metastases or if there is a high risk of metastases. Cytotoxic therapy is particularly recommended for premenopausal women with known lymph node involvement. A common regimen is six months of CMF (cyclophosphamide, methotrexate, and 5-fluorouracil in combination) given in 6–9 cycles as an outpatient treatment. Another popular cytotoxic regimen in breast cancer is MMM (mitozantrone, methotrexate, and mitomycin C). The side effects of the cytotoxic regimens used to treat breast cancer tend to be less than in other cancers.

Hormonal therapy

The importance of steroid hormones in some types of breast cancer has been known since 1896 when Beatson demonstrated that bilateral removal of the ovaries caused a regression of metastatic breast cancer. Oestrogen is of particular importance and over 30% of patients with breast cancer respond to treatment with the oestrogen antagonist tamoxifen. Tamoxifen is the modern equivalent of oophorectomy. Tamoxifen may be used to treat small tumours and as adjuvant therapy following surgery. Tamoxifen has a low toxicity and side effects are unusual. It can therefore be used as an adjuvant therapy in all postmenopausal women even if the lymph nodes are not involved.

Nursing management of the woman requiring surgery for breast cancer
The psychological impact of potential breast cancer should never be under-estimated. The patient will have all the fears and anxieties associated with cancer. These are likely to heighten as diagnosis can usually only be confirmed after biopsy. The patient will be dreading the worst and hoping for the best. This is likely to be compounded by the pyschosexual implications of breast surgery. In developed countries the breast is probably more associated with sexuality than with its biological function of lactation. The woman faces potential mutilation of one of the more obvious symbols of her femininity and sexuality. Given these two fears it is not surprising that women experience many symptoms of acute anxiety when a breast 'lump' is discovered. Whatever her age the woman may suffer considerable anxiety about how the operation may affect her body image and how she will be regarded by her family and friends. Careful assessment of physical, psychological, and psychosexual factors are critical in the investigation phase and when the patient is admitted for surgery.

Preoperative care
In addition to the usual admission assessment as outlined in Chapter 2 the nurse will need a comprehensive assessment of:

- The patient's reaction to her diagnosis and her fears and concerns about breast cancer.
- The family's reaction to the diagnosis and their fears and concerns about breast cancer.
- The patient's knowledge about her condition, surgical treatment, postoperative care, the wound and appearance after surgery, and any adjuvant therapy. It may be difficult to assess how much she knows or wants to know. Unless the diagnosis has been confirmed she may prefer to assume the lump is not malignant. In addition, until biopsy and exploration there may be some uncertainty about the exact nature and extent of the surgery or adjuvant treatment.
- Whether the patient has the necessary knowledge and understanding to give informed consent. She may be pulled by two opposing fears: fear of cancer may tend to favour more radical surgery, while fear of sexual mutilation may favour breast conservation.
- The patient's concerns about the effects of possible surgery on her body image, sexuality, and sexual relationships.
- The patient's husband's or partner's knowledge and need for support.
- Additional sources of stress for example divorce, bereavement, and job or financial worries.
- Any previous history of mental illness (i.e. anxiety or depression).
- Preoperative shoulder function if axillary node clearance is anticipated.

During the initial assessment, the nurse identifies the particular anxieties of her patient. The patient may have had to make decisions about the nature of her treatment and this can be very stressful. Anger, confusion, and denial associated with a diagnosis of breast cancer impair concentration, and any explanation and reassurance may have to be repeated. For some women, the realization that the operation will mean that the cancer will be taken away will afford some comfort, but despite this the sense of loss can cause feelings of hopelessness and depression. It is most important that throughout the period of care the patient is encouraged to freely express grief over her condition. The nurse must be prepared to help the patient explain breast cancer and the particular course of treatment the patient has chosen to follow to her family. However, the patient's right to privacy if she does not wish to discuss these issues with the nurse must be respected.

Preoperative preparation will include helping the patient learn deep breathing and arm and hand exercises. In particular, the patient should be encouraged to use the arm and hand of the affected side and to consider the potential problems that may arise at home and alternative ways of dealing with them. The nurse should remind the patient that exercise will be gradually introduced postoperatively to avoid stress on the healing tissues. Exercise will also help facilitate drainage in the arm. The patient should be warned that intravenous therapy or perhaps a blood transfusion may be required postoperatively. Pain control, the expected size and position of the wound, and the use of sutures and wound drains can all be explained. It is worth emphasizing that the breast bruises easily and that there may be extensive bruising and swelling immediately postoperatively. The appearance of the scar in the first few days will not reflect the final cosmetic outcome.

Postoperative care
Besides the usual postoperative care four main areas will require special attention after breast surgery:

- Wound management.
- Pain.
- Difficulty with arm movement and potential for lymphoedema.
- Altered body image and pyschosexual implications of mastectomy.

Wound management
The size and position of the wound will be determined by the procedure adopted. If lymph nodes have been resected, the wound will involve the auxillary area. The wound drains are inserted to prevent haematoma or seroma forming. Initially drains are observed half-hourly to ensure suction is maintained and drainage recorded. The wound is observed frequently for signs of haemorrhage or infection. Regular observations of vital signs are also required. The wound dressing will not need frequent changing unless blood staining or infection is apparent. Wound drains are likely to be left *in situ* for 2–5 days. Adequate

analgesia should be established before removal of the drains. Sutures are usually removed between 10–14 days postoperatively. It may take 2–3 months for oedema and swelling in the wound to fully resolve. The patient may need reassurance that any lumps felt in the wound will be seroma formation and not a recurrence of the cancer.

Pain
The site, nature, and degree of pain must be assessed regularly, and the use of the prescribed postoperative analgesia encouraged. As discussed in Chapter 7 psychological state can influence a patient's experience of pain. After mastectomy and axillary dissection shoulder pain on moving the affected arm is often the main source of pain. The arm on the affected side may be supported on a pillow, and gentle exercise can begin as soon as the patient is fully alert. Judicious use of analgesia while arm exercises are being established may help the patient overcome the association of arm movement with pain.

Shoulder and arm mobility and potential for lymphoedema
Axillary lymph node resection or radiotherapy can reduce shoulder mobility, particularly if pain is not adequately controlled. However, with the encouragement of postoperative exercises the full range of movement will return within a month of surgery. Encouraging the use of the affected arm for hygiene activities such as teeth and hair brushing can supplement the exercise regimen. Lymphoedema is a complication of axillary resection or radiotherapy and is experienced to some degree by about 25% of women after breast surgery. Lymphoedema may occur as a late complication, and women should be alert to this possibility and contact their general practitioner or outpatient clinic as soon as they notice any swelling.

Altered body image and pyschosexual implications of mastectomy
The patient may be reluctant to look at her incision at first. The nurse should gently encourage the patient to look at her operation site and a Polaroid photograph of the area may help the patient overcome her fears.

General nursing care
Throughout the postoperative period the nurse must be willing to listen to the patient about any fears for the future with regard to her diagnosis, for example in relation to body image and sexual function. The nurse should point out to the patient the problems to look for in relation to the incision, such as redness, heat, and pyrexia. If these occur the patient must inform her general practitioner. If radiotherapy, chemotherapy, or other adjuvant therapy are included in the treatment, the patient should be given comprehensive information about the side effects of treatment and how to combat them. She should be encouraged to protect the skin of the arm on the affected side by trying to avoid bruising, breaking the skin, or sunburn. Efforts to promote the patient's general health should be encouraged by the nurse. Information may be needed in relation to the

dangers of smoking, a high fat diet, and excessive alcohol. The dates and times of follow-up appointments should be clearly understood. The Breast Care Sister who has helped support the patient throughout her care will provide a telephone number to ring if further support is needed. She will also supply the patient with useful addresses such as the Mastectomy Society.

Radiotherapy

Radiotherapy may be used after surgical removal of a breast tumour to destroy migrant or remaining cancer cells. The usual treatment is 3500–4500 rads over a period of 3–5 weeks. A reaction may occur within a few days of the onset of treatment, which usually appears as a generalized erythema or redness of the irradiated area, and there may be tenderness and itching. Application of an emollient cream is helpful for lessening the irritation and preventing the breakdown of skin into moist desquamating areas. Lawton and Twoomey (1991) advocate avoiding perfumed and coloured soaps and suggest using a hair dryer on a cool setting to dry any areas of damp skin.

Breast reconstruction

Some women may wish to undergo breast reconstruction after mastectomy. According to Chaglassian and Sherman (1983), the latissimus dorsi muscle can be used and sometimes a silicone implant is placed under the muscle. However, this type of operation is not always successful and there are fears that the silicone gel inside the implants can cause connective tissue disorders.

Outpatient mastectomy

Morris *et al.* (1992) describe a modified radical mastectomy carried out in an American outpatient department. A carbon dioxide laser and modified anaesthetic techniques are used. However, the patient with invasive breast carcinoma having surgery in this way as an outpatient must have adequate support at home and must be free of any other condition that could complicate anaesthesia such as asthma or a heart condition. Adequate community services must be available before and after surgery to support the patient and to prepare the patient preoperatively. Preoperative medication such as sublingual haloperidol or a scopolamine patch is prescribed for the patient to take at home before admission. After admission, approximately one hour before surgery, the patient is prepared as usual and taken to theatre, and the anaesthetic is administered. The patient's breast and axillary contents are then removed using the laser. The stab wounds for inserting wound drains are infiltrated with local anaesthetic and the wound is closed with staples.

After the patient has been extubated and is awake, she is taken to the post-anaesthetic care unit where she is observed for 2–3 hours before going home. The patient and her carer are given full information about her treatment at home, including the management of the wound drain and the incision, and pain control. The patient is asked to return to hospital for drain removal and subsequent removal of the staples. She is also asked to limit arm movement on the affected side until the wound has healed as laser wounds tend to heal more slowly than scalpel wounds. These patients are also treated with tamoxifen and sometimes chemotherapy is necessary.

Conclusion

As Stein and Zera (1991) point out 'Breast cancer is an evolving process. Surgery will likely be a part of the therapy for the forseeable future.' They go on to emphasize that though the incidence of radical breast surgery is diminishing, many patients still choose mastectomy and it is essential that nurses ensure that as far as possible patients are allowed to continue to exercise their right to choose.

References

Beatson GT (1896) On the treatment of inoperable cases of carcinoma of the mamma: Suggestions for a new method of treatment with illustrative cases. *Lancet* **2**:104, 162.

Breast Cancer Services (1995) Vol. II, p. 243. HMSO, London.

Browse N (1978) *An Introduction to the Symptoms and Signs of Surgical Disease*, p. 268. Edward Arnold, London.

Chaglassian TA, Sherman JE (1983) Breast reconstruction after mastectomy. In *Breast Cancer*, Margolese RG (ed.), Chap. 7, pp. 157–171. Churchill Livingstone, New York.

DHSS (Department of Health and Social Security) (1987) *Breast Cancer Screening* (Report to the Health Ministers of England, Wales, Scotland and Northern Ireland by a working group chaired by Professor Sir Patrick Forrest), p. 9. HMSO, London.

Ellis H, Calne R (1993a) The breast. *Lecture Notes on General Surgery*, 8th Edition, Chap. 48, p. 343. Blackwell Scientific Publications, Oxford.

Ellis H, Calne R (1993b) The breast. *Lecture Notes on General Surgery*, 8th Edition, Chap. 48, p. 345. Blackwell Scientific Publications, Oxford.

Ellis H, Calne R (1993c) The breast. *Lecture Notes on General Surgery*, 8th Edition, Chap. 48, p. 345. Blackwell Scientific Publications, Oxford.

Early Breast Cancer Trialists' Collaborative Group (1992) Systematic treatment of early breast cancer by hormonal, cytotoxic or immune therapy. *The Lancet* **339(8785)**:71–85.

Fentiman IS (1991) Management of early breast cancer. *Br J Clin Psychol* **45(3)**:197–201.

Gaze H (1991) Europe against cancer. *Nurs Times* **87(47)**:16–17.

Haagensen CD (1986) The microscopical classification of breast carcinoma. *Diseases of the Breast*, 3rd edition, pp. 719–842. WB Saunders, Philadelphia.

Hirst S, Whitehead D (1984) A minor surgical procedure? *Nurs Times* **80(37)**:45–46.

Hollingworth H (1992) Choice without fear. *Nurs Times* **88(50)**:27–29.

Inglehart ID (1991) The breast. In *Textbook of Surgery. The Biological Basis of Modern Surgical Practice*. Sabiston D (ed.), Chap. 21, pp. 510–550. WB Saunders, Philadelphia.

International Union Against Cancer and the American Joint Committee on Cancer (1986) cited in Sabiston DC (ed) (1991) *Textbook of Surgery*, 14th edn, Chap 21, p. 527. WB Saunders, Philadelphia.

Lawton J, Twoomey M (1991) 'Skin Reaction to Radiotherapy.' Nursing Standard **6(10)**:53–54.

Morris PB, Piper R, Reinke B, Young JR (1992) Outpatient carbon dioxide laser mastectomy. *Association of Operating Room Nurses Journal* **55(4)**:984–992.

Novitskie Pool K, Judkins A (1990) A health investment that may save your life. *Cancer Nurs* **13(6)**:329-334.

Shapiro S, Venet W, Strax P *et al.* (1982) Ten to fourteen year effect of screening in breast cancer mortality. *J Natl Cancer Inst.* **69**:349–355.

Stein P, Zera R (1991) Breast cancer. *Association of Operating Room Nurses Journal* **53(4)**:938–964.

Tabar L, Faberberg CJG, Gad A *et al.* (1985) Reduction in mortality from breast cancer after mass screening with mammography. *Lancet* **1**:829–832.

Veronesi U, Banfi A, Salvadori B *et al.* (1990) Breast conservation is the treatment of choice in small breast cancer: long term results of a randomised trial. *Eur J Cancer* **26**:668–670.

Chapter 13
Thyroid Surgery

CONTENTS

- Anatomy and Physiology
- Thyroid Disorders
- Investigation of Thyroid Dysfunction
- Treatment of Goitre and Hyperthyroidism
- Thyroid Surgery
- Nursing Management
- Future Health Considerations
- Treatment of Thyroid Carcinoma
- Conclusion

Disorders of the thyroid gland are quite common. Thyroid hormones have wide ranging effects on the body, but thyroid symptoms are usually related to either hormone excess or deficit, and the complications produced by these imbalances. Treatment is usually by means of medication and, if necessary, surgical intervention.

ANATOMY AND PHYSIOLOGY

The thyroid gland is situated in the neck just below the larynx. It is highly vascular and weighs only 15–20 g, having a high rate of blood flow per gram of tissue. The thyroid consists of two conical lobes joined near the base by a narrow bridge of tissue called the isthmus (*Figure 13.1*). In about 30% of people, there is a smaller pyramidal lobe, which projects upwards from the isthmus. The isthmus crosses in front of the trachea at the level of the second to fourth cartilaginous rings, with the lobes extending laterally. The four parathyroid glands lie in pairs on the posterior aspect of the apex of each lobe of the thyroid. These glands secrete parathormone, which is a hormone with an important role in calcium metabolism. Decreased serum calcium (hypocalcaemia) can result in increased neuromuscular excitability, tetany, laryngospasm, flaccid heart muscle, and cardiac arrhythmia (Seeley *et al.*, 1992).

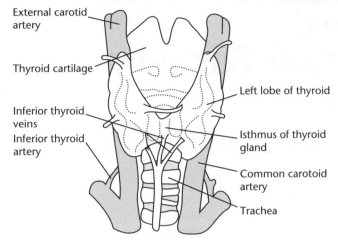

Figure 13.1 The thyroid gland.

Clinically it is important to understand that the thyroid gland:

- Lies near the airway.
- Is highly vascular.
- Shares innervation with the vocal cords.

Understanding the basic anatomy of the thyroid will help focus nursing assessment and interventions and anticipate potential postoperative difficulties (Litwack-Saleh, 1992).

Histologically the thyroid gland is made up of follicles (*Figure 13.2*), which synthesize the main thyroid hormones triiodothyronine (T_3) and tetraiodothyronine, which is more commonly known as thyroxine (T_4). Scattered between the follicles are parafollicular cells, which produce another hormone called

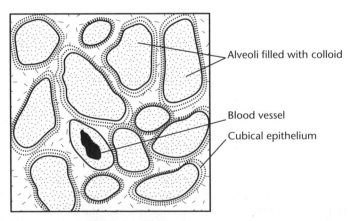

Figure 13.2 Microstructure of the thyroid gland.

calcitonin. Calcitonin has a role in reducing the calcium concentration in body fluids. Iodine obtained from the diet is essential for the synthesis of T_3 and T_4. The thyroid hormones (T_3 and T_4) are essential for:

- Regulating the basal metabolic rate (BMR).
- Normal growth and development.
- Potentiation of the action of other hormones.
- Normal lactation.

T_3 and T_4 increase the BMR of most body cells and this results in increased heat generation and a rise in body temperature. Physiological levels of T_3 and T_4 potentiate the action of insulin, and so promote the storage and correct use of glucose. T_3 and T_4 also assist in protein metabolism. At physiological levels these hormones help in the maintenance and repair of body tissues, but in large doses they can cause tissue breakdown. All aspects of lipid metabolism are influenced; the net effect is to encourage lipid utilization. The thyroid hormones are required for the conversion of carotene to vitamin A. In hypothyroid conditions, the serum carotene concentration increases and the skin may become yellow, but unlike jaundice, the eyes are not affected. T_3 and T_4 are also required for normal growth and maturation of the bones and development of the brain and other nervous tissues. In infant hypothyroidism, myelination and neuronal development in the brain are disrupted, and unless treated, mental retardation will occur (cretinism). The overall effect of the thyroid hormones is to increase catabolism and the BMR. The energy produced raises body temperature. Evidence suggests a strong link between thyroid hormones and the sympathetic nervous system. Hyperthyroidism can result in overactivity of the sympathetic division of the autonomic nervous system resulting in increases in blood flow, heart rate, motility of the gastrointestinal tract and increased activity of the nervous system generally (Porth and Hurwitz, 1994). These factors can be related to the overactivity of the gland and hyperthyroidism is discussed below.

THYROID DISORDERS

A euthyroid state is one where the thyroid hormones produced by the thyroid are within normal levels (Litwack-Saleh, 1992). Thyroid disease tends to result in either excessive secretion of thyroid hormones (hyperthyroidism) or a deficiency of the hormones (hypothyroidism or myxoedema). The main thyroid pathologies that may require surgical treatment include goitre and thyroid tumours.

Goitre

Goitre refers to any enlargement of the thyroid gland. It can result from hypertrophy of the gland or may be due to a benign or malignant thyroid tumour. Tumours of the thyroid will be discussed later. Most goitres are due to acquired disease and common causes are:

- Inflammation (thyroiditis).
- Neoplasia.
- Iodine deficiency (endemic goitre).
- Physiological or colloid goitre (cause unknown).
- Goitrogens (include some drugs and certain foods).

A goitre presents as a mass in the neck that moves on swallowing as the thyroid is attached to the larynx by fascia. Thyroid enlargement may be on one or both sides of the trachea. The trachea may be displaced and compression may alter tracheal, oesophageal, and vocal function. If surgery of the thyroid is required, it is important to assess functioning of the vocal cords so that changes in the voice after surgery can be recognized.

Occasionally a goitre may extend down into the upper mediastinum; this is known as a mediastinal, intrathoracic, or 'plunging' goitre. It may be asymptomatic and detected only after routine chest radiography. Displacement of the trachea can result and removal of the goitre may be advised to avoid potential pressure symptoms or malignancy developing later.

Ellis and Calne (1993) suggest a two-stage assessment of goitre:

- Stage 1: Is the enlarged thyroid smooth, is there a single nodule, or is the goitre nodular?
- Stage 2: Is the patient euthyroid, hyperthyroid, or hypothyroid?

By combining the findings of these two stages, the most common presentations are:

- Smooth non-toxic or physiological goitre.
- Nodular non-toxic goitre (single or multinodular).
- Smooth toxic goitre (Graves' disease).
- Toxic nodular goitre (secondary thyrotoxicosis).

Ellis and Calne (1993) also list Hashimoto's thyroiditis (a smooth firm goitre with myxoedema) and thyroid carcinoma as less common findings.

Nodular goitre occurs more commonly in females. At certain times in the patient's life there is an increase in thyroid activity accompanied by enlargement of the gland. After the period of increased activity, glandular enlargement may recede, but often there is a progressive build-up of nodular tissue within the thyroid. Increased activity often occurs during adolescence, pregnancy, and at the menopause. There may also be some fluctuation with each menstrual cycle. The hypothalamic and pituitary changes seen at puberty may contribute to the small goitres sometimes seen in prepubertal girls. The patient is usually euthyroid, but sometimes excess T_3 and T_4 are produced and a secondary thyrotoxicosis can develop. Over time, the periods of hyposecretion and hypersecretion cause an episodic and localized enlargement of the thyroid that may result in the formation of a multinodular goitre. Patients may complain of the sudden appearance of a lump in the neck due to haemorrhage into the nodules of a multinodular goitre. Complications of multinodular goitres include tracheal compression or displacement, acute haemorrhage, and hyperthyroidism, and rarely, cancerous change. Multinodular goitre may respond to medical treatment, but surgery is often required.

Colloid goitre results when the thyroid enlarges as atrophic follicles become filled with excess thyroglobin and is commonly due to iodine deficiency. The thyroid hypertrophies in an attempt to compensate for inadequate concentrations of serum thyroid hormone. One example is endemic goitre, which is found in parts of the world where the diet is deficient in iodine. Inadequate production of the thyroid hormones results in an increased concentration of serum thyroid stimulating hormone (TSH). TSH is produced by the anterior pituitary gland. Excess TSH causes hypertrophy of the thyroid gland with an accumulation of colloid in the follicles. Enlargement of the thyroid can then cause pressure symptoms on the trachea and laryngeal nerves. This condition used to be common in the UK (Derbyshire neck) until the iodination of table salt. However, it is still seen in regions where the iodine concentration in water and soil is low, for example Central Africa and the Himalayas.

In primary thyrotoxicosis or Graves' disease there is hyperplasia of the thyroid resulting in a smooth swelling of the gland and hypersecretion of the thyroid hormones. The gland becomes very vascular, the colloid is scanty, and there is lymphocyte infiltration. A lymphadenoid goitre may occur in Hashimoto's thyroiditis due to infiltration of the thyroid by lymphoid tissue and thyroid follicle hyperplasia. Unless the pressure symptoms are severe, lymphadenoid goitre is unlikely to require surgical treatment.

Hyperthyroidism (Thyrotoxicosis)

Hyperthyroidism or thyrotoxicosis is characterized by an excess secretion of thyroid hormones. When it is accompanied by exophthalmos (abnormal unilateral or bilateral protrusion of the eyeballs) and enlargement of the gland, it may be referred to as exophthalmic goitre. A number of conditions can result in hyperthyroidism (*Box 13.1*).

Grave's disease or primary thyrotoxicosis is the single most common cause of hyperthyroidism It is an autoimmune disorder and is eight times more common in women. Its onset is usually between 20–40 years of age and the condition shows a familial tendency. There is a toxic enlargement and inflammation of the thyroid with histological evidence of the deposition of immunoglobins and serum proteins, which stimulate inflammation. The exact cause of the disease is not known, but it involves the formation of autoantibodies to TSH. Long-acting thyroid stimulating immunoglobulins (LATS) are found in about 80% of patients with Graves' disease. LATS bind to thyroid follicle cell receptors for TSH, stimulating excessive production of the thyroid hormones. Other antibodies, for example antithyroglobulin antibodies, are also produced in Graves' disease. The main features of Graves' disease are central nervous system (CNS) disturbances and there may be exophthalmos.

Box 13.1 Causes of hyperthyroidism.

Common
- Graves' disease (diffuse toxic goitre)
- Toxic adenomas of the thyroid

Rare
- Thyrotoxicosis factitia
- Struma ovarii
- TSH-secreting pituitary tumour
- Metastatic functioning thyroid carcinoma

Toxic adenoma of the thyroid is the common cause of secondary thyrotoxicosis. The adenoma is a benign neoplasm and produces symptoms due to excessive secretion of the thyroid hormones and pressure effects. It may be single or part of a toxic multinodular adenoma. The onset of the condition is usually more gradual than in Graves' disease and in general it affects an older age group. LATS are not produced and tests for other antithyroid antibodies are usually negative. Exophthalmos is not seen and the main presenting features are cardiovascular system (CVS) changes. The CNS disturbances seen in primary thyrotoxicosis are less evident.

Clinical features of hyperthyroidism

The type and intensity of features (*Table 13.1*) varies between individuals, but patients with thyrotoxicosis are usually female. Symptoms include increased nervousness, restlessness, inceased sweating, heat intolerance, weakness, fatigue, weight loss (often accompanied by increased appetite), palpitations, muscle cramps, and diarrhoea. In severe cases the mental changes can be so extreme that a psychosis may be suspected. The clinical manifestations are due to the multiple effects of excess thyroid hormone secretion, but the main causitive mechanisms include:

- Increased catabolism and increased heat production.
- Autonomic lability and increased sensitivity to catecholamines.
- Increased gastrointestinal activity (increased motility).

Although goitre is a common presentation of hyperthyroidism, it may be absent in as many as 40% of older patients with the condition (Davis and Davis, 1974). The effect of Graves' disease on the eyes is one of the most distressing features of hyperthyroidism and ranges from the appearance of staring, to lid lag and exophthalmos. Exophthalmos or protrusion of the eyes and lid lag can result in visual loss from corneal ulceration or effects on the optic nerve. The cause is uncertain, but in severe cases patients may be unable to close their eyes and risk

Table 13.1 Clinical characteristics of hyperthyroidism.

Patient problems	Signs and symptoms
Altered nutrition and metabolism (negative nitrogen balance)	Weight loss and muscle wasting Increased appetite Increased heat intolerance Sometimes impaired glucose tolerance and glycosuria
Altered CVS activity	Tachycardia (rapid bounding pulse) Increased sleeping pulse Palpitations, atrial fibrillation (older patient) Increased cardiac output Increased blood pressure (but diastolic pressure may be lower than expected in younger patients) Older patient may present with congestive cardiac failure
Altered respiratory activity	Shortness of breath
Altered skin integrity	Skin warm and increased sweating
Altered activity patterns	Weakness and fatigue but may be hyperkinetic Hand tremor, altered tendon reflexes
Altered mental and emotional status	Emotional lability, increased anxiety Restlessness and increased irritability Insomnia
Altered elimination	Intestinal hurry (frequent defecation) Diarrhoea, nausea, and vomiting may occur
Altered patterns of sexuality	Impact of exophthalmos and goitre on body image Menstrual disorders (oligomenorrhoea, amenorrhoea)

corneal ulceration. Surgical decompression of the orbit may be needed for severe exophthalmos.

Hypothyroidism (Myxoedema)

Congenital hypothyroidism or cretinism occurs when a child is born with subnormal thyroid function. Adult hypothyroidism or myxoedema is caused by a variety of conditions, but usually affects middle-aged and elderly women. Hashimoto's thyroiditis is a condition marked by goitre and myxoedema. In hypothyroidism, the patient may present with slowing mental processes, lethargy, increased sleep, and mental disturbance. Speech becomes slow, monotonous, and hoarse. Metabolism is decreased, but despite poor appetite, weight gain is likely. Pulse rate, blood pressure, and respiratory rates are decreased, and reduced gastrointestinal motility may contribute to constipation. Hypothyroidism is likely to occur after extensive thyroid surgery including total thyroidectomy.

Thyroid Neoplasms

Thyroid neoplasms are either benign or malignant (*Box 13.2*).

Thyroid adenomas, which are benign encapsulated nodules in the gland, are common, but usually occur as part of a multinodular goitre. True benign thyoid adenomas are less common and generally of the follicular type. Thyroid carcinomas are rare, accounting for only 1% of all malignancies (Leight, 1991). Papillary adenocarcinoma is the most common thyroid malignancy and is a slow growing tumour with late lymphatic involvement. Follicular adenocarcinoma has a greater tendency for vascular invasion and a poorer prognosis. Bone, lung, brain, and liver are common sites for metastases.

Box 13.2 **Classification of thyroid neoplasms.**

Benign
- Adenoma (follicular, papillary, atypical)

Malignant
- Well differentiated (papillary adenocarcinoma, follicular adenocarcinoma)
- Undifferentiated (spindle and giant cell carcinoma, small cell carcinoma)
- Miscellaneous (lymphoma, squamous cell carcinoma, metatastic, others)

INVESTIGATION OF THYROID DYSFUNCTION

The thyroid gland can be assessed by a variety of laboratory and specialized imaging tests. A simple test for hyperthyroidism is the sleeping pulse rate. Ellis and Calne (1993) recommend the sleeping pulse rate as the simplest and most reliable way of clinically distinguishing between an acute anxiety state and hyperthyroidism. In acute anxiety states the sleeping pulse will be normal, but it remains elevated in hyperthyroidism. A series of tests can be carried out to estimate the thyroid hormone concentrations in the blood, and the uptake of iodine by the gland. Tests of thyroid function and imaging procedures are summarized in *Box 13.3*. If the patient has Graves' disease, a test for serum LATS concentration may be ordered, but there is no agreement on the clinical value of this test. Most of the tests of thyroid function are simple blood tests. The nurse will need to explain the reason for the tests to the patient and observe the venepuncture site for haematoma formation. Many drugs may interfere with tests for the thyroid hormones and medication may need to be withheld. If medication (e.g. thyroid supplements) must be continued, this should be noted on the request form. However, the radioactive iodine uptake test may cause more anxiety. This test requires fasting, and patients and their relatives are likely to be concerned about taking a radioactive substance. The nurse will need to reassure

> ## Box 13.3 Investigation of thyroid dysfunction (adapted from Wheeler, 1994).
>
> **Serum tests** (used to evaluate thyroid function and distinguish between hyper- and hypothryroidism)
> - T_4 concentration (raised in hyperthyroidism)
> - T_3 concentration (raised in hyperthyroidism)
> - Thyroid stimulating hormone (TSH) concentration (raised in primary hypothyroidism)
> - Thyroid releasing hormone (TRH) concentration
> - T_3 resin uptake
> - Free T_4 and T_3 concentrations
>
> **Radioactive scanning procedures**
> - Radioactive iodine uptake test
> - Radionuclide thyroid imaging
>
> **Other imaging procedures**
> - Thyroid ultrasonography
> - Computerized tomography (CT)
> - Magnetic resonance imaging (MRI)
>
> **Biopsy**
> - Fine-needle aspiration or closed biopsy (can be useful in diagnosing thyroiditis and some malignancies)
>
> **Other tests**
> - Serum cholesterol (normal or slightly low in hyperthyroidism, usually raised in myxoedema)
> - Electrocardiogram (ECG) (will confirm cardiac problems – atrial fibrillation – in hyperthyroidism or myxoedema)

patients that they will not be exposed to dangerous levels of radiation from either the radiochemical or imaging equipment. These tests are contraindicated in pregnancy and lactation.

TREATMENT OF GOITRE AND HYPERTHYROIDISM

The treatment of non-toxic goitre depends on the size of the goitre, the presence of pressure effects, and the age of the patient. Thyroidectomy will be considered for cosmetic reasons in the younger patient because of the danger of haemorrhage into a thyroid cyst and the slight risk of malignant change. Thyroidectomy will be advised if there are pressure symptoms. A longstanding goitre in an elderly patient is unlikely to require surgical treatment. Ellis and Calne (1993) recommend investigation and removal of any solitary thyroid nodule.

Hyperthyroidism requires treatment and four forms of therapy are available:

- Antithyroid drug treatment.
- Beta-adrenocepter blocking drugs.
- Radioactive iodine therapy.
- Surgery.

Antithyroid drugs are used to control thyrotoxicosis. They interfere with the synthesis of the thyroid hormones and are used to produce remission and to prepare the patient for thyroid surgery. Carbimazole is the drug of choice in the UK, but propylthiouracil may be used if the patient is sensitive to carbimazole. Antithyroid drug therapy generally lasts for 12–18 months and produces a permanent remission in only a minority of patients. The beta-adrenoceptor blocking drugs, notably propranolol, are used to provide rapid relief from some of the major effects of thyrotoxicosis. However, the use of a beta-adrenoceptor blocking drug is contraindicated if the patient has suspected myocardial dysfunction as it may cause heart failure.

It is important that the nurse informs the patient that because thyroid hormone stores in the body take up to one month to become depleted, the drug dose may need adjusting to find the correct dose required to maintain a euthyroid state. This may take some time and patient compliance is essential. The toxic effects of the prescribed medication must be explained by the nurse. Problems such as rashes, sore throats, or any pain must be reported immediately to the patient's general practitioner or practice nurse. Regular checks of serum T_4 concentration are necessary to detect hypothyroidism caused by overtreatment. It must be emphasized that relapses can still occur once a euthyroid state has been achieved.

Radioactive therapy is an effective treatment that avoids prolonged drug therapy or the need for surgery. The patient simply swallows a solution or capsule of gamma-emitting radioactive sodium iodide, which destroys thyroid tissue and therefore reduces T_3 and T_4 production. The treatment can be given on a day case or outpatient basis. The nurse must be aware of the anxieties and fear any treatment associated with radioactive substances can cause. The patient needs to fast for three hours after taking the radioactive iodine; it is then important to drink at least three litres of fluid over the next 24 hours to rid the body of excess radioactive iodine not taken up by the gland. Patients may be asked to isolate themselves from their families for 3–4 days to avoid infection. Behi (1989) asserts that patients should also minimize contact with children for a week in order to protect them from the risk of radiation. The nurse needs to explain that the treatment can cause transient discomfort in the glands of the neck. It usually takes 2–3 months to achieve a euthyroid state, and antithyroid drugs may be required during this period. It must be emphasized that radioactive iodine therapy may not be successful the first time and subsequent treatment may be necessary. Despite successful treatment, recurrences may occur in up to 10% of cases, and 40–70% of cases show permanent hypothyroidism after ten years (Lyerly, 1991). Hypothyroidism requires thyroid replacement therapy. Radioactive iodine therapy is particularly suitable for older patients, especially those with cardiomyopathies or problems with compliance. Children and women in their reproductive years are not considered suitable for radioactive iodine therapy, which is usually used only for patients over 45 years of age.

THYROID SURGERY

If other therapies are unsuitable or have failed, a subtotal thyroidectomy will be required. Antithyroid drugs will be used to achieve a euthyroid state and a subtotal thyroidectomy, which leaves the posterior portion of each lobe intact, is performed. This procedure leaves sufficient thyroid tissue to provide an adequate supply of hormones. The nursing management of a patient requiring subtotal thyroidectomy is considered in the next section. Thyroid surgery (total or subtotal thyroidectomy) is indicated if:

- Antithyroid drugs and radioactive iodine therapy have failed.
- There is a risk of haemorrhage or pressure effects from the goitre.
- There are cosmetic reasons in the younger patient who is not suitable for antithyroid drugs or radioiodine.

Surgery will be essential if:

- There are pressure effects or haemorrhage.
- An operable carcinoma is suspected.

NURSING MANAGEMENT

Preoperative Care

A patient requiring subtotal thyroidectomy will be admitted for elective surgery after a period of antithyroid drug therapy aimed at achieving a euthyroid state. The patient is usually admitted 1–2 days before surgery. Although euthyroid, the patient may be overanxious about surgery. The patient's preoperative needs are likely to include maintenance of the euthyroid state, promotion of rest, quiet, and freedom from emotional stress, provision of adequate nutrition, preoperative information, general preoperative preparation, assessment of the voice and trachea, and surgical preparation.

Maintenance of euthyroid state

Regular monitoring of vital signs and the degree of anxiety, restlessness, or agitation will help identify possible thyrotoxicosis. A check on the sleeping pulse may be requested; if it is regularly more than 80 beats per minute, the patient's suitability for immediate surgery may need reassessing. It is critical that anti-thyroid drug therapy is administered as prescribed.

Promotion of rest, quiet, and freedom from emotional stress

Anxiety related to the patient's history of thyrotoxicosis may be identified and it is important to promote a calm relaxed atmosphere. The patient should be allocated a bed in a quiet area of the ward and interaction with visitors observed. A tachycardia or increased agitation after visitors may suggest that visiting needs to be limited. Night sedation may be required to enable the patient to have rest and adequate sleep.

Provision of adequate nutrition

The hyperthyroid patient requires a high-protein high-calorie diet and adequate fluids. However, for elective surgery, the patient should be euthyroid with no additional nutritional needs. A nutritional assessment and daily weighing are important to detect any signs of hyper- or hypothyroidism.

Preoperative information

Patients may need help to understand their condition, drug therapy, and the forthcoming operation. The likely length of stay in hospital should be discussed with the patient and relatives. Hospitalization may not exceed four days, and patients may have to arrange for assistance in the convalescent period for themselves and perhaps in looking after their family. It is also important that the nurse liaises closely with the patient's family in the time before and after surgery. The patient's family may have experienced difficulties in coping with the patient, who due to the condition may have been anxious and irritable. This can have a serious effect on family relationships and it is important that the nurse listens, explains, and reassures relatives that successful treatment will enable the patient to maintain a stable body weight and have sufficient energy to participate in normal activities and achieve restful sleep at night. The relatives can be of tremendous help in reinforcing this information for the patient.

General preoperative preparation

As well as the general preoperative care discussed in Chapter 2, patients undergoing thyroid surgery require some specific preparation. The nurse should demonstrate how to support the neck with the hands; hands placed behind the neck will ease strain on the neck muscles, which will minimize stress on the incision. This teaching can be reinforced by a chance to practise the manoeuvre. The patient may wish to discuss the operation scar and can be reassured that the incision is made taking the natural folds of the neck into consideration. When healing is complete, the scar will be barely noticeable. The nurse can suggest the patient wears a scarf or necklace until the scar has faded. A drain may be used and the wound is closed with clips or sutures, and this should be explained to the patient. The patient will need to sit upright and oxygen may be prescribed for a few hours postoperatively; intravenous fluid replacement therapy is likely.

Assessment of the voice and trachea

The enlarged thyroid gland may be causing pressure on nearby structures. A chest radiograph is taken to ensure that the enlarged gland is not constricting the trachea or causing its deviation to one side. The recurrent laryngeal nerve supplies the vocal cords and it may be damaged by pressure from the enlarged thyroid or during surgery. Unilateral damage will result in a hoarse voice and bilateral injury can cause permanent debilitating hoarseness. To assess for postoperative damage, the nurse must first assess the voice preoperatively, and laryngoscopy may be required to assess the state of the vocal cords. Indirect laryngoscopy is an uncomfortable procedure and the patient may need considerable support. Some patients are reassured by the fact that the procedure will be repeated after the operation to ensure that the cords have not been damaged by the operation.

Surgical preparation

The thyroid is a vascular gland and antithyroid drugs may have caused additional compensatory vascularization. Potassium iodide and iodine (Lugol's solution) may be prescribed for ten days preoperatively to reduce vascularization of the gland and help maintain the euthyroid state (Lyerly, 1991). Blood typing and crossmatching are of course essential. An ECG will be obtained to check cardiac status. Thyroid function tests will be repeated and basal parathyroid function will be determined from serum calcium and phosphate concentrations. Care may be required in the management of the antithyroid therapy in the final preoperative days in view of the danger of postoperative hypothyroidism after surgery has removed most of the gland.

Care of the Patient after Subtotal Thyroidectomy

Thyroid surgery carries the same hazards and risks of postoperative complications as any surgical operation (i.e. pain, haemorrhage, postoperative infection). However, thyroidectomy is also associated with particular problems, and nursing management needs to address these besides the more general postoperative problems. Specific problems may relate to hormonal disruption or damage to related anatomical structures.

Hormonal disruption includes:

■ Tetany due to damage or removal of the parathyroid glands.
■ Hypothyroidism due to extensive removal of thyroid tissue.
■ Recurrence of hyperthyroidism due to inadequate removal of toxic goitre.
■ Thyroid crisis (thyroid storm).

Damage to related anatomical structures includes:

- Unilateral or bilateral damage to the recurrent laryngeal nerve causing hoarseness or loss of voice.
- Tracheal damage.
- Haemorrhage into the thyroid bed.

It should be noted that these complications of thyroid surgery are now comparatively rare, mainly due to improved techniques and preoperative preparation. However, the complications are serious and the nurse must be alert for early indications of a developing problem.

Nursing Considerations – Special Problems

Potential for obstructed airway

Respiration may be compromised by injury to the trachea, compression of the trachea due to haematoma, irritation, and an increase in tracheal and bronchial secretions due to the effects of the anaesthetic, immobility, and pain in the head and neck inhibiting breathing and expectoration.

Occasionally oedema of the glottis causes difficulty in respiration with the development of cyanosis and noisy breathing. Regular assessment of the respiratory system for dyspnoea and noisy breathing or stridor is vital. The patient will need to be helped into a sitting position as soon as possible, with the head supported carefully to avoid tension on the wound site. Patients should be taught to support their own head and neck when moving. Frequent encouragement should be given to deep breathe to allow full oxygenation of the lungs and prevent atelectasis. Coughing should be minimized to prevent tissue damage and stress to the incision. Any drainage tube and bag must be carefully positioned. Humidified oxygen may be prescribed for a few hours after surgery and suction equipment should be available. The risk of damage to the laryngeal nerve is discussed later.

Potential for haemorrhage

Modern thyroid surgery entails careful preoperative preparation and the risk of haemorrhage is low. However, haemorrhage into the thyroid bed is particularly dangerous as it can compress an already swollen trachea and rapidly obstruct the airway. The nurse must observe for dyspnoea or stridor and be alert for signs of shock. The patient's blood pressure and pulse should be monitored carefully, half hourly at first, and any increase in pulse rate and fall in blood pressure must be reported immediately. It is important for the nurse to be alert for any complaint from the patient of a sensation of pressure at the wound site as this may indicate haemorrhage and must be reported immediately. The wound site must be inspected frequently to ensure free drainage and to note for signs of fresh bleeding. Blood may be visible through the dressing, but it is important to inspect the side and back of the patient's neck where blood may have collected. If a haematoma occurs, it may be necessary to quickly remove a clip or suture to release the clot, and for this reason, a clip or suture removal pack should be kept by the patient's bed. After this emergency measure, the patient would be returned to theatre for resuturing. Crossmatched blood should be available for emergency transfusion.

Potential for tetany
Trauma or accidental removal of the parathyroid glands during surgery can result in hypoparathyroidism and the patient may develop tetany within a few days of surgery. The parathyroid glands release the hormone parathormone, which has a role in maintaining plasma calcium concentration. Decreased secretion of this hormone causes hypocalcaemia. Early signs of hypocalcaemia are numbness or tingling in the fingers and toes, but the most obvious sign is carpopedal spasm. Trousseau's and Chovstek's signs can be used to check for hypocalcaemia. Trousseau's sign is a characteristic contraction of the hand due to carpopedal spasm induced by a tourniquet around the upper arm. It is most usually seen when measuring the blood pressure. Chovstek's sign is a spasm of the facial muscle in response to a gentle tapping of the patient's face over the zygoma. Hypocalcaemia is confirmed by checking plasma concentration and initial treatment is with intravenous calcium gluconate. Traumatized parathyroids may recover and the tetany will be temporary. However, if the glands are removed, permanent treatment will be needed with oral calcium supplements.

Risk of damage to the laryngeal nerves
Traumatic damage to the laryngeal nerves during thyroid surgery can result in alteration or loss of phonation and paralysis of the larynx leading to respiratory problems. Observe for respiratory problems and changes in the patient's voice. Vocal cord spasm and laryngeal paralysis can cause a serious narrowing of the airway and require tracheostomy. Emergency tracheostomy equipment must be available on the ward. If the injury is incomplete, some function may return, but occasionally the tracheostomy will be permanent. Sometimes the patient experiences a sore throat and some hoarseness of the voice because of the anaesthetic intubation. In this case the patient should be reassured that the problem is transitory and cool drinks should be encouraged.

Potential for thyroid crisis
Thyroid crisis or thyroid storm is an acute thyrotoxic condition that is probably caused by massive release of thyroid hormones into the blood during surgery. The patient may complain of a sudden onset of breathlessness, palpitations, and a feeling of great heat. This is very frightening and will cause great distress and agitation. There is an uncontrolled rise in metabolic rate, hyperpyrexia, a marked tachycardia, and raised blood pressure. The patient may develop mania, and death can result from heart failure. Thyroid storm can occur during the operation, but has been known to appear 6–24 hours after surgery, and is abrupt in

onset. Careful monitoring of the patient's temperature, pulse, respirations, blood pressure, and mental state are essential. Intravenous fluids are given to correct dehydration and control hyperthermia. The patient is nursed in a cool environment and prescribed sedatives, and oxygen are administered. High doses of intravenous beta-adrenoceptor blocking drugs (propranolol), antithyroid drugs (carbimazole), and glucocorticosteroid therapy (intramuscular hydrocortisone) are instituted as emergency treatment. Thyroid crisis is now extremely rare due to improved preoperative preparation to establish a euthyroid state. Frequent postoperative observations of respiratory, cardiovascular, and mental status allow its early identification.

Nursing Considerations – General

Potential problem of pain in the neck wound

This is minimized by the administration of regular prescribed analgesia at first, the effects of which must be carefuly evaluated. Patient Controlled Analgesia (PCA), which allows patients to control their own pain relief, is helpful. Various narcotic drugs can be used, including diamorphine, papaveretum, pethidine, and dihydrocodeine tartrate. A change to non-narcotic drugs can be made when the patient indicates that the pain is less severe. A comfortable position – upright with the head well supported with pillows to avoid tension of the neck – is very important because the neck muscles are then allowed to relax and tension on the wound is relieved. Drainage tubes should be adequately supported and the patient's glass of water and personal belongings such as tissues should be within easy reach. The upright position may cause sacral discomfort, and the patient should be helped and encouraged to move from side to side. Reassurance can be given that the wound drain and intravenous infusion will most likely be removed within 24 hours, and the patient can then be helped into a chair. Regular monitoring for signs of haemorrhage, pain, and shock is necessary.

Potential problems associated with the wound and wound drainage

The incision is made along a natural skin fold so that the scar will be less visible when healing has taken place. The wound is closed with clips or small sutures and drained through a separate stab incision. The drain is usually connected to a decompression drainage container. The main aims of decompression drainage in the clean wound are:

■ Removal of fluid.
■ Reduction in seroma and haematoma formation.
■ Obliteration of dead space.

These are particularly important considerations in a compact structure such as the neck. Wound drainage must be observed carefully, and the nature and amount of fluid recorded; this is necessary to detect haemorrhage and note the amount of fluid loss. The drainage tube must be checked for patency and to ensure suction is adequate. The wound drain and any pressure dressing are usually removed on the day after surgery if drainage is minimal. The wound is inspected within 36 hours of surgery. Between then and the discharge of the patient on the fourth day after operation, the clips or sutures are removed providing the wound is healing satisfactorily. Not every surgeon will use drains after thyroid surgery. There is some evidence from trials of suction drainage after thyroid surgery that 'no drain' treatment has no more complications than the 'with drain' treatment (Torrance, 1993).

Eating and drinking

Intravenous therapy is usually discontinued when the risk of haemorrhage is over and the patient is taking sufficient fluids orally. However, swallowing can be uncomfortable after thyroidectomy, and the patient may be reluctant to eat and drink. Cool drinks and soft food of the patient's choice should be offered to encourage progression to a normal diet. It should be explained to the patient that fluid and food intake containing adequate levels of protein and vitamin C are essential for successful wound healing and recovery.

Ambulation

Early ambulation and gentle neck movements should be encouraged. Complications are rare, and the usual pattern of recovery after subtotal thyroidectomy is uneventful. By the fourth day after operation, the patient is usually up and about, eating and drinking normally and ready for discharge home. It is important that time and encouragement are given for patients to question the nurse with regard to rest, exercise, or any other issue related to their recovery. Patients may need to be reminded that it may take 2–3 months before recovery is complete. An appointment is usually made for the patient to be seen in the outpatient clinic, and serum thyroxine concentrations are monitored.

FUTURE HEALTH CONSIDERATIONS

A long term problem after subtotal thyroidectomy is the risk of developing hypothyroidism. Within 1–2 years postoperatively, 5–50% of patients develop a degree of myxoedema (Lyerly, 1991). Patients may complain of tiredness, feeling cold, thickening of the skin, and thinning hair after surgery. They can become overweight and apathetic, and speech becomes slow, monotonous, and hoarse. Bradycardia, constipation, and a tendency to feel cold in hot weather are additional indicators of myxoedema. The condition requires assessment of thyroid function, and treatment with oral thyroxine is likely to be required for the rest of the patient's life.

TREATMENT OF THYROID CARCINOMA

A localized thyroid carcinoma may require removal of the affected lobe and lymph node dissection. Well-differentiated localized tumours may respond to treatment with radioactive iodine. They may also regress when large doses of thyroxine are given to suppress TSH release. A radical thyroidectomy is indicated for anaplastic carcinoma, but patients with this condition often present late with an inoperable mass. Radiotherapy and chemotherapy may be used, but often treatment is palliative. Pressure effects on the trachea may necessitate a tracheostomy. Nusing management is similar to that required after subtotal thyroidectomy. In anaplastic carcinoma, prognosis is often poor and palliative terminal care may be the priority.

CONCLUSION

Thyroid disorders can often prove complex to diagnose and difficult to treat. Careful assessment and vigilant observation on the part of the nurse is essential to ensure a patient's successful recovery from thyroid surgery. To facilitate this, it is essential that the nurse has a clear understanding of the anatomy and physiology involved to be able to target postoperative assessment towards the detection of complications specific to this type of surgery.

References

Behi R (1989) Treatment and care of thyroid problems. *Nursing* **3(41)**:4–6.

Davis PJ, Davis FB (1974) Hyperthyroidism in patients over the age of 60. *Medicine* **53(3)**:161.

Ellis H, Calne R (1993) *Lecture Notes on General Surgery*. 8th edition, pp. 323–326. Blackwell Scientific Publications, Oxford.

Leight Jr GS (1991) Nodular goitre and benign and malignant neoplasms of the thyroid. In *Textbook of Surgery*. Sabiston Jr DC (ed.), 14th edition, pp. 579–590. WB Saunders, Philadelphia.

Litwack-Saleh K (1992) 'Practical points in the care of the patient post thyroid surgery'. *J Post Anaesthetic Nurs* **7(6)**:404–406.

Lyerly HK (1991) Hyperthyroidism. In *Textbook of Surgery*. Sabiston Jr DC (ed.), 14th edition, pp. 568–576. WB Saunders, Philadelphia.

Porth CM, Hurwitz LS (1994) Alterations in endocrine control of growth and metabolism. *Pathophysiology. Concepts of Altered Health States*. 4th edition, Chap. 45, p. 907. JB Lippincott, Philadelphia.

Seeley RS, Stephens TD, Tate P (1992) *Anatomy and Physiology*. 2nd edition, p. 889. Mosby-Year Book, St. Louis.

Torrance C (1993) Introduction to surgical drainage. *Surg Nurse* **6(2)**:19–23.

Wheeler MH (1994) Investigations of the thyroid. *Surgery* **12(7)**:145–147.

Chapter 14

Surgery of the Gastrointestinal Tract

This chapter opens with an account of the anatomy of the abdomen and its contents. The part played by the nurse in the physical examination and investigations required for patients with disorders of the gastrointestinal tract and anorectum is discussed. Finally, the preparation, surgical management and nursing care of acute and chronic conditions relating to the gastrointestinal tract and anorectum are described.

ANATOMY OF THE ABDOMEN

The abdominal cavity (*Figure 14.1*) contains structures such as the liver, spleen, kidneys, ureters, abdominal aorta, vena cava, terminal portion of the oesophagus, stomach, and small and large intestines. *Table 14.1* lists the main muscles of the abdomen. The anterior wall of the abdominal cavity is formed from three layers of muscle and their aponeuroses. The outer layer, formed by the external oblique muscle runs at an angle across the abdomen from its lateral superior origins to its inferior medial insertions (*Figure 14.2*). The internal oblique muscle forming the middle layer runs mainly perpendicular to the external oblique, from its inferior lateral origins to superior medial insertions. The transverse

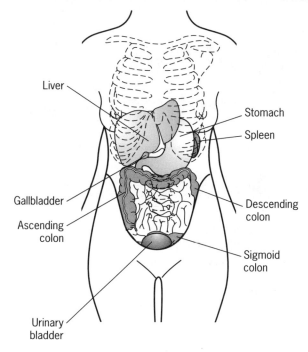

Figure 14.1 Structures within the abdominal cavity.

Table 14.1 The main muscles of the abdomen.

Name	Origin	Insertion
Anterior		
External oblique	Ribs 5–12	Iliac crest Inguinal ligament
Internal oblique	Iliac crest Inguinal ligament Lumbar fascia	Ribs 10–12 Rectus sheath
Transversus abdominis	Costal cartilages 7–12 Lumbar fascia Iliac crest Inguinal ligament	Xiphoid process Linea alba Pubic tubercle
Rectus abdominis	Pubic crest Symphysis pubis	Xiphoid process Lower ribs
Posterior		
Quadratus lumborum	Iliac crest Lower lumbar vertebrae	Rib 12 Upper lumbar vertebrae

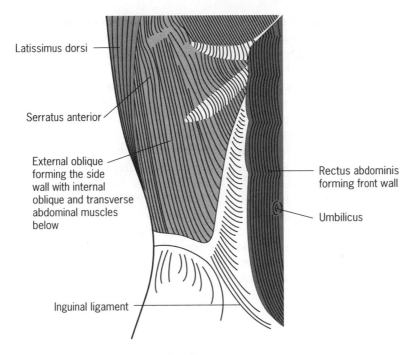

Latissimus dorsi

Serratus anterior

External oblique
forming the side
wall with internal
oblique and transverse
abdominal muscles
below

Rectus abdominis
forming front wall

Umbilicus

Inguinal ligament

Figure 14.2 Muscles of the abdominal wall.

abdominal muscle forms the inner muscle layer and runs horizontally across the abdominal wall. This criss-cross arrangement of muscle layers results in a strong but flexible abdominal wall. However, weakness can develop with resulting herniation of abdominal organs (see Chapter 17).

The abdominopelvic cavity, the largest of the body cavities, lies within the abdomen. The abdominal cavity lies within the abdomen proper and the pelvic cavity within the bony pelvis. The abdominal cavity contains most of the major abdominal organs, the pelvic cavity contains the bladder, other urogenital organs, some loops of small intestine, and the sigmoid colon. However, there is no anatomical barrier dividing these two cavities; functionally they act as a single cavity. Conditions affecting the kidneys and urogenital organs are considered in Chapter 16.

The peritoneum is a continuous serous membrane that lines the abdomino-pelvic cavity and covers many of the abdominal organs. The parietal peritoneum represents the innermost layer of the abdominal wall. It completely encloses the cavity in the male, but in the female the fallopian tubes enter through openings in the parietal peritoneum and can act as a route for infection of the peritoneum (i.e. peritonitis). The visceral peritoneum covers the viscera, and the mesenteries are layers of peritoneal tissue that bridge the visceral and parietal peritoneum, providing support for blood vessels, nerves, and the abdominal organs. The greater omentum is a mesentery connecting the stomach to the transverse colon, and the lesser omentum connects the stomach at the lesser curvature to the liver. The serous layers support and protect the abdominal contents, but at the same time allow some mobility and expansion. The peritoneum secretes a small amount of serous fluid that helps lubricate the peritoneal membranes and allows movement without friction. However, if the peritoneum becomes inflamed or infected fluid production increases and fluid may build up in the cavity causing ascites.

In surgery the distinction between peritoneal and retroperitoneal structures can be important. *Figure 14.3* illustrates the relationship between peritoneum, mesentery, and peritoneal and retroperitoneal structures.

In general the gastrointestinal (GI) tract can be viewed as a continuous, muscular tube lined with epithelium. At various points the tube is structurally adapted for different functions. The epithelial lining moderates ingestion of digested particles, while peristaltic movement of the smooth muscles mixes and moves food within the tract. At various points specialized muscle areas, sphincters, control movement along the GI tract.

The gut is insensitive to stimuli such as cutting, but sensitive to distension, muscle spasm, ischaemia, and tension on the mesentery. These produce pain impulses, which are carried by the sympathetic nerve supply to the abdominal organs. The sympathetic nerves also supply the visceral layer of the peritoneum.

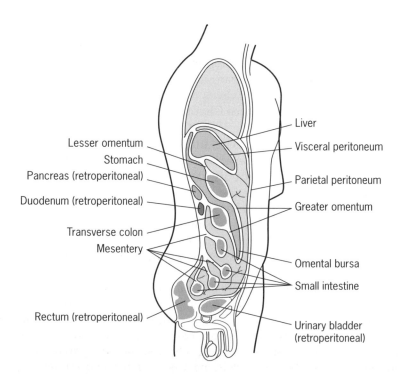

Figure 14.3 Perioneal cavity, peritoneum, and mesenteries.

The parietal layer of the peritoneum is supplied by the spinal nerves to overlying muscles and subcutaneous segments of the body wall. The nature and site of abdominal pain described by the patient are significant in clinical diagnosis.

Much general surgery is concerned with conditions affecting the abdominal organs and this chapter will review surgical interventions and nursing management of conditions affecting the stomach, small intestine, colon, rectum, and anal canal. Conditions affecting the liver, biliary system, pancreas, and spleen are considered in Chapter 15.

PHYSICAL EXAMINATION OF THE ABDOMEN

When examining the abdomen it is important to be familiar with surface landmarks and the position of underlying organs. It is also useful to be familiar with the system of quadrants and regions used to describe the location of abdominal structures. *Figure 14.4* shows some of the major hard and soft tissue landmarks. The xiphoid process and costal margins help define the upper limit of the abdomen, although it should be remembered that the diaphragm is dome-shaped and the superior surfaces of the liver and spleen lie slightly higher than

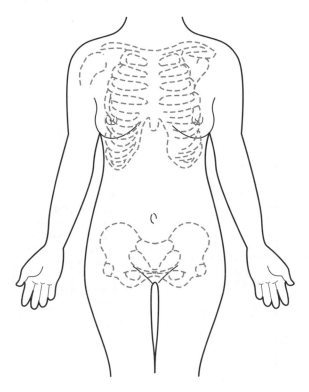

Figure 14.4 Major hard and soft tissue landmarks.

the costal margins. The lower limits are located by finding the iliac crest and anterior superior iliac spine and following the line of the inguinal ligament as it runs downwards and medially to the tubercle of the pubic bone. On the abdominal surface the linea alba forms the midline, extending from the xiphoid process to the symphysis pubis. It represents the fusion of the aponeuroses of the major anterior abdominal muscles. The linea semilunaris may also be visible (especially if the abdominal muscles are tensed) as a curved line or groove on either side of the linea alba. The linea semilunaris represents the lateral border of the rectus abdominis muscles.

For descriptive purposes the abdomen can be divided into four quadrants or nine regions (*Figure 14.5*). The position of the abdominal organs or symptoms can then be described in relation to these regions and quadrants. The abdomen can be examined by inspection, palpation, percussion, and auscultation.

Inspection

The position of any abdominal incisions or scars should be noted (*Figure 14.6*) and the abdomen observed for signs of distension, visibly pulsating vessels, or peristaltic waves. The contour or shape of the abdomen should be noted. Is it symmetrical? Is there any sign of ascites? Are there abnormal lumps or hernias? Is the skin colour normal? Are there any stretch marks?

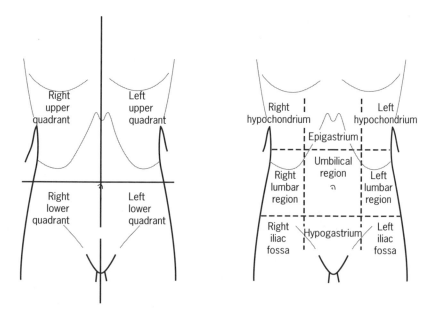

Figure 14.5 Abdominal quadrants and regions.

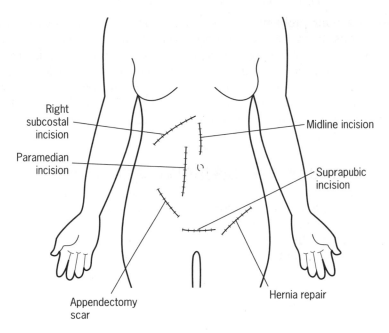

Figure 14.6 The position of common abdominal scars.

Palpation

Abdominal palpation may indicate areas of tenderness or confirm the appearance of muscle rigidity. Rigidity may be due to apprehension or to guarding, an involuntary muscular contraction that can be an indication of peritoneal irritation.

Percussion

This consists of gently tapping the part of the abdomen under examination. As a hollow area emits a more resonant sound than a solid one, this may reveal the presence of gas, fluid, or a tumour, or organ enlargement.

Auscultation

Altered sounds may be heard in the presence of the exaggerated peristalsis, which may occur in obstruction of the intestine. Normal sounds may be absent when mobility is inhibited by inflammation of the intestines or paralytic ileus following surgery.

Problems Relating to Abdominal Examination

Problems such as anxiety, fear, or embarrassment may be identified by the nurse. Explanations and reassurance should be offered, and patients given the opportunity to express their problems and describe their symptoms in their own way. Every effort must be made to ensure privacy and avoid exposure of the patient. It should be explained that it may not be possible to provide analgesia until a diagnosis has been made as important diagnostic points can be masked. The patient should lie supine with one pillow. Physical support may be necessary, for example to sustain the patient in the left lateral position for rectal examination. The patient may require a vomit bowl, tissues, a urinal, or a bedpan.

INVESTIGATIONS OF THE GASTROINTESTINAL TRACT

If the patient is admitted as an acute surgical emergency, investigations other than a plain abdominal radiograph may not be possible. However, in elective surgery the patient is likely to have undergone a range of clinical investigations. Investigations for abdominal and GI disorders include:

- Radiological investigations.
- Other imaging techniques.
- Endoscopic investigations.
- Blood and biochemical investigations.

Radiological Investigations

Plain radiography

An upright chest radiograph is essential in cases of abdominal pain to rule out conditions such as pneumonia, but may also show gas under the diaphragm, which can result from a perforated bowel. Plain abdominal radiography can identify abnormalities of bony structures, abnormal collections of air, signs of obstruction or distension, and abnormal calcifications. It will also demonstrate distended loops of an obstructed intestine. Air can commonly be seen in the colon and stomach, but is not normally present in the small intestine. If air is localized within one region of the small intestine it suggests a paralytic ileus. Mechanical obstruction may be indicated by air and fluid-filled loops of bowel before the obstruction and decompressed bowel after the obstruction. Plain abdominal radiography may also identify air outside the GI lumen. For example, the presence of air in the peritoneal cavity suggests perforation of the bowel, while gas in the biliary system may indicate cholangitis or a sinus connecting the GI and biliary tracts. Plain radiography may also help identify kidney stones, gall stones, faecaliths in the appendix, and other types of calcification.

Contrast radiography

Contrast media such as barium sulphate or meglumine diatrizoate (Gastrografin) can be used to improve the information provided by radiography. Procedures commonly used to investigate GI function include:

- Barium swallow, meal or follow-through.
- Barium meal and follow-through.
- Barium enema.

A barium swallow is used primarily to identify oesophageal problems such as hiatus hernia (see Chapter 17), varices (see Chapter 16), and diverticula. The patient is fasted and given a flavoured solution of barium sulphate solution to drink. The patient is then secured on a tilt table and radiographs are taken in various positions. The procedure takes about 15 minutes and will not usually be uncomfortable. In a barium follow-through patients take barium and lie on their right side. The barium is delivered to the small intestine in a single bolus or column and radiographs are taken at regular intervals until the barium reaches the large intestine. A barium meal will be used to investigate suspected upper GI problems such as dyspepsia, weight loss, or upper GI bleeding. In the single-contrast method only barium sulphate is used. In the double-contrast method the patient is first asked to swallow a solution that releases carbon dioxide (CO_2) gas and then a high-density barium solution. The patient is tilted so that the barium coats the stomach mucosa and the gas distends the stomach. This technique allows better visualization of mucosal abnormalities.

A barium enema will be requested to investigate lower GI problems. It is mainly used in the diagnosis of colorectal cancer, polyps, diverticula, and other diseases of the colon and rectum. To prepare the colon the patient will be prescribed laxatives or enemas or both and a low-residue or fluid-only diet may be ordered for 24 hours before the test. The patient will be fasted. The patient is placed on a tilt table and a rectal tube inserted for administration of the barium. Radiographs will be taken as the barium fills the bowel. The patient may experience cramping pain as the barium enters and will need to resist the urge to evacuate the bowel. It is important that the patient retains the barium so that the intestinal walls are adequately coated. After the procedure the patient is taken to the toilet or given a bedpan and asked to evacuate as much of the barium as possible. A check radiograph may then be taken to assess the mucosa and the efficiency of defaecation. As with the barium meal a single- or double-contrast technique may be used.

After barium studies the patient needs to be aware that the stool may be chalky and pale coloured for 24–72 hours. Barium residues in the GI tract can harden and cause obstruction or faecal impaction so it is important to record and describe the amount and type of stool for 2–3 days. An enema may be prescribed to cleanse the colon after a barium enema.

Other Imaging Techniques

Computerized tomography (CT) and ultrasound scanning can be used in assessing the abdomen and GI tract. CT allows the relationships and densities of a patient's anatomy to be seen by producing a picture of a transverse slice through the patient's body at a given level. It is particularly useful for imaging the accessory organs of digestion such as the liver and pancreas. Ultrasonography is not generally applied to investigations of acute abdominal pain, but is useful in investigations of the biliary system, liver, and pancreas. For a proctogram an ultrasound probe is inserted into the rectum to detect lower rectal tumours.

Endoscopy

Endoscopy allows direct visualization of the GI tract using a flexible endoscope. The mucosal surface can be inspected and biopsy samples taken for histological investigations. In many cases therapeutic interventions can be carried out via the endoscope. Oesophagogastroduodenoscopy is the visual inspection of the mucosal lining of the oesophagus, stomach, and duodenum. It is indicated in patients with haematemesis, malaena, or epigastric or substernal pain, and can identify tumours, inflammation or ulceration, varices, hiatus hernia, polyps, and obstruction. The endoscope has several channels, which allow fine instruments to be used to obtain biopsy specimens, to coagulate bleeding points, and remove polyps. Colonoscopy is the endoscopic examination of the rectum, sigmoid colon, and colon. It offers the same opportunities for inspection and treatment as upper GI endoscopy. Colonoscopy can be used as a primary diagnostic method or as a screening process for recurrence in patients previously treated for colonic cancers. For colonoscopy the bowel must be prepared and free from faecal material so a clear diet, laxatives, and enemas may be prescribed.

Endoscopy is generally a safe procedure, but perforation is a rare complication. It may be contraindicated in cases of severe GI bleeding and requires a cooperative patient. The nurse will need to provide support and encouragement during the procedure and observe the patient closely for some hours afterwards.

Other Investigations

Routine and specialized blood tests may be required and in addition specimens of the patient's vomit, aspirate, and urine may be tested. Faeces may be collected for testing for the presence of occult blood or fat. Some of the investigations mentioned may be undertaken before the patient is admitted to hospital. In order to avoid having to repeat the investigation, it is important that clear, preferably written, instructions are given to patients so that they are correctly prepared. If patients are returning home soon after investigations they must be fully recovered, comfortable, and safe. The patient can be told that the results of their investigations will be sent to their general practitioner or discussed at an out-patient appointment.

ACUTE ABDOMINAL CONDITIONS

There are four main causes of acute, potentially life-threatening conditions requiring emergency abdominal surgery:

- Acute abdomen.
- Acute haemorrhage.
- Perforation.
- Obstruction.

Acute Abdomen

Acute abdominal pain is one of the commonest surgical emergencies and accounts for about 1% of hospital admissions in the UK (de Dombal, 1990). Severe abdominal pain is the main presenting symptom in acute abdomen. Abdominal pain may have a surgical or nonsurgical origin (*Figure 14.7, Box 14.1*) and it is important that the history and examination permit an accurate diagnosis. General symptoms may include:

- Pain.
- Anorexia, nausea, and vomiting.
- Altered bowel function.
- Signs of sepsis.

Pain

Pain may present in different forms and these can be important clues in diagnosing the problem (*Figure 14.8*). Gradual pain in the periumbilical region

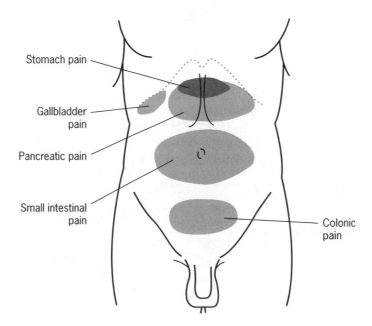

Figure 14.7 Abdominal pain. (Reproduced with kind permission from Sabiston DC (1991) *Textbook of Surgery*, 14th edn. WB Saunders, Philadelphia.)

Box 14.1 Conditions causing acute abdominal pain (after de Dombal, 1990).

General causes
- Appendicitis
- Diverticular disease
- Perforated peptic ulcer
- Nonspecific abdominal pain
- Acute cholecystitis
- Intestinal obstruction
- Acute pancreatitis
- Renal colic
- Dyspepsia

In the elderly
- Colorectal cancer
- Vascular disease

In women
- Pelvic inflammatory disease
- Urinary tract infection
- Ectopic pregnancy
- Ovarian cysts

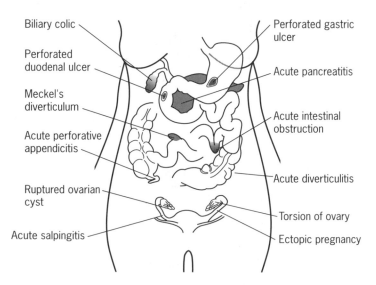

Figure 14.8 Common causes of abdominal pain. (Reproduced with kind permission from Sabiston DC (1991) *Textbook of Surgery*, 14th edn. WB Saunders, Philadelphia.)

indicates visceral peritoneal irritation, as occurs with inflammatory conditions, appendicitis, and diverticula. The pain may become more localized as the disease process develops. Perforation of the bowel or other hollow structures will be suggested by severe, sudden, or explosive pain caused by contact of organ contents with the parietal peritoneum. A more progressive severe pain, either local or general, may indicate progressive worsening of an abdominal condition such as necrosis of strangulated bowel. If a localized pain becomes more generalized there is the risk that an inflamed organ has perforated. Bowel obstructions are associated with a repeating pattern of cramping pain. The abdominal cramps build up to a crescendo and slowly reduce, and may then be followed by a pain-free period. If cramping pain develops into a continuous severe pain it may indicate ischaemic necrosis of the bowel.

Anorexia, nausea, and vomiting

These symptoms are seen in many of the conditions causing acute abdomen. They are common in conditions requiring surgical intervention, but also occur regularly with nonsurgical causes of acute abdominal pain. Armenti and Jarrel (1996) note that in conditions such as gastroenteritis the nausea and vomiting commonly precedes abdominal pain.

Bowel function

Changes in bowel habit are common in most abdominal conditions and may be of little help in differential diagnosis. However, in intestinal obstruction the patient may have noticed that they have not moved their bowels or passed flatus for the last 1–2 days. If the abdominal pain is accompanied by bloody diarrhoea an intestinal infection, colitis, or ischaemic colon may be suspected. A rectal examination is routine in cases of acute abdomen.

Sepsis

Patients with acute abdomen need to be carefully monitored for indications of developing sepsis. Conditions such as simple appendicitis may only result in a mild pyrexia, but an increase in temperature can indicate perforation. Other abdominal conditions may be accompanied by fever, chills, or rigors.

With an acute abdomen it is important to look for specific as well as general symptoms. Previous surgical history can be important and may suggest a cause such as adhesions or recurrence of malignancy. At the same time it can eliminate other likely causes. If the pain has occurred before, the results of previous investigations will be invaluable and the patient may have learned manoeuvres that limit the pain and are characteristic of certain conditions. For example, a patient with a peptic ulcer may have found that taking antacids or some types of food relieves the pain. Previous medical conditions can be important, particularly urinary tract disease, gynaecological problems, and cardiovascular disease. A gynaecological examination is recommended for all women presenting with abdominal pain.

Management

The history, clinical examination, and investigations are critical in allowing a speedy diagnosis and treatment. Immediate investigations will include blood and biochemical tests, plain radiography, and perhaps ultrasound. It may be necessary to perform an investigative laparoscopy. During this period the patient will be fasted, intravenous fluids will be commenced, and pain control will be important. However, it should be noted that a complete history of the pain is important for diagnostic purposes and should be obtained before the pain is masked by analgesia. The nurse will have an important role in supporting and informing the patient during this period. Treatment will ultimately depend on the diagnosis. Individual conditions that can cause an acute abdomen are considered in more detail later in this chapter.

Gastrointestinal Haemorrhage

Gastrointestinal haemorrhage is generally considered as either upper or lower GI tract bleeding. *Box 14.2* lists the main causes of upper and lower tract bleeding. As with an acute abdomen, the history and physical examination are important, but diagnosis may depend on endoscopic identification (and sometimes treatment) of bleeding points. Armenti and Jarrell (1996) make the point that while a diagnosis of GI tract haemorrhage may be obvious the type of bleeding can help to localize the source.

■ Haematemesis is the vomiting of fresh or coffee-grounds blood. Coffee-grounds haematemesis indicates that the blood has mixed with the stomach acids long enough to alter the haemoglobin.

Box 14.2 The main causes of upper and lower GI tract bleeding.

Upper GI tract
- Duodenal ulcer
- Gastric erosions
- Gastric ulcer
- Benign and malignant tumours
- Oesophageal varices
- Mallory–Weiss tears
- Undiagnosed causes

Lower GI tract
- Diverticular disease
- Colorectal carcinoma
- Small bowel lesions
- Angiodysplasia
- Miscellaneous

- Haematochezia is the rectal passage of frank blood and does not help localize the bleeding.
- Melaena is the passage of black tarry stools due to the presence of blood in the GI tract for some time.
- 'Currant-jelly stool' is a mixture of blood, stool, and mucus and suggests Meckel's diverticulum.

GI haemorrhage requires rapid assessment and treatment, which will depend on the cause and the extent of blood loss. Ambrose and Wedgwood (1990) reviewed lower GI tract haemorrhage and suggested that minor bleeds (less than two units in 24 hours) can be managed either on an in- or outpatient basis while investigations are carried out to identify the cause. Intermediate bleeding, more than two but less than four units of blood in 24 hours requires immediate hospitalization, investigation, and treatment. Major haemorrhage of more than four units in 24 hours should be considered a life-threatening emergency. Fluid resuscitation measures will be required with transfusion to replace blood loss.

Perforation and Peritonitis

Perforation
Perforation of an abdominal organ can result in its contents spilling out into the peritoneal cavity and causing inflammation of the peritoneum (i.e. peritonitis). The content of the digestive organs, for example stomach, small intestine, and colon, may be highly irritant due to their content of digestive juices and enzymes. The risk of infection is considerable. Causes of perforation include:

- Peptic ulcer.
- Appendicitis.
- Diverticulitis.
- Inflammatory disease of the colon.
- Malignancy.
- Penetrating wound or surgical trauma.

Peritonitis
Peritonitis may result from a number of causes including:

- Perforation.
- Penetrating wounds.
- Postoperative infection (e.g. after laparoscopy).
- Postoperative leakage from anastomosis or suture lines.
- Acute salpingitis or puerperal infection.
- Septicaemia.

Ellis and Calne (1993a) identify the three main causes as postoperative complications (30%), acute appendicitis (20%), and perforated peptic ulcer (20%).

Peritonitis presents with severe pain. Characteristically the patient wants to lie still as movement aggravates the pain. Nausea and vomiting are common and pyrexia and tachcardia develop as the condition progresses. The abdominal wall will be rigid and guarding will be noted. In severe peritonitis the abdomen will become distended, vomiting may be faeculent, and the patient can rapidly become toxic and develop shock. Treatment depends on the underlying cause, but immediate measures include pain control with opioid analgesics, fasting, nasogastric intubation and aspiration, intravenous fluid support, and antibiotic therapy. Surgery will be necessary if a perforation or defect requiring closure or drainage is identified. The patient with peritonitis is very ill and needs constant supportive care. The relatives also need constant explanation and reassurance as the outcome of this serious condition is sometimes difficult to predict.

Obstruction

Intestinal obstruction can develop due to mechanical or functional impairment of intestinal mobility. Functional impairment may result from irritation (as in peritonitis) or after handling of the bowel during surgery (paralytic or adynamic ileus). It can also be caused by conditions damaging the nerve supply to the gut. Mechanical obstruction may be due to:

- Faecal impaction.
- Adhesions (adherence of loops of gut caused by fibrous tissue scarring from a previous inflammatory response or surgery).
- Volvulus (a twisting of a section of bowel so as to occlude the lumen).
- Intussusception (one portion of the gut is telescoped into a distal portion).
- Abdominal mass (e.g. tumour).
- Hernia (strangulated hernia, see Chapter 17).

Adhesions, hernias, and intestinal tumours are the three most common causes of intestinal obstruction.

Fluid, intestinal contents, and gas collect in the gut in front of the obstruction. This results in distension, which stimulates gastric secretion and vomiting. The absorption of fluids is reduced. Peristalsis increases as the bowel attempts to force material through the congested bowel, causing severe pain. Eventually the increasing distension will cause peristalsis to cease. Meanwhile the circulating blood volume is reduced and the percentage of red cells in the volume of blood rises, increasing the risk of thrombosis. Shock may occur due to hypovolaemia and toxaemia (Brunt, 1982).

THE STOMACH AND DUODENUM

Anatomy

The stomach is a muscular organ located in the left hypochondrial and epigastric regions of the abdomen. It is distensible and can accommodate approximately two litres or more and is involved in the storage and digestion of food. *Figure 14.9* shows the four main regions of the stomach and the greater and lesser curvatures. The oesophagus merges with the stomach at the cardiac sphincter and the stomach empties into the duodenum via the pyloric sphincter. The stomach wall is made up of three layers of smooth muscle – an oblique inner layer, a circular middle layer, and a longitudinal outer layer – and the gastric mucosa. The gastric mucosa is thrown into folds or rugae. The stomach receives its arterial supply via the left and right gastric arteries, the right and left gastroepiploic arteries, and vasa brevia or short gastric arteries. The stomach is drained by both portal and systemic venous vessels and there is extensive lymphatic drainage. Due to the extensive venous and lymphatic drainage cancers of the stomach can frequently spread to other regions. The stomach has both sympathetic and parasympathetic innervation. The parasympathetic supply is via the vagus nerves and sympathetic supply is via the greater splanchic nerves.

The gastric mucosa is highly modified compared to the simple columnar epithelium seen in the oesophagus. It features millions of gastric pits and glands, which increase the surface area. The gastric mucosa secretes:

- Pepsinogen (a precursor of pepsin secreted by the peptic cells).
- Gastrin (secreted by enteroendocrine cells).
- Hydrochloric acid (secreted by parietal cells).
- Intrinsic factor (secreted by parietal cells).
- Mucus (secreted by the numerous mucus-secreting cells spread through the mucosa).

The peristaltic waves churn the stomach contents, mixing food with gastric secretions to produce chyme. Periodic peristaltic waves pass the chyme through the pyloric sphincter into the duodenum.

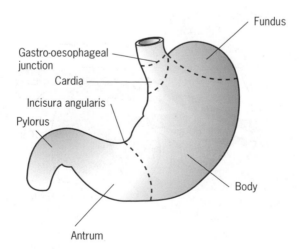

Figure 14.9 The stomach.

The duodenum (*Figure 14.10*) is the first and smallest portion of the small intestine. It is about 12 cm long and is essentially a curved muscular tube. The final portion of the duodenum is held in position by the ligament of Treitz at the duodenojejunal flexure. The head of the pancreas lies within the curve of the duodenum and the common bile and pancreatic ducts empty into the duodenum at the ampulla of Vater. The accessory pancreatic duct enters about 2 cm above the pancreatic duct. The duodenum receives its blood supply from the superior and inferior pancreaticoduodenal arteries. The walls of the duodenum are made up of four layers – inner mucosa, muscularis mucosa, muscle layer (longitudinal and circular muscle), and outer serosa – except the posterior wall, which is retro-peritoneal and has no serosa. The mucosa of the proximal duodenum contains Brunner's glands, which are specialized glands that secrete an alkaline mucus to help protect the mucosa from the acidity of the stomach contents.

The functions of the stomach include:

■ Storage of food.
■ Mixing of food with gastric juice to produce chyme.
■ Controlled release of food into the duodenum.

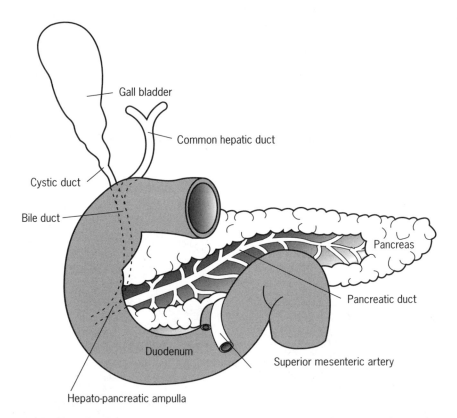

Figure 14.10 The duodenum.

- Secretion of gastrin, which facilitates gastric digestion by increasing gastric acid secretion, stomach motility, and pepsinogen secretion.
- Production of gastric acid, which destroys bacteria and solubilizes food.
- Secretion of intrinsic factor, which is required for vitamin B_{12} absorption.

The duodenum receives chyme from the stomach, bile from the liver, and pancreatic secretions.

DISEASES OF THE STOMACH AND DUODENUM

Conditions affecting the stomach and duodenum in the adult that may require surgical intervention include:

- Haemorrhage.
- Peptic ulcer.
- Gastric and duodenal tumours.
- Obstructions.
- Mallory–Weiss syndrome.
- Bezoars.

About 85% of cases of haemorrhage from the stomach and duodenum are due to peptic ulceration (discussed below), but other causes include Mallory–Weiss tears, tumours, and drugs (e.g. aspirin or indomethacin). Mallory–Weiss syndrome is a condition in which there is acute GI haemorrhage due to mucosal tearing at the gastro-oesophageal junction. However, surgery to oversew the tears is only required in about 10% of cases. Two types of bezoar requiring surgical removal may be seen. Trichobezoars are masses of hair (hairballs) found in the stomach and are seen most commonly in children and young women. Phytobezoars are agglutinated masses of vegetable fibres and are most often seen in older men after partial gastrectomy. Gastric and duodenal obstruction are usually secondary to peptic disease, but rare causes include gastric volvulus and superior mesenteric syndrome. Peptic ulcer disease and tumours represent the commonest gastro-duodenal conditions requiring surgery and these will be considered in more detail.

Peptic Ulceration

Peptic ulceration tends to occur where there is disturbance in the balance between the secretion of gastric acid and pepsin and the mucosal defence mechanisms. Peptic ulceration can affect the stomach or duodenum. Gastric ulcers commonly affect the body of the stomach, but may be found at the pylorus and at the gastro-oesophageal junction. 95% of duodenal ulcers are found in the first portion of the duodenum. Gastric ulcers at the pyloric outlet tend to mimic duodenal ulcers and may be treated in a similar fashion. Peptic ulceration results when the mucosa of the stomach or duodenum is eroded by acid or pepsin despite protective mechanisms (*Box 14.3*). Peptic ulceration appears to be a modern disease. It was unusual in Britain in the nineteenth century, rose rapidly to a peak in the 1950s and early 1960s and has declined since then (Williams and Fielding, 1993). The pattern of the disease has also altered. It used to be four times more common in men than women, but there is now little difference between the sexes (Kurata *et al.*, 1985a). The condition occurs most often in people aged 20–60 years, but where it once commonly presented in people in their forties there is now an increasing incidence in the older age group (Kurata *et al.*, 1985b).

The cause of peptic ulcer disease appears to be multifactorial although the role of *H. pylori* is under intense investigation. *H. pylori* is found in about 90% of patients with peptic ulcer or chronic gastritis. Williams and Fielding (1993) suggest that the organism may produce toxins that produce local mucosal damage or may cause increased gastrin production and alter gastric motility. In acute peptic ulceration the lesions are often multiple, but shallow, but in chronic ulceration a single, deep scirrhous lesion is common (Thompson, 1991). Increased gastric acid secretion has been identified in about 40% of patients with duodenal ulcer (Grossman *et al.*, 1963), but gastric and stress ulcers are not associated with increased acid secretion.

Diagnosis and investigations
Peptic ulceration often presents with a history of burning epigastric pain relieved by eating. The pain may recur an hour or two after meals and is often aggravated

---

Box 14.3 Aetiology of peptic ulceration (Williams and Fielding, 1993).

Protective mechanisms
- Soluble mucus layer
- Insoluble mucus layer
- Bicarbonate secretion (pancreas, duodenum)
- Gastroduodenal motility
- Mucosal blood flow
- Prostaglandins

Damaging factors
- Acid
- Pepsin
- *Helicobacter pylori*
- Drugs such as non-steroidal anti-inflammatory drugs (NSAIDs), glucocortico-steroids
- Smoking
- Stress
- Alcohol

by spicy foods and relieved by milk or alkali preparations. Heartburn, nausea, vomiting, and weight loss may occur, but weight gain due to increased milk intake may also be noted. Investigations may include:

- Barium swallow and meal.
- Gastroscopy and biopsy.
- CT scan.
- Faecal occult blood test.
- Full blood count and haemoglobin estimation.
- Basal and maximal gastric acid output.
- Serum gastrin.
- *H. pylori* detection.

Gastric washing and cytology may be used in addition to biopsy to rule out gastric cancer.

Complications

The three main complications of peptic ulcer are:

- Perforation
- Haemorrhage.
- Gastric outlet obstruction.

Perforation can complicate both gastric and duodenal ulcers, but gastric perforations are less common. Perforation most commonly occurs on the anterior surface of the duodenum. Although there has been a decline in hospital admission for uncomplicated duodenal ulcer, the incidence of perforated duodenal ulcer has remained stable and the associated mortality rate remains unchanged (Williams and Fielding, 1993). Nonsurgical treatment is occasionally used, but surgical intervention is usually required. Haemorrhage remains the commonest cause of death in peptic disease, and Williams and Fielding (1993) noted that the risk of mortality is increased when:

- There is a large haemorrhage (needing four or more units of blood).
- Haemorrhage recurs while in hospital.
- The patient is aged over 65 years.

Gastric outlet obstruction is a less common complication of peptic ulceration that may be suspected if the patient presents with a history of prolonged or projectile vomiting. The stomach may be dilated and radiographic studies will indicate outflow obstruction. The patient may lose large volumes of fluid and electrolytes. Electrolyte disorders, for example hypokalaemic metabolic alkalosis, can develop. A nasogastric tube will be inserted to decompress the stomach. The ulcer will be treated and the obstruction may resolve as oedema decreases. If the obstruction is caused by chronic scarring then endoscopic balloon dilation may be attempted. Surgery to relieve gastric outflow obstruction usually involves truncal vagotomy and pyloroplasty or gastrojejunostomy if the duodenum has become heavily scarred or deformed (*Figure 14.11*). A combination of pyloric dilation with selective vagotomy has also been used.

Treatment

Treatment of peptic ulcer disease has two main aims:

- To heal the ulcer.
- To treat predisposition and prevent recurrence.

Currently medical management is the mainstay of treatment and surgery the exception rather than the rule. Drugs may be prescribed to neutralize acid secretion, to decrease acid production, to improve mucosal protection, or to eradicate *H. pylori*. Management will also involve recommending lifestyle changes; the nurse can help educate the patient in stress reduction techniques and the importance of adequate rest, stopping smoking, alcohol reduction, and eating sensibly. Aspirin and NSAIDs should be avoided. Although there is little evidence that strictly controlled diets will improve ulcer healing, avoidance of

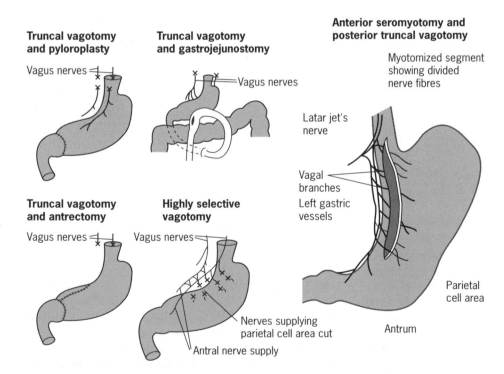

Figure 14.11 The surgical procedures for duodenal ulcer (Reproduced from Williams & Fielding, 1993 by kind permission of The Medicine Group (Journals) Ltd).

gastric irritants such as alcohol, tobacco, certain drugs, and some highly spiced foods may be recommended. Antacid therapy, the use of alkali preparations to neutralize gastric acids, is often prescribed to relieve symptoms and can help heal the ulcer. However, it is not clear whether antacids are superior to placebo in ulcer healing (Gillum, 1996).

Histamine receptor (H_2)-antagonists are the main group of drugs used in ulcer therapy. Using H_2-antagonists such as cimetidine, ranitidine, famotidine, and nizatidine, ulcer healing can be achieved in as little as eight weeks. H_2-antagonists are effective for both gastric and duodenal ulcers and act to reduce gastric acid output by blocking the H_2-receptor. The H_2-receptor has been associated with gastric acid secretion. H_2-antagonists are generally well tolerated and have few common side effects, and some have now been licensed for over-the-counter sales. Long-term maintenance with H_2-antagonists can prevent recurrence in about 80% of patients (Williams and Fielding, 1993). H_2-antagonists may be less effective in treating ulcers associated with NSAID use and an alternative is omeprazole, a proton pump inhibitor that also reduces acid secretion. Omeprazole is a very effective treatment, healing about 90% of duodenal ulcers within four weeks, but is considerably more expensive. Sulcralfate is an effective treatment for peptic ulceration that appears to act by protecting the mucosa from acid–pepsin attack. The drug has an aluminium base, but does not have an antacid action. Misoprostol, a prostaglandin analogue with both protective and antisecretory actions, can also be used for treating ulcers associated with NSAIDs. It is particularly recommended for treating elderly patients when NSAID therapy cannot be discontinued.

The recognition of the importance of *H. pylori* has introduced a new approach to treatment. Studies have shown that antibiotic treatment can reduce ulcer recurrence rates from around 80% to 0–20% in individuals infected with *H. pylori* (Williams and Fielding, 1993). A variety of different antibiotic regimens in combination with omeprazole are currently in use for the long-term eradication of *H. pylori*. These are effective, but an ideal treatment regimen has not yet been identified. *Table 14.2* illustrates three common regimens.

Surgery

Surgical intervention will be necessary when the ulcer proves intractable or when malignancy cannot be ruled out. The complications of peptic ulceration (i.e. haemorrhage, perforation, or obstruction) are also indications for surgery. The definition of 'intractable' is unclear and may vary between centres and surgeons. Some form of hemigastrectomy and reconstruction with vagotomy is the normal approach. A Billroth I gastrectomy is used to treat a gastric ulcer. The ulcer is removed, together with the gastric-secreting zone of the antrum and a gastroduodenal anastomosis is formed (*Figure 14.12*). For a duodenal ulcer a vagotomy with drainage or Polya gastrectomy may be used (see *Figure 14.12*). Laparoscopic approaches are also being developed and include truncal vagotomy and pyloric stretching, highly selective vagotomy, and posterior truncal vagotomy with selective anterior seromyotomy.

Table 14.2 Common regimens for treating *Helicobacter pylori*.

Treatment type	Regimen	Drugs (list of alternatives)
Triple therapy	One week	Amoxycillin + Metronidazole + Omeprazole Clarithromycin + Metronidazole + Omeprazole Amoxycillin + Clarithromycin + Omeprazole

Triple therapy	Two weeks	Tetracycline + Metronidazole + Tripotassium
		  dicitratobismuthate
		Amoxycillin + Metronidazole + Ranitidine
		Ranitidine bismuth citrate + Amoxycillin or
		  Clarithromycin

Dual therapy	Two weeks	Clarithromycin + Omeprazole Amoxycillin + Omeprazole

British National Formulary (1996) No. 32, pp. 34–35

Haemorrhage can be an immediate complication of gastric surgery. Late complications of hemigastrectomy and vagotomy procedures include:

- Dumping syndrome.
- Diarrhoea.
- Bilious vomiting.
- Chronic gastritis.
- Small stomach syndrome.
- Anaemia.
- Steatorrhoea.

Dumping syndrome consists of episodes of pallor, fainting, sweating, vertigo, and colic occurring after food. The stomach acts as an osmoregulator: it mixes food with the stomach acids and regulates movement into the duodenum. After gastrectomy there is a risk that the sudden passage of a large volume of hyperosmolar food into the intestine will cause a rapid fluid shift resulting in a temporary reduction in circulating fluid volume. The effect may be sufficient to produce transient changes in serum potassium levels that can be detected by alterations in the electrocardiogram (ECG). The patient may need to lie down and rest for half an hour after meals.

Nutritional disturbances and weight loss can result from 'small stomach syndrome'. The patient feels full after even a modest meal and appetite is impaired. Steatorrhoea, the loss of more than 7% of ingested fat in the stool, may occur if the anastomosis bypasses the duodenum and there is inadequate mixing of food with bile and pancreatic secretions. Diarrhoea may occur after vagotomy, but the exact mechanism is uncertain. The reduction in acid production and a deficiency of intrinsic factor may result in anaemia. Anaemia is inevitable after total gastrectomy. Bilious vomiting is more common after Polya gastrectomy, and if serious may require further surgery to convert the repair into a Billroth gastrectomy.

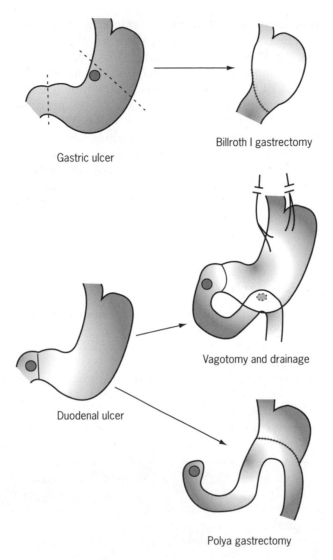

Gastric ulcer

Billroth I gastrectomy

Duodenal ulcer

Vagotomy and drainage

Polya gastrectomy

Figure 14.12 Surgical interventions for peptic ulcer.

Nursing care

In most cases the initial treatment for peptic ulcer disease will be medical and patient education and information giving is central to the nursing care. The patient needs to understand the condition, drug treatment, and any alterations required in lifestyle. When surgery is required the patient is facing a major abdominal procedure and requires careful preoperative preparation and post-operative care.

For an elective procedure the patient will have been assessed as an out-patient and will be admitted on the day before surgery. A full preoperative assessment will be required with particular emphasis on nutritional status and assessing for anaemia. Encouraging the patient to stop smoking is especially important in this condition. In the immediate postoperative period the usual postoperative observations will be required and the nurse should be particularly alert for the risk of haemorrhage. A nasogastric tube will be *in situ* to allow free drainage and decompression of the stomach. If copious drainage persists it may indicate paralytic ileus. Intravenous fluids will be used to maintain hydration for the first 24 hours, and when bowel sounds have returned, oral fluids and a light diet are slowly introduced. Adequate analgesia and early mobilization are essential. After the immediate postoperative period the nurse should be alert for the later complications of partial gastrectomy and vagotomy (listed above). Nutritional intake and fluid balance may be monitored and the patient encouraged to report any problems. In uncomplicated cases the patient will be ready for discharge within a week, although older or debilitated patients may take longer to recover.

Cancer of the Stomach

Box 14.4 lists benign and malignant gastric tumours. Benign tumours are relatively rare. Between 90–95% of gastric tumours are malignant and of these 95% are carcinomas (Gillum, 1996). This section will focus on carcinoma of the stomach, causes, treatment, and nursing care.

Carcinoma of the stomach is common, with an annual mortality rate of about 9500 per year in England and Wales. The incidence of gastric cancer has fallen in Europe and the USA, but now appears to have stabilized. It is an international problem, but is more common in some races, notably the Japanese. However,

---

Box 14.4 **Benign and malignant gastric tumours (adapted from Ellis and Calne, 1993b).**

Benign (uncommon)
- Gastric polyps (hyperplastic, adenomas)
- Leiomyoma
- Fibroma
- Neurofibroma
- Haemangioma

Malignant
- Adenocarcinoma
- Leiomyosarcoma
- Lymphoma
- Hodgkin's disease
- Secondary tumour

studies of Japanese–Americans suggest that environmental rather than genetic factors may be the key to regional distribution. The cancer also seems to be linked to social class, sex, and genetic factors. It is more common in social classes III and IV, men are twice as likely to be affected as women, and there is an increased incidence in people with blood group A. Pernicious anaemia is associated with a threefold increase in gastric cancer and hypogammaglobulinaemia with a 50-fold increase (Fielding, 1990). Gastric surgery also appears to be associated with a 3–4-fold increase 30 years after the surgery. Atrophic gastritis, intestinal metaplasia, dysplasia, and gastric polyps may be precursors of gastric cancer. Smoking, alcohol, and dietary factors such as increased salt consumption have been implicated, but their role remains uncertain.

Adenocarcinoma of the stomach can develop anywhere in the stomach. Ellis and Calne (1993b) suggest that about 33% are diffuse, involving a large area of the stomach, 25% arise in the pyloric region, and the remainder are distributed throughout the stomach. Stomach cancers may be described as fungating (least common type), ulcerating (most common type), or diffusely infiltrating (linitis plastica) with extensive submucosal infiltration. Ellis and Calne (1993b) describe four main types of adenocarcinoma in terms of their macroscopic appearance.

- Malignant ulcer with raised everted edges.
- Polypoid tumour.
- Colloid tumour (a massive gelatinous growth).
- 'Leather-bottle' stomach or linitis plastica (infiltrating fibrous tumour with minimal surface erosion).

Direct spread of gastric cancer can involve the duodenum, spleen, diaphragm, colon, and other adjacent structures. Lymphatic spread can involve the mediastinal or subpyloric and hepatic nodes. Distant spread via the bloodstream may involve liver, lungs, and bone. Gastric cancer can also spread transcoelomically to the ovaries or the pouch of Douglas. It may be classified using the TNM system or a simpler system such as the Birmingham staging system (*Table 14.3*).

Presentation and investigations

Patients with gastric carcinoma tend to present late in the course of the disease because the initial symptoms are fairly nonspecific. Symptoms include pain, anorexia, weight loss, and anaemia. Pain is often epigastric, but may radiate to the back suggesting pancreatic involvement. Vomiting may be a feature indicating a pyloric tumour or pyloric obstruction. Dysphagia may result from tumours in the cardiac region. Perforation and haemorrhage are occasional complications of gastric cancer. Metastatic spread may be indicated by jaundice, abdominal distension, and ascites.

Barium studies, CT scanning, endoscopy, biopsy, and gastric cytology are common investigations that help in diagnosis. Plain chest radiography may reveal mediastinal metastases, and CT scanning may also be used to identify distant spread. Laparoscopy may be used to investigate extensive disease, and

Table 14.3 Birmingham staging system for gastric cancer (Fielding, 1990).

Stage	Clinical findings	Pathological findings
I	Radical resection	Muscularis propria – Serosa – Node – $(T_1N_0M_0)$
II	Radical resection $(T_{2-4}N_0M_0)$	Muscularis propria + Serosa + – Node – $(T_{2-4}N_0M_0)$
III	Radical resection $(T_{x-4}N_1M_0)$	Muscularis propria + – Serosa + – Node + $(T_{x-4}N_{1-3}M_0)$
IVa	Palliative resection $(T_{x-4}N_{x-3}M_{0-1})$	Residual disease $(T_{x-4}N_{0-3}M_{0-1})$
IVb	No resection $(T_{x-4}N_{x-3}M_{0-1})$	Positive histology $(T_4N_{0-3}M_{0-1})$

Few patients are suitable for curative surgery (stages I–III); most patients present with advanced disease.

laparotomy is recommended as it allows investigation of the peritoneal cavity for evidence of metastastes.

Surgical treatment

Surgical treatment depends on nodal involvement and distant spread. Depending on the location of the tumour, cancer limited to the stomach may be treated by partial or total gastrectomy (curative surgery). Due to the late presentation of patients only about 20% are suitable for curative surgery (Fielding, 1990). However, it is hoped that better guidelines for the investigation of dyspepsia may improve the rates of early diagnosis of gastric carcinoma. If the tumour is in the fundus or cardia, the spleen may also have to be removed. Total gastrectomy has the advantage in terms of preventing tumour recurrence, but is associated with an increase in postoperative morbidity and mortality related to the surgery. Partial gastrectomy reduces the surgical risks, but may increase the chance of tumour recurrence. In gastric cancer surgery is usually palliative and palliative resections may be carried out to relieve obstruction or bleeding. Adjuvant treatment such as radiotherapy and chemotherapy have not been shown to have major benefits after gastrectomy, but may be used to treat inoperable tumours.

Nursing care

The immediate postoperative care after gastrectomy for cancers is similar to that following gastric procedures for peptic ulcer disease. Particular care is required in identifying and dealing with postgastrectomy complications as listed above. Particular aspects of long-term care after palliative procedures relate to the progressive increase in symptoms associated with the cancer. Care will include:

- Dealing with any psychosocial distress.
- Relieving pain.
- Ensuring the patient has suitable nutrition.
- Assisting the patient to deal with excretion needs.

- Ensuring the patient's hygiene needs are met.
- Assisting in the relief of any ascites.

Patients and their families will need support from hospital and community staff from the moment of diagnosis. If treatment is palliative it can be useful to involve specialist agencies, for example the Macmillan nursing services. It is important to be honest about the benefits and limitations of palliative surgery. As the condition progresses, pain control is important, and metastases in the liver and abdomen may cause jaundice and ascites. Abdominal paracentesis may be required to remove excess fluid and relieve symptoms. Nutritional disorders are a risk after any gastric surgery and the effects of cancer may increase anorexia and weight loss. Diarrhoea can be a problem after gastrectomy, but equally constipation may occur due to the use of opiate analgesia. Cancer can increase susceptibility to infection. Oral hygiene can be particularly important for patients with terminal cancer.

THE SMALL INTESTINE

Anatomy

The small intestine (*Figure 14.13*) extends approximately 3 m from the pylorus of the stomach to the caecum of the large intestine. It is made of three sections: duodenum, jejunum, and ileum. The duodenum is the first and smallest section extending from the pylorus to the ligament of Treitz. It is retroperitoneal. The jejunum makes up the first two-fifths of the peritoneal portion of the small intestine, the ileum the last two-fifths. The middle fifth may have characteristics of both jejunum and ileum. The jejunum and ileum are supported by the mesentery, and arterial supply is from jejunal and ileal branches of the superior mesenteric artery. The intestinal lymphatics transport absorbed triglycerides to the thoracic duct and thence into the circulation. Venous drainage is via the superior mesenteric vein, which is the largest of the veins contributing to the hepatic portal vein. The wall of the small intestine is made up of four layers: the mucosa, submucosa, muscle, and serosa. The mucosa and submucosa form folds known as the plicae circulares. Intestinal villi increase the surface area of the mucosa, which is covered by a columnar epithelium with goblet cells. The mucosa also features intestinal glands known as the crypts of Lieberkühn. Lymphoid tissue called Peyer's patches are found in some areas. The functional distinctions between the duodenum, jejunum, and ileum are summarized in *Table 14.4*.

The main functions of the small intestine are digestion and absorption. Ingested food is mixed with biliary, pancreatic, and intestinal secretions within the small intestine. About 9 l will move through the small intestine each day, but most of this is reabsorbed and only a small volume is normally lost in the faeces. The smooth muscles of the small intestine produce two forms of contraction, which mix and move food within the gut. To-and-fro movement mixes chyme with digestive juices and facilitates contact with the absorptive surface of the

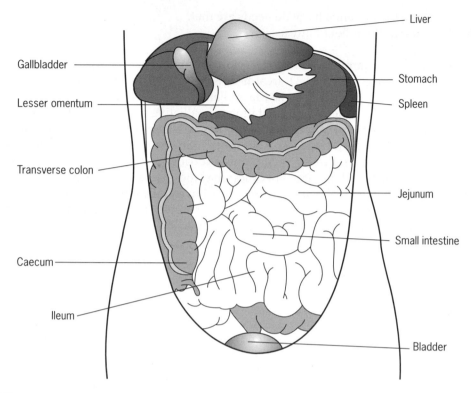

Figure 14.13 The small intestine.

Table 14.4 Functional distinctions between the duodenum, jejunum, and ileum.

Distinguishing feature	Duodenum	Jejunum	Ileum
Mucosal folds	High	High, narrow, and branching	Broad and low
Villi	Long	Long, narrow	Short and thick
Lymphatic tissue	Solitary mucosal nodules	Solitary mucosal nodules	Peyer's patches (submucosal aggregations)

small intestine. Peristaltic contractions act to move food along the tract towards the colon. Water and all major and minor nutrients are absorbed from the small intestine.

Surgical Problems Affecting the Small Intestine

Diseases affecting the small intestine include peptic ulcer disease, benign and malignant neoplasms, diverticular disease, and Crohn's disease. Peptic ulcer disease has been reviewed above, while diverticular disease and Crohn's disease, which may involve both the small and large intestine, are considered below. Meckel's diverticulum is an embryonic remnant that can survive to form an ileal diverticulum in about 2% of the adult population. It is located about 0.6 m from the ileocaecal valve and measures about 5 cm in length. Meckel's diverticulum is generally asymptomatic, but occasionally problems are seen in adults. These include bleeding, bowel obstruction, and acute inflammation, which can be difficult to distinguish from appendicitis. Tumours of the small intestine (*Box 14.5*) are surprisingly rare, with benign conditions being ten times more common than malignant tumours. Adenocarcinomas account for about 40% of malignant growths, carcinoid tumours 30%, and lymphomas about 20%. The remainder

---

Box 14.5 Tumours of the small intestine (after Studley and Williamson, 1991).

Common benign tumours
- Tubular adenoma
- Lipoma
- Haemangioma

Rare benign tumours
- Neurogenic neoplasm
- Brunner's gland adenoma
- Fibroma
- Lymphatic neoplasm

Common intermediate tumours
- Leiomyoma
- Carcinoid

Rare intermediate tumours
- Gastrinoma
- Villous adenoma

Primary malignant tumours
- Adenocarcinoma
- Lymphoma
- Sarcoma

Secondary malignant tumours
- Carcinoma
- Melanoma
- Lymphoma

Acquired immunodeficiency syndrome (AIDS) related tumours
- Kaposi's sarcoma
- Lymphoma

include sarcomas and secondary deposits from other malignancies. Adenocarcinomas are more common in the duodenum and proximal jejunum, and because of late presentation and diagnosis there are usually metastases. Adenocarcinoma of the small intestine is more common in patients with Crohn's disease. Carcinoid tumours arising from enterochromaffin cells are more common in the appendix, but also occur in the small intestine. These tumours may cause carcinoid syndrome (see the section on the appendix, p. 290). Further information on tumours of the small intestine can be found in an article by Studley and Williamson (1991).

THE APPENDIX

The vermiform appendix is a thin tube-like structure found on the posterior medial aspect of the caecum about 2–3 cm from the ileocaecal valve. On average it is about 9 cm long, but the length can vary from 0.5–25 cm. The appendix is a blind-ended muscular structure with a narrow irregular lumen. It has abundant folds of lymphoid tissue and some mucus-secreting glands. The appendix also has an abundant blood supply. Its blood supply and lymphoid tissue tend to atrophy with age (Krukowski, 1990).

Acute Appendicitis

Acute appendicitis is one of the most common abdominal emergencies. Appendicitis is caused by obstruction, subsequent inflammation, and infection. In about 60% of cases this appears to be linked to a hyperplasia of the lymphoid folds. Other causes include the presence of a faecalith or foreign body in the appendix or obstruction by a tumour of the appendix or caecum. Inflammation can vary from minor inflammation that resolves spontaneously to a suppurative condition that can cause general peritonitis and even death. Bacterial infections of the appendix are usually aerobic or anaerobic species found in the colon. Dietary and genetic factors may influence the development of appendicitis. In Europe up to 16% of the population may undergo appendectomy, but the incidence is much lower in Africa and Asia. In developed countries the incidence has decreased over the last 35 years, but is increasing in developing countries as they adopt a Western-style diet.

Presentation and diagnosis
Classically appendicitis starts with a colicky, periumbilical pain with anorexia, nausea, and one or two episodes of vomiting. After about 6 hours, usually after the vomiting, the pain becomes localized in the right iliac fossa and is aggravated by movement or coughing. Constipation generally develops, although about 20% of patients may present with diarrhoea due to irritation of the bowel by the inflamed appendix. On questioning, the patient may report a history of similar, but less severe episodes. The patient will usually present for emergency

treatment within 24 hours. This pattern is seen in about 55% of patients, but the other 45% have an atypical pattern of pain. The pain may be localized in the lower right quadrant from the start or may fail to localize and remain diffuse. Older patients are more likely to have an atypical pattern. Pain localization may reflect the position of the appendix. Nausea and anorexia are features in about 90% of cases, but vomiting is more common in younger patients and about 20% of patients never vomit. Vomiting is often absent in the elderly patient with appendicitis. However, appendicitis can be difficult to diagnose and Condon and Telford (1991) caution that about 75% of patients with an initial diagnosis of appendicitis are later found to be suffering from some other condition. Other causes of abdominal pain should be excluded. These can include other abdominal diseases, urinary or renal problems, gynaecological conditions, and right lower lobe pneumonia.

An attack of acute appendicitis may resolve spontaneously, but further attacks are then likely. If untreated the appendix will often become gangrenous and may perforate carrying the risk of causing a generalized peritonitis or a localized abscess. The rate of perforation is 25% in patients with a history of pain of less than 24 hours and 35% for those with a history of pain for more than 48 hours (Krukowski, 1990). Perforation of a gangrenous appendix greatly increases the risks of morbidity and mortality.

On examination the patient may be flushed with a tachycardia and pyrexia. Abdominal examination is important. The point of localized tenderness (*Figure 14.14*) is established and there is generally abdominal guarding. Tenderness revealed by rectal examination will indicate that the appendix occupies a pelvic position or that there is pus in the pouch of Douglas. Urinalysis is required to rule out a urinary tract infection or other urinary problems. Extensive investigations are not generally justified. A careful history and physical examination are usually sufficient. Investigations such as the leukocyte count, plain radiography, and CT

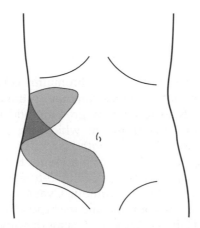

Figure 14.14 Point of maximal tenderness in acute appendicitis (Krukowski, 1990).

scanning have a very low specificity, especially in the early stages, and as the condition becomes more acute the need to treat becomes urgent.

Treatment

In the vast majority of cases the treatment for appendicitis is appendectomy. An incision is made in the area of maximal tenderness, the aponeurosis and muscles of the abdominal wall are split, and the peritoneum is entered to expose the appendix. The appendix is mobilized and resected and the appendiceal stump is sutured. After removal of the appendix the wound is closed; wound drains are not usually necessary or desirable. The mortality associated with appendicitis and appendectomy is low at less than 1%, but it is higher if perforation occurs. The associated mortality is most common in the elderly. Other complications of surgery include peritoneal sepsis and wound infection. If the appendix appears normal at operation the ileum should be checked to exclude a Meckel's diverticulum. Occasionally tumours of the appendix are discovered. These are usually carcinoid tumours (see below). For tumours of less than 2 cm in diameter appendectomy may be sufficient to remove the tumour, but for larger tumours a hemicolectomy would be considered. In the case of advanced peritonitis, surgery may be delayed until the patient's condition is improved by using an intravenous infusion, nasogastric suction, and antibiotics. MacFadyen et al. (1992) assert that laparoscopy can be a useful aid in the diagnosis of appendicitis and that laparoscopic appendicectomy can be easily performed.

Nursing care

As appendicitis often presents as an emergency situation nursing care will focus on preparation for emergency abdominal surgery, but it should not ignore the psychosocial aspects of care. In the postoperative period pain relief and early mobilization are important, but most patients will have an uneventful recovery.

Carcinoid Tumours

Carcinoid tumours derived from enterochromaffin cells affect the appendix, small bowel, and rectum, but are more common in the appendix. The primary tumour and secondaries tend to be slow growing and the prolonged survival times are good. Carcinoid syndrome in which the patient has a red-faced appearance and experiences flushing, with attacks of cyanosis, diarrhoea with borborygmus (rumbling caused by gas moving through the bowel), and bronchospasm. These symptoms are caused by 5-hydroxytryptamine and other vasoactive substances released by the tumour. Cyanosis is caused by pulmonary stenosis. Liver secondaries are common and may cause hepatomegaly. Treatment is by resection of the primary tumour. Chemotherapy may be required for secondaries.

THE COLON AND RECTUM

Anatomy and Physiology

The colon or large intestine (*Figure 14.15*) is about 1.5 m long, extending from the ileocaecal junction to the anus. The main functions of this final segment of the intestine are conservation of water and electrolytes, formation of semisolid faeces, and storage of faeces until voluntary evacuation. The colon receives up to 1.5 l of fluid from the ileum, but only 100–200 ml of fluid is normally lost in the faeces. Intestinal fluid and electrolyte loss in severe diarrhoea can become a life-threatening condition. Bacterial activity in the colon may provide some nutrients (i.e. short-chain fatty acids and vitamins). Bacteria form about one-third of the dry weight of faeces. *Bacteroides* is the most common anaerobic species in the colon, while *Escherichia coli* is the most common aerobic organism. Gas in the colon consists of nitrogen, oxygen, carbon dioxide, hydrogen, and methane, and is formed from swallowed air, bacterial activity, and diffusion from the blood.

The colon is divided into several sections: caecum, ascending colon, transverse colon, descending colon, and sigmoid colon. The rectum extends from the sigmoid colon to the anus. The vermiform appendix arises from the caecum (see

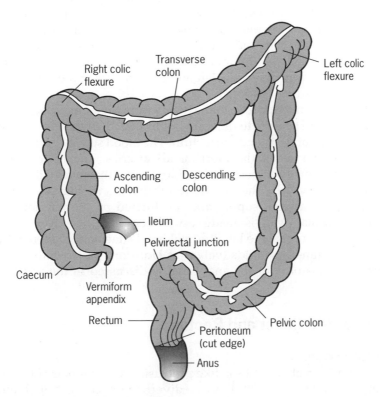

Figure 14.15 The colon or large intestine.

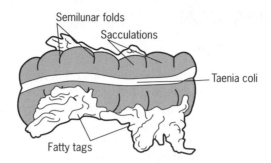

Figure 14.16 The taenia coli and epiploic appendages.

above). The colonic wall is made up of the usual four layers: mucosa, submucosa, muscularis and the serosal layer of peritoneum. However, the outer layer of longitudinal muscle is incomplete and forms three distinct bands called the taenia coli (*Figure 14.16*). Fatty tags (the appendices epiploicae) are found scattered over the surface of the colon. The colon is distensible and the muscle layer produces contractions, which move faeces along the colon to the rectum. Branches of the superior mesenteric artery serve the caecum, ascending colon, and the proximal part of the transverse colon. The distal transverse colon, descending colon, and sigmoid colon are served by branches of the inferior mesenteric artery. The inferior and superior mesenteric veins, respectively, provide the venous drainage of the left and right halves of the colon. Lymphatic vessels parallel the arterial supply.

The rectum is about 13 cm long and extends from the sigmoid colon to the anal canal (*Figure 14.17*). The urge to defecate is stimulated when faeces stored in the sigmoid colon enter and distend the rectum. The blood supply is via the superior, middle, and inferior rectal (haemorrhoidal) arteries. The upper and middle rectum are drained by the superior and middle rectal (haemorrhoidal) veins, and the anal canal is served by the middle rectal (haemorrhoidal) vein. Lymphatic vessels parallel the arterial supply and are filtered by the inferior mesenteric nodes. The muscular wall is made up of complete layers of circular and longitudinal muscle unlike the longitudinal bands (taenia coli) seen in the rest of the colon. Three transverse folds (valves of Houston) project into the lumen of the rectum. The anatomy of the anal canal is discussed in the section on anal conditions.

Disorders of the Colon and Rectum

Diverticular disease

A diverticulum is an abnormal sac-like protrusion at some point of weakness in the abdominal wall (*Figure 14.18*). A true diverticulum consists of all four layers of the abdominal wall and is rare, while the more common false diverticulum

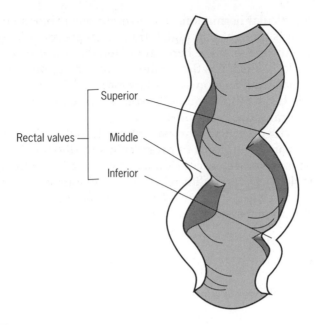

Rectal valves —

Superior

Middle

Inferior

Figure 14.17 The rectum.

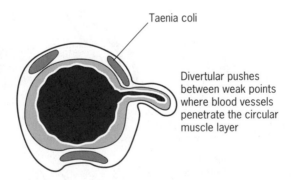

Taenia coli

Divertular pushes
between weak points
where blood vessels
penetrate the circular
muscle layer

Figure 14.18 Diverticula.

lacks a portion of the wall. Diverticulosis is the presence of diverticula, and diverticulitis is infection or inflammation associated with diverticula. Diverticulosis is especially prominent in the sigmoid colon. The sigmoid colon is involved in 90% of cases and is the only part of the colon affected in 50% of cases (Whittaker, 1994). Diverticulitis is a disease of modern living and is the most common colonic condition in developed countries. However, it was unknown before the Industrial Revolution and remains rare in less industrialized nations. The condition appears to be associated with a decrease in the intake of dietary fibre. The incidence is low in populations that eat a high-fibre low-sugar diet. The condition is rare before the age of 30, but is present in about 75% of those over 80 years of age. Diverticular herniations tend to occur where blood vessels cross the abdominal wall. It is thought that high intraluminal pressures associated with a low-fibre diet are the cause of the herniations and that the pressures are highest in the sigmoid colon, which has the smallest radius (by application of Laplace's Law, pressure equals wall tension divided by radius). With ageing, alterations in the collagen and elastin of the wall of the colon reduce its ability to expand and withstand high intraluminal pressures.

Most patients with diverticula are asymptomatic, but 10–30% may eventually develop the signs and symptoms of diverticulitis or diverticular haemorrhage. After the first episode of diverticulitis about two-thirds of patients will experience further problems. Diverticulitis results from inflammation and infection of a diverticulum or diverticula. *Figure 14.19* illustrates the possible sequence of events in the inflammatory process. The complications of diverticular disease include:

- Perforation.
- Peritonitis.
- Abscess and fistula formation.

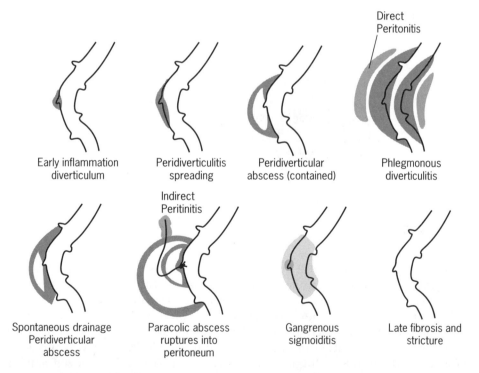

Figure 14.19 The sequence of events in the inflammatory process. (Reproduced from Whittaker MG (1994) Colonic diverticular disease. *Surgery* **12(1)**: 13 by kind permission of The Medicine Group (Journals) Ltd.)

- Systemic infection.
- Haemorrhage.
- Scar formation.

Perforation of a diverticulum permits free communication between the bowel lumen and the peritoneal cavity. Leakage of bowel contents can result in a local, pelvic, or generalized peritonitis. The peritonitis may be serous, purulent, or faecal in nature. Perforation of a pericolic abscess may result in the formation of a fistula. These complications also increase the risk of systemic disease because bacteria or endotoxins gain access to the blood. Systemic effects include bacteraemia, septicaemia, and endotoxic shock. Haemorrhage occurs in about 15% of patients with diverticulosis and varies from sudden acute haemorrhage to chronic blood loss. It is thought that blood vessels in the wall of the colon close to the neck of the diverticulum may erode. Arterial bleeding can result in a sudden profuse haemorrhage. The sequence of inflammation and resolution seen in diverticulitis can result in fibrous scarring of the colon and cause narrowing of the lumen or stricture formation. The fibrous thickening may mimic the appearance of colonic cancer radiologically.

Clinical presentation and investigation
Diverticulosis most commonly presents with acute-onset central abdominal pain, which relocates to the left iliac fossa, earning the condition the nickname of 'left-sided appendicitis'. Pain may radiate to the suprapubic area, groin, and back. Fever and leukocytosis are common and there may be an abdominal or pelvic mass. An ileus may develop with abdominal distension and vomiting. Chronic diverticulosis tends to mimic the effects of cancer of the colon. There may be alternating bouts of diarrhoea and constipation. Chronic haemorrhage may cause anaemia. Formation of adhesions between the small bowel and the affected colon can result in small bowel obstruction. Less common presentations include sudden rectal haemorrhage and pneumaturia (air bubbles in the urine), dysuria, pyuria, or faecaluria due to a vesicocolic fistula. Abdominal and rectal examination are important and investigations may include:

- Sigmoidoscopy and colonoscopy.
- Barium enema.
- CT or ultrasound scan.
- Leukocyte count.
- Chest radiography.

Sigmoidoscopy is indicated to exclude colonic cancer, but oedema and inflammation may block passage of the endoscope. Sigmoidoscopy and colonoscopy may be carried out at a later stage when the acute episode has resolved. Abdominal and pelvic CT scanning is helpful, and if an intravenous contrast agent is given before the procedure the urinary system can also be visualized. CT or ultrasound-guided percutaneous drainage is sometimes used to treat any abscesses. A barium enema can also be useful in visualizing the colon, but may increase the risk of contrast media and faeces entering the peritoneum if perforation has occurred. Leukocyte counts should be monitored to assess the progress of the condition and a chest radiograph helps identify subdiaphragmatic air, which occurs in about 3% of cases. Cytoscopy may be indicated if there is suspicion of a vesicocolic fistula.

Treatment

Treatment depends on the severity and history of the condition, the presence of complications, and the general state of the patient. An acute attack may be managed conservatively. Intravenous fluid therapy is started and either nil orally or a fluid-only diet is prescribed. Broad-spectrum intravenous antibiotic therapy is instituted and metronidazole with gentamicin or a cephalosporin is a common combination. A nasogastric tube may be required if ileus is present. Abscesses can also be managed conservatively or percutaneous drainage may be attempted using ultrasound or CT guidance. A laparotomy is necessary if there is obstruction to confirm the diagnosis and to construct a temporary colostomy. Resection of the affected section of colon and closure of the colostomy can be carried out when the acute condition has settled. If perforation has occurred and there is a purulent or faecal peritonitis the condition is serious and laparotomy and resection of the affected section of colon is required. A defunctioning colostomy will be fashioned as it is not safe to create an anastomosis while the bowel is infected. A few weeks later the colostomy can be closed and the colon attached to the rectum after the patient has recovered from the peritonitis and emergency surgery. Vesicocolic fistula will be treated by a temporary colostomy followed by resection of the affected segment of bowel. Mild chronic diverticular disease is managed conservatively once the diagnosis has been confirmed. A high roughage diet is prescribed and lubricant laxatives can be used to prevent constipation. However, if the symptoms are severe elective laparotomy and resection of the sigmoid colon may be indicated.

Inflammatory bowel disease

Ulcerative colitis and Crohn's disease are the two major types of inflammatory bowel disease. They mainly affect the colon, but Crohn's disease may also affect the small intestine. These conditions are particularly prevalent in the USA and northern Europe. Stebbing and Mortensen (1995) report that in these areas ulcerative colitis has an incidence of 5–8 per 100,000 per year and a prevalence of 80–90 per 100,000. The incidence of Crohn's disease is 2–5 per 100,000 per year and the prevalence 40 per 100,000. For both conditions the peak age at onset is 20–35 years. Region, gender, race, occupation, and social class have little effect on the distribution of these conditions. There is an indication that smoking may be protective against ulcerative colitis, but it increases the risk of Crohn's disease. The cause of these diseases is not well understood. They appear to result from immune-related trauma to the intestinal wall that causes recurrent episodes of intestinal inflammation. It is thought that the conditions arise in response to a complex interaction of trigger factors, modifying factors, and genetic predisposition. *Table 14.5* summarizes the differences between the two conditions.

Ulcerative colitis
Ulcerative colitis is characterized by extensive damage to the epithelial lining of the colon and rectum with crypt abscess formation. Sometimes pseudopolyps are present. The affected area becomes oedematous and ulcerated, and infection follows, resulting in a loss of fluid, blood, and electrolytes. The underlying mechanism appears to be autoimmune. There is a marked influx of neutrophils and other inflammatory cells into the mucosa. Damage to the epithelium may then increase permeability to bacterial products with further amplification of the inflammatory response. Genetic factors may be involved as there is some evidence of a familial incidence of the disease. Hypersensitivity to certain foods and emotional stress have also been suggested as causes.

Ulcerative colitis appears to begin in the rectum, and in about 30% of cases is confined to the rectum. However, it normally extends proximally for variable distances. Inflammation extends in a continuous manner; it does not skip areas. In about 20% of patients the whole of the colon is affected. The disease is colon specific. The small bowel is not involved and there is usually no anal or perianal disease. Perianal complications such as fistulae, anal abscesses, and fissures are uncommon. There is an increased incidence of cancer of the colon and this increases as the disease progresses. Ulcerative colitis is also associated with a number of extraintestinal manifestations affecting the skin, joints, eyes, and hepatobiliary system (*Box 14.6*).

Clinical presentation and investigations
The most common symptom is bloody diarrhoea. In rare cases rectal haemorrhage can be severe and life-threatening. Loose stools may be accompanied by the passage of mucus and pus. In mild to moderate cases abdominal pain is

Table 14.5 Inflammatory diseases of the colon (after Fry, 1996).

Feature	Ulcerative colitis	Crohn's disease
Location	Rectum, left colon	Any part of the colon, usually ileocolic
Rectal bleeding	Common, continuous	Less common, intermittent
Rectal involvement	Almost always	About 50%
Fistulas	Rare	Common
Ulceration	Continuous distribution; shaggy, irregular ulcer	'Cobblestone' appearance, patchy distribution
Stricture	Rare	Common
Carcinoma	Increased incidence	Increased incidence, but much less than with ulcerative colitis

> **Box 14.6** **Extraintestinal manifestations of ulcerative colitis (Stebbing and Mortensen, 1995).**
>
> **Skin**
> - Erythema nodosum
> - Pyoderma gangrenosum
> - Aphthous stomatitis
>
> **Joints**
> - Peripheral arthritis
> - Ankylosing spondylitis
>
> **Eyes**
> - Uveitis
> - Episcleritis
> - Conjunctivitis
>
> **Hepatobiliary**
> - Fatty liver
> - Sclerosing cholangitis
> - Chronic active hepatitis

seldom a problem, but in severe cases cramp-like abdominal pains will accompany the diarrhoea. In severe cases the patient may suffer from urgency and tenesmus (painful straining at stool). Malaise, fever, anorexia, weight loss, and anaemia are common in patients with severe disease. The severity of the condition can range from episodic diarrhoea to fulminant colitis with toxic megacolon. Fulminant colitis is characterized by:

- Dilatation of the transverse colon.
- Abdominal pain, tenderness, and distension.
- Toxaemia with fever, leukocytosis, and hypoalbuminaemia.
- Increased risk of perforation.

Investigations depend on the extent of the disease. Mild to moderate cases can be investigated on an outpatient basis. Investigations may include abdominal radiography, sigmoidoscopy and colonoscopy with biopsy, barium enema, and stool examination. However, fulminant colitis with toxic megacolon represents an emergency condition requiring rapid assessment, intensive medical resuscitation, and emergency surgery if the condition fails to respond to medical treatment. Colonoscopy and sigmoidoscopy with mucosal biopsy and barium enema will usually confirm the diagnosis, but should be avoided in fulminant colitis as they can exacerbate the condition. Abdominal radiography may be used to check for colonic dilatation, and barium studies of the small intestine to check for inflammatory involvement indicative of Crohn's disease.

Treatment

The aim of medical management is to induce and maintain remission of symptoms. Fluid and electrolyte resuscitation will be required in acute episodes. The patient may present with metabolic acidosis and a marked reduction in extravascular volume due to fluid and electrolyte losses. Drug therapy is the mainstay of medical treatment. Glucocorticosteroids (prednisolone or hydrocortisone) can be given orally or as suppositories, enemas, or in foam preparations. They are effective in the short term, but side effects prevent long-term therapy. Sulphasalazine and newer alternatives such as mesalazine or olsalazine are the main therapeutic agents for inducing and maintaining remission. Their mode of action is uncertain. Side effects include blood disorders and the Committee for the Safety of Medicines (CSM) recommend that patients are advised to report any unexplained bruising, bleeding, purpura, sore throat, malaise, or fever. Immunosuppressive agents such as cyclosporin are also used, but their role needs further clarification. Broad-spectrum antibiotics are indicated in patients with severe or fulminating colitis. As patients can become very debilitated, total parenteral nutrition may be required to prepare them for surgery. Surgery is indicated for:

- Haemorrhage.
- Perforation leading to faecal peritonitis.
- Unresponsive fulminant colitis or toxic megacolon.
- Failure to respond to medical treatment.
- Colonic stricture.
- Dysplasia or cancer.

Figure 14.20 illustrates some of the principle surgical procedures described by Stebbing and Mortensen (1995) for ulcerative colitis. Total colectomy with temporary ileostomy and mucus fistula is usually performed as an emergency procedure. It provides time for pathological confirmation of the disease, patient counselling, and preparation for a more definitive surgical solution. Panproctocolectomy with permanent ileostomy or Kock pouch formation may be used for those with poor anal canal function. Its main disadvantage is the formation of a permanent ileostomy. Currently the treatment of choice is restorative proctocolectomy with ileal pouch–anal anastomosis. This is a staged procedure. The diseased colon is removed and a temporary ileostomy formed. After about ten weeks the patient returns to surgery and an ileal pouch is formed and anastomosed to the anal canal. It has the advantage of a normally functioning anal sphincter.

Crohn's disease

Crohn's disease is characterized by a patchy inflammation affecting the whole of the bowel wall. The regional lymph nodes may be enlarged. It is seen in the

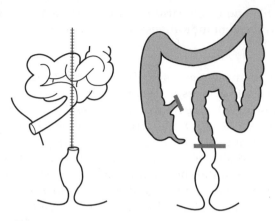

Total colectomy with ileostomy and mucous fistula

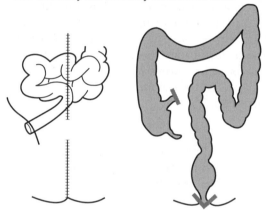

Panproctocolectomy with ileostomy or Kock pouch

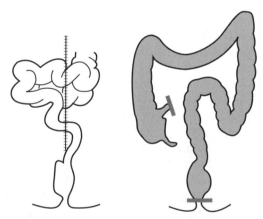

Restorative proctocolectomy with ileal pouch – and anastomosis

Figure 14.20 Procedures performed for ulcerative colitis (Reproduced from Stebbings and Mortensen, 1995 by kind permission of The Medicine Group (Journals) Ltd).

terminal ileum and the colon, but the rectum is often spared. Granulomas are evident in 30–50% of cases, and anal and perianal disease (fissures, fistula, abscesses) affect about 35% of patients. There is an increased risk of colonic cancer, but to a much lesser extent than with ulcerative colitis. Similar extra-intestinal manifestations are associated with Crohn's disease and affect about 30% of patients, but sclerosing cholangitis is much less common. The cause of the disease is uncertain, but it is linked to chronic T lymphocyte activation, an abnormal immunological response to viral or bacterial agents has been suggested (Stebbing and Mortensen, 1995).

Clinical presentation and investigations
As in ulcerative colitis, Crohn's disease presents with diarrhoea, abdominal pain, malaise, fever, weight loss, and leukocytosis can occur. In Crohn's disease, fistulae may develop between the bowel and bladder, vagina, or skin. Anal abscess or fistula is the presenting condition in about 5% of cases. Fulminant colitis can develop and may be severe, but does not usually develop into mega-colon. The risk of perforation is about the same as for ulcerative colitis and the need for vigorous treatment is unchanged. Investigations are similar to those for ulcerative colitis.

Treatment
Medical treatment is broadly similar to that for ulcerative colitis (i.e. gluco-corticosteroids for acute disease, broad-spectrum antibiotics, and immuno-suppressive agents). Metronidazole may be useful for the treatment of anal disease. Total parenteral nutrition is also useful in some cases and produces a higher rate of remission than in patients with ulcerative colitis. Surgical treat-ment will not cure Crohn's disease as it is so diffuse and can extend beyond the colon. The recurrence rate after surgery is high and is 50% after five years. Surgery is therefore aimed at symptom relief or to treat complications and to conserve the bowel. Only grossly affected bowel is resected: usually the affected area is removed and an anastomosis is formed between the healthy bowel sections. Indications include:

- Perforation with generalized peritonitis.
- Massive haemorrhage.
- Cancer.
- Fulminant or unresponsive colitis.
- Obstruction.
- Abscesses.
- Fistulas.
- Anorectal disease.

Nursing care in inflammatory bowel disease
The impact of inflammatory bowel disease on the patient depends on the history and severity of the disease and individual responses. Nursing care focuses on

the symptoms and individual experiences of the condition. The nurse needs an acute awareness of the anxiety and despair experienced by many patients with this disabling condition. It is important that the nurse establishes a rapport with the patient and gets to know the patient's lifestyle and sources of anxiety or stress. When inflammatory bowel disease has been confirmed the patient will need even more support and information to deal with this additional stress. Patients and families may benefit from contact with the *National Association for Colitis and Crohn's Disease*. Pain relief and the promotion of comfort will improve rest and help with the patient's emotional state. The physical effects of the condition, particularly the alterations in bowel habit, will be a source of stress and potential embarrassment. Patients need privacy and easy access to toilet facilities due to the faecal frequency and the often offensive nature of the stool. Soft toilet paper, handwashing facilities, and if necessary, deodorants should be readily available. Ensuring adequate nutrition is also important. Small frequent meals or snacks will improve calorie intake. A high-protein diet with added vitamins, iron, and potassium may be required to replace nutrients lost due to diarrhoea.

In acute episodes the patient may be very ill, and observation and management of fluid intake and output is essential. Dehydration and electrolyte imbalances can be life-threatening. The surgical nurse should monitor vital signs, looking for pyrexia and signs of dehydration or shock such as hypotension or reduced urine output. Fluid intake and output should be recorded, and the volume of liquid diarrhoea or fistula drainage assessed. The frequency and nature of stools must be recorded. Pre- and postoperative care follows the same general pattern as for other major abdominal surgery, but stoma care (see section on stoma care, p. 308) is an important aspect of the postoperative period.

Tumours of the colon and rectum

Benign and malignant tumours affecting the colon and rectum are listed in *Box 14.7*. Polyps are the most common benign and carcinoma the most common malignant colorectal conditions.

Colorectal polyps

A polyp may be defined as any circumscribed lesion projecting from the surface of the intestinal mucosa. Colonic polyps are usually the result of epithelial overgrowth, although occasionally they may be caused by proliferation of connective tissue. In a sessile polyp the epithelial growth results in a flat raised lesion with no stalk. The sessile polyp will often develop into a pedunculated polyp attached to the intestinal wall by a stalk. Polyps can be classified on histological appearance:

■ Hyperplastic polyps are the most common type affecting about 50% of the adult population. They are small, thickened, mucosal lesions with a normal cellular appearance and no malignant tendency. Treatment is not usually required.

Box 14.7 Benign and malignant tumours of the colon and anorectum.

Benign tumours
- Polyp
- Adenoma
- Endometrioma
- Papilloma
- Lipoma
- Neurofibroma
- Haemangioma

Malignant tumours
- Carcinoma
- Squamous cell carcinoma of the anal canal
- Basal cell carcinoma
- Lymphoma
- Melanoma
- Carcinoid tumour
- Rodent ulcer of the anal margin
- Secondaries

- Adenomatous polyps are the second commonest type in adults. They are neoplastic polyps, by definition benign, but with the potential of developing malignant changes. They are characterized by epithelia dysplasia and three types are recognisable: tubular adenomas account for 75%, and are usually pedunculated and have a smooth firm appearance; villous adenomas account for about 10%, are soft sessile polyps with frond-like projections into the intestinal lumen, and if large may cause watery diarrhoea and potassium loss; the remaining 15% are tubulovillous adenomas with a variable mix of both tubular and villous elements.
- Inflammatory polyps result from inflammatory reactions and include the pseudopolyps found in ulcerative colitis.
- Hamartomatous polyps are a group of developmental polyps that mainly affect children.

The importance of neoplastic colorectal polyps lies in their association with carcinoma. There appears to be a definite relationship between adenomatous polyps and carcinoma of the colon. It has been estimated that 95% or more of colorectal carcinomas arise from neoplastic polyps. The peak age for discovery of polyps is 50 years, the peak for colorectal cancer is 60 years. There is also a condition, familial adenomatous polyps, which when untreated develops into cancer. Removal of the polyps (polypectomy) results in a demonstrable decrease in the risk of colorectal carcinoma. The malignant potential of neoplastic polyps appears to be related to size, structure, and grade of dysplasia. Fry (1996) suggests that about 15% of polyps less than 1 cm in size, 10% of those 1–2 cm in size, but 50% of polyps greater than 2 cm in size will become malignant. Tubular adenomas are associated with a 5% malignancy rate, tubulovillous adenomas have a 20% malignancy rate, and villous adenomas show a 40% malignancy rate. The risk of malignancy is also increased with the degree of epithelial dysplasia.

The risk of malignant transformation is an indication for removal of neoplastic polyps. Colonoscopy or sigmoidoscopy with polypectomy is suitable for pedunculated polyps and for small superficial sessile polyps. Rectal polyps may be removed by the transanal route. A partial or segmental colectomy may be required for sessile polyps that cannot be excised cleanly and for any polyps with malignant changes. A pedunculated malignant polyp can be removed by endoscopic polypectomy provided:

- The cancer is confined to the head of the polyp.
- The cancer is moderately or well differentiated.
- There is no evidence of lymphatic or venous invasion.

Luchtefeld *et al.* (1993) describe laparoscopic colon surgery, emphasizing that patient selection is a crucial factor, and that ideally the tumour should be benign. One example is for large benign adenomatous polyps that cannot be removed endoscopically. The use of a laparoscopic technique for malignancy is controversial. Patients undergoing laparoscopic colon surgery are prepared preoperatively as for conventional laparotomy. Potential advantages of laparoscopic colon surgery are the avoidance of an incised wound and a shortened recovery period. However, the procedure takes longer to complete in theatre.

Colorectal carcinoma

Carcinoma of the colon and rectum is the most common GI cancer and is the second most common cause of cancer death in the UK after lung cancer. Colorectal tumours can arise at any age, but most occur in people over 50 years of age, and the incidence increases with age. In one study of over 800 people with cancer only 3.6% were under 41 years of age (Pitluk and Poticha, 1983).

The causes of colonic cancer are not clear, although neoplastic polyps and a familial predisposition may have a role. Ulcerative colitis, and to a lesser extent Crohn's disease, also increase risk. Dietary and environmental factors may have a role. The incidence is much higher in countries such as the USA and the UK where the consumption of animal fat, protein, and refined carbohydrate is high, than in countries such as Japan, parts of South America, and Africa where meat intake is reduced and vegetable fibre intake is higher. Such variation is not likely to be genetic because immigrant groups, for example Japanese–Americans tend to develop the same colonic cancer rate as their host nation. There is a suggestion that a diet high in saturated fats increases the risk of colorectal cancer, while a high fibre diet is protective. Increased calcium consumption may also have a protective effect. The risk of colorectal cancer is increased two-fold for heavy beer drinkers. The sigmoid is the most common site for colonic carcinoma, but about one-third of large bowel cancers occur in the rectum.

Clinical presentation and investigations
The effects of colorectal tumours can be separated into local effects, general effects, and the response to secondaries. Local effects depend on the location and size of the tumour. A right-sided tumour will cause a right-sided mass, iron deficiency anaemia, and melaena, while a left-sided tumour produces more alteration in bowel habit, the passage of blood per rectum, and possibly abdominal cramps due to partial obstruction. Altered bowel function may be constipation or diarrhoea or a pattern alternating between the two. Diarrhoea may be accompanied by the passage of excess mucus or frank or occult blood. Less common problems are obstruction, perforation, and fistula formation. General effects include anaemia, weight loss, and anorexia. Secondary deposits may result in jaundice, abdominal distension, and ascites. Abdominal and rectal examination are important and specific investigations may include:

- Proctoscopic examination.
- Endorectal ultrasonography.
- Colonoscopy and sigmoidoscopy with biopsy.
- Barium enema.
- Chest radiography.
- CT scan.
- Check for anaemia and occult blood loss in the stool.

If the diagnosis remains uncertain a laparotomy may be indicated. Carcino-embryonic antigen (CEA) is a glycoprotein produced by intestinal cells during embryonic development. The production of this protein stops before birth, but it may reappear with colorectal carcinoma. However, production of CEA can also be restarted by biliary disease, heavy smoking, alcohol hepatitis, and other malignant diseases, and its presence or absence is not diagnostic. It can, however, provide useful additional information for staging colorectal carcinoma and for monitoring the effectiveness of treatment. *Box 14.8* illustrates the TNM classification system for the staging colorectal cancer.

Treatment
Surgical resection is the treatment of choice. Key aspects of surgical treatment include appropriate patient preparation, thorough bowel preparation, and extensive exploration of the abdomen to identify metastases or other abdominal complications. In general there will be a wide resection of the affected segment and its regional lymph nodes. It is important that a viable anastomosis without tension and with an adequate blood supply can be formed. Surgery may involve fashioning a temporary colostomy or, in cases where anastomosis is not viable, a permanent colostomy. Surgical procedures include:

Box 14.8 The TNM classification system for colorectal cancer (Fry, 1996).

Primary tumour (T)
- T_x Primary tumour cannot be assessed
- T_0 No evidence of primary tumour
- Tis Carcinoma *in situ*
- T_1 Tumour invades submucosa
- T_2 Tumour invades muscularis propria
- T_3 Tumour invades through muscularis propria into submucosa or into non-peritonealized pericolic or perirectal tissues
- T_4 Tumour perforates the visceral peritoneum or directly invades other organs

Regional lymph nodes (N)
- N_x Regional lymph nodes cannot be assessed
- N_0 No regional lymph node metastasis
- N_1 Metastasis in 1–3 pericolic or perirectal lymph nodes
- N_2 Metastasis in four or more pericolic or perirectal lymph nodes
- N_3 Metastasis in any lymph node along the course of a named vascular trunk

Distant metastasis (M)
- M_x Unable to assess presence of distant metastases
- M_1 No distant metastases
- M_2 Distant metastases

- Right hemicolectomy for carcinoma of the caecum, ascending colon, and hepatic flexure.
- Transverse colectomy for carcinoma of the transverse colon.
- Left hemicolectomy for carcinoma of the splenic flexure and descending colon.
- Sigmoid colectomy for cancer of the sigmoid colon.
- Abdominal–perineal resection for carcinoma of the rectum and anal structures.

If the bowel is obstructed it may be necessary to relieve the obstruction and schedule an elective procedure for when the patient has recovered. Even if the cancer is not curable by surgery a resection may be required to relieve symptoms. Adjuvant therapy, cytotoxic drugs, and radiotherapy may also be employed. The use of these is controversial in colorectal cancer, although they may be recommended for palliative effects. Surveillance is essential after surgery for colorectal cancer. Physical examination may not identify early recurrence and check colonoscopy is recommended one year after surgery and then every 3–5 years.

CEA is a sensitive indicator of colorectal cancer, but cannot usually be detected until the tumour has penetrated the intestinal wall.

Nursing management in colorectal cancer

Nursing management of the patient requiring surgery for colorectal cancer provides an opportunity to examine the nurse's role in GI surgery in more detail. The principles applied can be generalized to most types of intestinal surgery. The surgery requires extensive bowel preparation and often includes stoma formation.

Preoperative care

All patients requiring intestinal surgery need to be physically and mentally pre-pared to meet the demands placed upon them before, during, and after surgery. Patients need accurate and relevant information about the nature of their con-dition and the options for treatment. The patient may be very distressed. Seemingly minor symptoms such as diarrhoea or constipation have turned out to be cancer. If the condition has presented late, a cure may be in doubt. The surgical nurse needs to offer psychological support to the patient and their family. Although medical staff will have explained the condition and surgical treatment to the patient, information and explanations may need to be repeated several times and in different ways. Time must be spent allowing the patient and families to express and talk through their fears and concerns. Bysshe (1988) asserts that most patients use information constructively to help themselves deal with and reduce their anxiety. However, a few patients will simply not want to know, and will show no interest in any attempt to educate them about their operation.

Extensive abdominal surgery may have an effect on body image, particularly if a stoma is likely to be required. Thinking about the site, care, and appearance of a stoma can be a major source of stress. The nurse should attempt to foster a positive environment, and to help in this it may be useful to involve a specialist stoma care nurse or a representative from one of the ostomy associations. It is important that the patient knows what the stoma will look like, where it will be located, and how it will function. The type and frequency of the drainage expected should be discussed. If the patient is receptive, diagrams and photographs should be used to explain and clarify the nature of the stoma, and the patient should be shown and allowed to handle the available drainage bags. It is often useful to introduce the patient to someone who has had a similar operation and appears to be coping well.

A careful assessment must be made of the additional fluid that may be required according to the patient's history, symptoms, general appearance, and haematological findings. The nurse must monitor fluid and blood replacement carefully, explaining all procedures to the patient and ensuring that all anxieties the patient may have in relation to the safety of a blood transfusion have been alleviated. If time and the patient's condition allow, a high-calorie low-residue diet is given for several days before operation.

Bowel preparation is an important aspect of care with some procedures and one that may cause patients some anxiety or embarrassment. If the bowel is to be opened, bowel preparation is required to reduce the risk of infection and to empty the bowel to aid handling. Cleansing of the bowel is commonly carried out using laxatives and enemas. Oral antibiotic preparations may be prescribed to help prepare the bowel by reducing bacterial activity. An iso-osmotic cleansing solution may be used to clear the bowel of faecal residues. Klean-Prep is a polyethylene glycol and electrolyte preparation used for this. Four sachets are made up with 4 L of water and the patient is encouraged to drink 250 mL every 10–15 minutes. Patients may find the solution unpalatable, even after the addition of flavourings and have difficulty consuming such high volumes.

Deep breathing and coughing exercises are important with abdominal surgery. Simple movement that can be helpful after the operation should also be taught by the nurse. Pugh (1989) emphasizes how the complications of immobility after surgery can be overcome by simple measures such as teaching the patient how to turn from side to side and how to relax the abdomen. It is important to reassure the patient that any postoperative pain can be controlled, and the method to be used to control the pain should be agreed with the patient. Patient-controlled analgesia is often the method of choice.

Postoperative care

Observation, pain relief, ensuring adequate fluid and nutritional intake, and monitoring output are all essential. The abdominal incision may limit movement and breathing, but this can be avoided with good pain control and follow-up of preoperative teaching. Postoperative analgesics, which might cause constipation should be avoided. The wound and wound drains must be observed for drainage. A nasogastric tube will be in place and the nurse should listen for the return of bowel sounds and observe for any signs of abdominal distension. The nurse will need to care for the indwelling urinary catheter, which is used to prevent urinary retention. If there is a perineal wound it must be closely monitored for bleeding and later for necrosis of tissue. The perineal drains or packing are removed gradually by the sixth day following surgery. The patient should be helped in moving from side to side in order to prevent pressure on the perineum, which might cause pain and delay healing.

If the surgery is curative the discharge planning will be directed towards the need for health promotion and the importance of attending outpatients for regular screening. If the surgery is palliative the patient and family need to be prepared to use the hospital and community services to maximize independence and quality of life.

Ostomy care

To form a colostomy a loop of colon is mobilized and divided and the proximal portion is brought to the surface of the abdominal wall. A colostomy may be temporary or permanent. A temporary colostomy may be formed:

- In an acute emergency such as intestinal obstruction.
- If there is a tumour that is not immediately resectable.
- If it is necessary to rest the colon.
- In conditions such as diverticular disease where there may be fistula formation.

Both the proximal and distal loops of the colon are brought to the surface, the latter as a defunctioning colostomy. Once the underlying condition has been treated, the colostomy is closed. If the rectum or distal portion of the bowel is totally removed or the patient's condition precludes a successful anastomosis a permanent colostomy is necessary. Although mainly dictated by surgical necessity it is important that the siting of a stoma is discussed with the patient.

The contents of a colostomy are less fluid than those of an ileostomy and the patient has some control over its function, especially if the stoma is sited in the sigmoid colon. The nurse must monitor the patient for signs of:

- Prolapse or retraction of the stoma.
- Faecal impaction.
- Skin irritation surrounding the stoma.

The nurse should encourage the patient to get out of bed on the first post-operative day and teach the patient to care for the colostomy. The patient should also be encouraged to return to a normal diet as soon as they are able and as far as possible to live as they did before the operation. Once the stoma wound has healed and any oedema has disappeared the stoma care nurse will discuss the various appliances available with the patient.

The patient should be taught to protect the peristomal skin by frequently washing the area with a mild soap. A skin-protecting barrier is applied around the stoma and the drainage pouch is securely attached. The stoma is measured to determine the correct size for the bag. The pouch opening needs to be 0.6 cm larger than the stoma. The drainage appliance is changed when it is one-third full so that the weight of its contents does not cause the bag to separate from the adhesive flange and spill the contents. The nurse should encourage the patient to discuss any problem relating to the care of the stoma. One problem, for example, may relate to the control of odour from the excreta in the appliance bag. Chlorophyll solution or deodorizing tablets will help to control odours, while crushed charcoal will help to absorb the odours.

The patient may be unsure about returning to normal activities including sexual activity. There may be direct or indirect clues about their fears. Some may fear odour leakage from the bag, others have more complex fears relating to body image. The stoma care nurse can be consulted to advise about adaptations to the ostomy bag that will facilitate more freedom of movement. Many of the patient's problems relating to loss of body image can be relieved by the nurse's use of appropriate counselling skills. Taylor (1994) refers to some of the specific problems relating to sexuality that may be encountered by people with a stoma.

Dyspareunia may be relieved by a change of position during intercourse. A substitute for the natural body lubricant may be needed. Impotence can be treated by the use of a vacuum device to encourage penile blood flow or by surgically implanting silicone rods into the corpus cavernosum to create an erection. Careful preoperative counselling is essential for both partners in a homosexual relationship who practice anal intercourse. The stoma must not be used as a substitute for the anus as it may become damaged necessitating further surgery.

Care of the patient with an ileostomy

An ileostomy will be fashioned when a total colectomy is performed as surgical treatment for conditions such as ulcerative colitis. The ileum is divided and the proximal portion brought to the surface of the abdominal wall as a spout about 4 cm long covered with mucous membrane. The contents of the ileum are fluid and contain enzymes, which damage the surrounding skin. In addition, the discharge is not under voluntary control and may occur without warning. Immediately after surgery a temporary plastic bag with an adhesive facing is placed over the ileostomy and firmly pressed onto the surrounding skin. After the ileostomy has healed, a permanent appliance is chosen with help from the stoma nurse. The stomal size is reassessed some weeks later when any oedema should have subsided. The size and type of the bag may have to be changed again some months later when the stoma has shrunk.

Nasogastric aspiration is required postoperatively to prevent build-up of fluid in the intestines causing pressure on the suture line. Intravenous fluids are given until bowel sounds return. Thereafter clear fluids progressing to a low-residue high-calorie diet will be given. The perineal wound may need to be irrigated two or three times daily until the wound is healed. Because there is loss of a body part, the patient may pass through the various phases of grieving and it is important that the nurse recognizes the patient's need for empathy and support at this time. The Ileostomy Association is able to offer advice and useful information, and the stoma therapist can also prove to be a valuable resource for the ileostomy patient.

THE ANAL AND PERIANAL REGION

Anatomy

The anal canal and anus form the final section of the GI tract. The anal canal (*Figure 14.21*) is essentially a short (3–4 cm) muscular and membranous tube surrounded by the internal and external sphincters. The levator ani muscle, which forms the bulk of the pelvic floor, clasps the anal canal at the anorectal junction. The muscle acts like a 'rectal sling' holding the rectum at an angle to the anal canal. The maintenance of this angle is important in the maintenance of faecal continence. The internal sphincter is a continuation of the rectal circular smooth muscle layer and as an involuntary muscle is not under voluntary

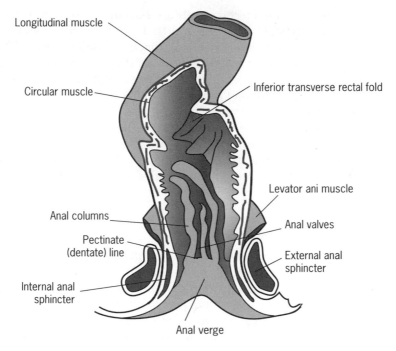

Longitudinal muscle

Circular muscle

Inferior transverse rectal fold

Levator ani muscle

Anal columns

Anal valves

Pectinate (dentate) line

External anal sphincter

Internal anal sphincter

Anal verge

Figure 14.21 The anal canal.

control. The approach of a peristaltic wave will result in relaxation of this muscle. The external sphincter, however, is made up of a striated muscle innervated by rectal branches of the pudendal nerve and is under voluntary control. The anus is the external opening of the anal canal. Specialized sweat and sebaceous glands, the circumanal (Gay's) glands, are found around the anus.

The upper two-thirds of the anal canal is lined by a columnar epithelium and has splanchic innervation: it is therefore essentially a visceral organ and is relatively insensitive to touch. The mucosa is thrown into longitudinal folds, the anal columns. The anal columns join at the base to form the anal valves, which are small semilunar folds of tissue. Rudimentary circumanal glands, the anal glands, are found between the bases of the anal columns. These glands can become infected and cause fistula formation. The anal valves mark the dentate line, which marks the division of the visceral and somatic portions of the anal canal. Below the dentate line the mucosa of the lower third of the canal has a squamous epithelium and a somatic innervation (rectal branches of the pudendal nerve) and is therefore touch sensitive. An understanding of this division can be important. Anal disorders such as haemorrhoids, which occur above the dentate line, will not be painful. These 'silent' haemorrhoids can become large and even dangerous. They may only become evident when they haemorrhage or are large enough to prolapse via the anus. Haemorrhoids below the dentate line are likely to be noticed at an early stage as they are often very painful.

The tissues of the anal canal receive their arterial supply from branches of the superior middle and inferior rectal (haemorrhoidal) arteries (Thomson, 1994). Venous drainage is via the inferior rectal (haemorrhoidal) veins. The anal mucosa and submucosa has an extensive venous (haemorrhoidal) plexus with dilatations or sacculations. Thomson (1994) suggests that these are normal and congenital and not an indication of pathology as has been previously assumed, and that the submucosal smooth muscle and dense elastic tissues support and surround the sacculations of the venous plexus. Thomson also describes three separate structures, the anal cushions, which are pads of tissue composed of the venous plexus and supporting tissue, and suggests that the internal sphincter squeezes the pads together to seal the anal outlet, preventing the escape of gas and liquid.

Disorders of the Anal Canal

Figure 14.22 summarizes some of the main conditions affecting the anal canal. Tumours of the anorectum are considered above in the section on the colon. Pruritus ani or anal and perianal itching is a common problem in adults. It can vary from a minor annoyance to a severe problem that reduces quality of life. It is most often related to poor hygiene, but is of interest because secondary causes include surgical conditions such as haemorrhoids, fissures, fistulas, and anorectal tumours.

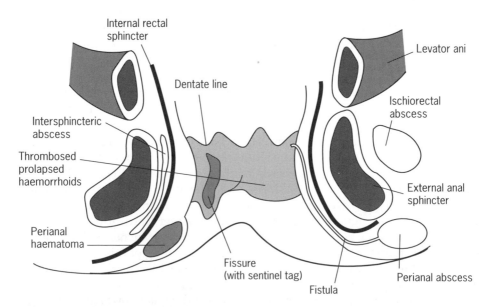

Figure 14.22 Disorders of the anal canal (Reproduced from Dyke and Ambrose, 1995 by kind permission of The Medicine Group (Journals) Ltd).

Anal fissure

An anal fissure is a split in the skin at the anal margin. It typically presents as severe pain that lasts 20–30 minutes and is brought on by defaecation. There may be slight bleeding. The pain often results in the development of constipation. Approximately 98% of fissures in men and 90% in women are found near the posterior midline of the anus. The remainder are found near the anterior midline. The fissure will be evident if the anus is everted, and there is often an associated hypertrophic skin tag (sentinel tag or pile). About 40% of fissures heal with conservative treatment including local anaesthetic suppositories or applications, stool softeners, and anal dilation (Dyke and Ambrose, 1995). Surgical treatment includes manual dilatation of the anus and sphincterotomy.

Anorectal abscess and fistula

Infection of the perianal skin or the circumanal glands can develop into a perianal abscess. It presents as a continuous throbbing pain and upon examination the skin will be red and tender and there will be a localized area of swelling. Treatment is by drainage, and a sample of pus is sent for culture. If the results show enteric organisms, further investigations may be necessary to exclude a fistula. Other anorectal abscesses include intersphincteric and ischiorectal abscess.

Fistula-in-ano is a general term used to describe fistulas or sinuses affecting the anal canal. They usually result from abscesses, but more rarely occur in tuberculosis, Crohn's disease, ulcerative colitis, and rectal carcinoma. Fistulas are usually treated by identifying both openings and opening the tract to promote healing by granulation. If the upper opening is above the anorectal ring, only the lower portion of the tract is opened as surgery above the ring could cause incontinence.

Haemorrhoids

Haemorrhoids (piles) is a condition classically described as presenting with three features that usually occur together, but can exist independently:

- Prolapse of the upper anal and lower rectal mucosa.
- Venous enlargement in the anal submucosa.
- Protrusions at the anal margin (commonly called skin tags or external haemorrhoids).

However, external haemorrhoid is not an accurate term and Ellis and Calne (1993) recommend that it is abandoned. The term has been used to include sentinel skin tags (see features of haemorrhoids above). The common belief that haemorrhoids are simply varicose veins is challenged by Thomson (1994) who contends that while anal varices may be a complication of portal hypertension they are rare and quite different in appearance from haemorrhoids and that the dilatation of the haemorrhoidal plexuses seen is normal. Thomson proposes that the submucosal smooth muscle normally supports the anal cushions during defaecation, but in haemorrhoids this mechanism fails and the cushions are dragged downwards with the stool until eventually they may protrude outside the anal canal. The causes of haemorrhoids are not clear. Straining at defaecation may be a factor. This could impede venous flow and cause oedema and swelling of the anal cushions, which would then be more prone to damage from the passage of a hard stool. Repetition of this pattern could result in permanent damage and descent of the anal cushion. Pregnancy is associated with the development of haemorrhoids.

Clotting of blood in the venous sacculations can cause a painful dark lump in the anal rim, which is often described as a perianal haematoma. This may resolve spontaneously, but can recur. Incision and evacuation may be required if it is large and painful.

The symptoms of haemorrhoids include bleeding, mucus discharge, prolapse, and pruritus. Bleeding is characteristically bright red, suggesting that it is from damaged capillaries in the swollen anal cushion. Strangulation, clotting, and thrombosis of haemorrhoids are complications that may cause necrosis and require a debridement haemorrhoidectomy. Haemorrhoids may be classified as:

- First degree (bleed, but do not protrude outside of the anal canal).
- Second degree (bleed and protrude, but reduce spontaneously).
- Third degree (bleed and protrude, but can be manually reduced).
- Fourth degree (prolapsed haemorrhoids that cannot be manually reduced).

Treatment

Before starting treatment it is important to exclude possible predisposing factors such as an associated lesion (e.g. carcinoma of the rectum). Conservative treatment involves dietary advice, the addition of fibre to the diet, stool softeners, and patient education to avoid straining and constipation. This may be sufficient for first degree haemorrhoids. First and second degree haemorrhoids can be treated on an outpatient basis by band ligation or sclerotherapy. Injection of a sclerosing agent such as 5% phenol in almond oil can be successful, but further similar injections may be needed at monthly intervals to completely eradicate the problem. It is important for the nurse to emphasize that as the injection is placed high in the anal canal it is painless. Infrared photocoagulation can also be used in the treatment of first and second degree haemorrhoids.

Elastic band ligation via the proctoscope is the mainstay of modern therapy. It can be used with first and second degree haemorrhoids and in selected cases of third and fourth degree lesions. A small rubber band is placed over the base of the haemorrhoid, though must be placed above the dentate line to avoid severe pain. The rubber band will occlude the blood supply to the pile, which should fall off in 5–10 days. The nurse must provide written instructions on the patient's discharge emphasizing the following points:

- There may be some slight bleeding for 4–5 days; this is quite normal.

- Paracetamol may be taken for the mild discomfort that may be experienced, but aspirin should be avoided as it can increase the risk of bleeding.
- Increase fruit and fibre in the diet to prevent constipation.
- Avoid strong laxatives, enemas, or suppositories.
- Excessive alcohol and strenuous exercise should be avoided for two weeks.
- Any excessive bleeding, fever, difficulty in passing urine, or anal swelling should be reported to the general practitioner immediately.

Third and fourth degree haemorrhoids are treated by ligation and excision of all haemorrhoidal tissue. It is important that the nurse is aware that the specific complications of this operation include:

- Pain.
- Haemorrhage, which is often related to infection.
- Acute retention of urine.

Patient education should emphasize the need to increase dietary fibre, ensure adequate physical activity, and maintain a high fluid intake.

References

Ambrose NS, Wedgwood KR (1990) Bleeding from the lower gastrointestinal tract. *Surgery* **October**(85): 2027–2033.

Armenti VT, Jarrel BE (1996) Common life-threatening disorders. In *Surgery* Jarrell BE, Carabasi RA (eds), pp. 161–174. Williams & Wilkins, Baltimore.

Brunt M (1982) *Physiology in Nursing*, p. 152. Harper and Row, London.

Bysshe JE (1988) The effects of giving information to patients before surgery. *Nursing*, **3**(3): 36–39.

Condon RE, Telford GL (1991) Appendicitis. In *Textbook of Surgery*. Sabiston DC (ed). pp. 884–898. WB Saunders, Philadelphia.

de Dombal FT (1990) Acute abdominal pain. *Surgery* 82: 1967–1971.

Dyke GW, Ambrose NS (1995) Painful perianal conditions and pruritus ani. *Surgery* **13**(3): 68–72.

Ellis H, Calne R (1993a) *Lecture Notes on General Surgery*, 8th edition, p. 214. Blackwell Scientific Publications, London.

Ellis H, Calne R (1993b) *Lecture Notes on General Surgery*, 8th edition, p. 164. Blackwell Scientific Publications, London.

Fielding JWL (1990) Gastric cancer. *Surgery* **85**: 2033–2038.

Fry RD (1996) Colon, rectum and anus. In *Surgery* Jarrell BE, Carabasi RA (eds), pp. 201–230. Williams & Wilkins, Baltimore.

Gillum DR (1996) Stomach and duodenum. In *Surgery* Jarrell BE, Carabasi RA (eds), pp. 183–194. Williams & Wilkins, Baltimore.

Grossman MI, Kirsner JB, Gillespie IE (1963) Basal and histolog-stimulated gastric secretion in control subjects and in patients with peptic ulcer or gastric cancer. *Gastroenterology* **45**: 14–26.

Krukowski ZH (1990) Appendicitis. *Surgery* **86**: 2044–2048.

Kurata JH, Haile BM, Elashoff JD (1985a) Sex differences in peptic ulcer disease. *Gastroenterology* **88**: 96–100.

Kurata JH, Honda GD, Frankl H (1985b) The incidence of duodenal and gastric ulcer in a large health maintenance organization. *Am J Pub Health* **75**: 625–629.

Luchtefeld MA, Palasek MB, Pobojewski BJ (1993) Laparoscopic bowel resection. *Today's OR Nurse* **15(1)**: 5–8.

MacFadyen BV, Wolfe BM, McKernan JB (1992) Laparoscopic management of the acute abdomen, appendix and small and large bowel. *Surg Clin N Am* **72(5)**: 1169–1183.

Pitluk H, Poticha SM (1983) Carcinoma of the colon and rectum in patients less than 40 years of age. *Surg Gynecol Obstet* **157**: 335–337.

Pugh J (1989) Nursing management for mobility: pre-operative phase. *Surg Nurse* **2(3)**: 24–27.

Stebbing JF, Mortensen N (1995) Ulcerative colitis and Crohn's disease. *Surgery* **13(4)**: 73–80.

Studley JGN, Williamson R (1991) Small bowel tumour. *Surgery* **April**(95): 2263–2267.

Taylor P (1994) Beating the taboo. *Nurs Times* **90(13)**: 51–53.

Thomson WHF (1994) Haemorrhoids. *Surgery* **12(12)**: 285–288.

Thompson JC (1991) The stomach and duodenum. In *Textbook of Surgery*. Sabiston DC (ed), pp. 756–787. WB Saunders, Philadelphia.

Williams JG, Fielding, JWL (1993) Duodenal ulcer. *Surgery* **11(12)**: 558–562.

Whittaker MG (1994) Colonic diverticular disease. *Surgery* **12(1)**: 11–18.

Chapter 15
Surgery of the Liver, Biliary Tract, Pancreas, and Spleen

This chapter considers surgical problems of the liver, biliary tract, pancreas, and spleen. The treatment and nursing management of some common surgical problems are discussed. However, it is not possible to consider every condition or surgical procedure affecting these organs and only major common conditions are discussed in detail.

THE LIVER, PORTAL HYPERTENSION, AND THE BILIARY TRACT

The liver is the largest of the abdominal organs, accounting for approximately 2% of body weight. It is the largest gland in the body, secreting up to 1 l of bile a day, and is situated in the abdominal cavity just under the ribs underlying the right hypochondriac and epigastric regions (see *Figure 14.5*). The liver is divided into a right and left lobe, and each lobe is in turn made up of two segments (*Figure 15.1*). Each lobe has a separate blood supply and biliary drainage. The falciform ligament marks the boundary between the medial and lateral segments of the left lobe. The right lobe has two smaller rudimentary lobes, the quadrate and caudate lobes, on its inferior surface (*Figure 15.2*). The liver receives oxygenated blood via the hepatic artery and its branches, but is also supplied with nutrient-rich blood via the hepatic portal vein (*Figure 15.3*).

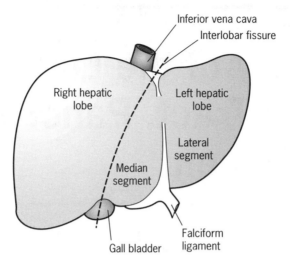

Figure 15.1 Anterior view of the liver.

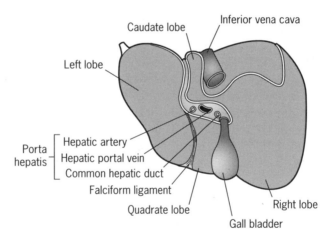

Figure 15.2 Inferior surface of the liver.

The role of the liver is primarily metabolic, although it also has secretory and storage functions. Briefly the principle functions of the liver include:

■ Formation and secretion of bile.
■ Metabolism and storage of protein, fats, and carbohydrates.
■ Synthesis of plasma proteins and clotting factors.
■ Storage of vitamins (A and D) and iron.
■ Inactivation of hormones (steroids, insulin, gastrin) and other endogenous substances.

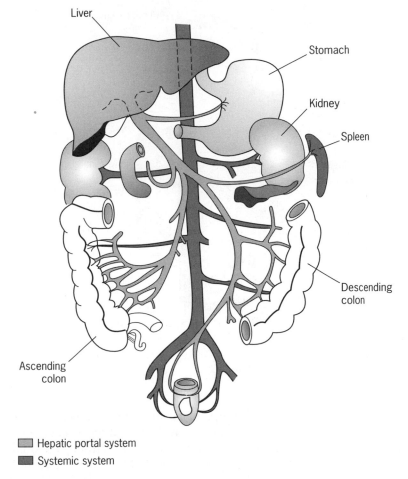

Figure 15.3 Hepatic blood supply and the portal system.

- Detoxification of drugs and other exogenous substances.
- Filtration of portal venous blood (all nutrient-enriched blood from the gastro-intestinal (GI) tract enters the liver's sinusoids).
- Heat production.

At the microscopic level the liver is made up of a system of about one million functional units, the hepatic lobules. The hexagonal lobule (*Figure 15.4*) features a central vein and a portal triad at each corner. The triad consists of branches of the hepatic portal vein and hepatic artery and the hepatic ductules. Bile drains from the canaliculi into the hepatic ductules, which unite to form the right and left hepatic ducts (*Figure 15.5*). The hepatic ducts leave the liver and converge to form the common hepatic duct. The cystic duct from the gall bladder joins the common hepatic duct at an acute angle to form the common bile duct. The

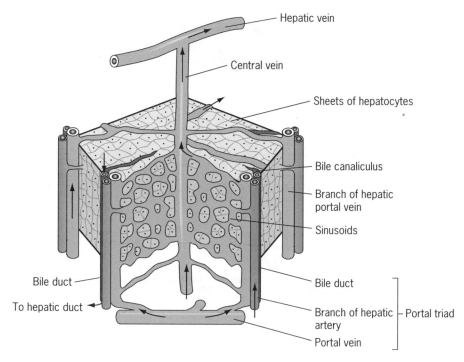

Figure 15.4 Hepatic lobule and portal triad.

common bile duct passes behind the pancreas and enters the duodenum at the ampulla of Vater. At the ampulla the common bile duct is encircled by the sphincter of Oddi, which controls bile flow. The gall bladder is a small organ about 6–10 cm long, located on the inferior aspect of the liver between the right and quadrate lobes (see *Figure 15.2*). It has a capacity of about 45 mL and its function is to store and concentrate bile. Contraction of the gall bladder and relaxation of the sphincter of Oddi releases bile. Release of bile is mainly under hormonal control, although vagal and splanchnic nerves may also have an influence. Cholecystokinin (CCK), a hormone secreted by the mucosa of the small intestine, is the main stimulus for gall bladder contraction.

DISORDERS OF THE LIVER AND BILIARY SYSTEM

Disorders of the liver include benign and malignant tumours, abscesses, cysts, and portal hypertension. Due to its size and position the liver is frequently involved in traumatic injury. Benign tumours include haemangioma, hepatocellular adenoma, and focal nodular hyperplasia. These are relatively rare conditions, although due to the use of oral contraceptives there has been a slight increase in the incidence of benign primary liver tumours in women (Neal *et al.*,

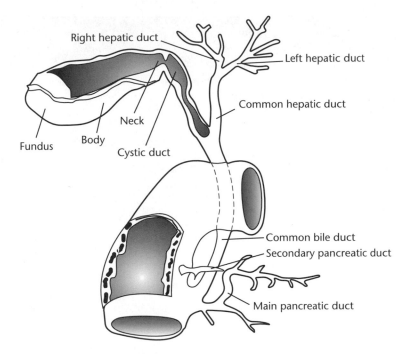

Figure 15.5 Biliary tree and gall bladder.

1996). Primary malignant tumours of the liver (i.e. hepatoma, hepatoblastoma, angiosarcoma) are also rare in the UK. However, the liver is the second most common site after the regional lymph nodes for metatastic spread from other abdominal tumours. Bacterial, viral, amoebic, and parasitic infections of the liver can cause abscesses and cysts. Cirrhosis of the liver can obstruct the portal circulation causing portal hypertension and this condition is considered in more detail below.

Neoplasia and trauma of the biliary system are relatively rare. The main problems seen in adult surgical practice are cholecystitis and cholangitis (i.e. infection of the gall bladder and bile ducts, respectively) and cholelithiasis and choledocholithiasis (i.e. stones in the gall bladder and common bile duct, respectively). The management of gall stones is discussed as the most common surgical problem of the biliary tract.

CIRRHOSIS AND PORTAL HYPERTENSION

Portal hypertension is an abnormal rise in the portal venous pressure above the normal level of 5–6 mm Hg. The causes of portal hypertension are listed in *Box 15.1*. Worldwide postviral hepatitis is the most common cause, but in developed societies alcoholic cirrhosis is the primary cause. Cirrhosis results from a group of

Box 15.1 Causes of portal hypertension (adapted from Sutton and Shields, 1995).

Prehepatic causes (rare)
■ Portal vein thrombosis or obstruction
■ Splenic vein thrombosis
■ Arteriovenous fistula
■ Tropical splenomegaly

Intrahepatic causes
■ Alcoholic cirrhosis
■ Postviral hepatitis cirrhosis
■ Schistosomiasis
■ Wilson's disease
■ Hepatic fibrosis
■ Haemochromatosis

Posthepatic causes (rare)
■ Budd–Chiari syndrome
■ Constrictive pericarditis
■ Venocclusive disease

conditions that cause chronic liver injury. The liver heals by regeneration and fibrosis and the fibrosis causes further injury and disruption of liver structure and function. This results in liver failure and portal hypertension. Cirrhosis causes a progressive narrowing and distortion of the sinusoidal (liver capillaries) and postsinusoid blood vessels. Ellis and Calne (1993) identify four main pathological changes in portal hypertension:

■ Development of collateral portosystemic circulation of the portal system.
■ Splenomegaly.
■ Ascites (except in prehepatic obstruction).
■ Liver failure.

The collateral veins that develop are fragile and when portal hypertension exceeds 20 mmHg varices (dilated veins) develop. Oesophageal varices develop at the gastro-oesophageal junction (due to the presence of collateral vessels between the gastric and oesophageal veins), while varices of the superior and inferior rectal veins present as haemorrhoids. Haemorrhage of oesophageal varices, and to some extent haemorrhoids, represents the most acute and serious complication of portal hypertension. Haemorrhaging oesophageal varices will present as sudden massive haematemesis and can cause cardiovascular collapse. With less profuse bleeding melaena may be the main presenting symptom.

Table 15.1 The Child's classification system of liver disease.

	Child Group		
	A	**B**	**C**
Serum bilirubin (μmol L^{-1})	< 35	35–50	> 50
Serum albumin (g L^{-1})	< 35	30–35	< 30
Ascites	None	Easily controlled	Refractory
Encephalopathy	None	Minimal	Advanced
Nutrition	Excellent	Moderate	Poor
Operative mortality rate (%)	2	10	50

From Sutton and Shields (1995)

Variceal haemorrhage can be a life-threatening emergency. Sutton and Shields (1995) note that although variceal haemorrhage accounts for only about 5% of acute upper GI tract bleeding it is responsible for over 50% of the associated deaths. The severity of chronic liver disease can be classed using Child's grading systems (*Table 15.1*), which takes into account the degree of liver failure, ascites, encephalopathy, and nutrition.

The liver is the main organ for detoxifying a range of endogenous and exogenous substances. These include substances produced by the intestinal flora and related to protein. Hepatic encephalopathy develops when liver disease, variceal haemorrhage, or shunting procedures prevent the detoxification of these substances, which enter the systemic circulation and travel to the brain. Hepatic encephalopathy presents as disorientation with bizarre neurological abnormalities and, occasionally, seizures. Investigations for patients with oesophageal varices are listed in *Box 15.2*.

Treatment

Haemorrhage due to oesophageal varices may require immediate resuscitation and control of the bleeding. Measures to control bleeding include:

- Pharmacotherapy.
- Balloon tamponade.
- Transjugular intrahepatic portosystemic shunting (TIPSS).
- Injection sclerotherapy.
- Surgical control.

Pharmacotherapy
Drugs can be used in an attempt to reduce portal pressure. Vasopressin (also known as antidiuretic hormone) produces a generalized vasoconstriction, which

> **Box 15.2** Investigations for patients with oesophageal varices (from Sutton and Shields, 1995).
>
> **Immediate**
> - Full blood count
> - Blood grouping and crossmatching
> - Clotting indices
> - Liver function tests
> - Urea and electrolytes
> - Screening for hepatitis
> - Fibreoptic endoscopy
>
> **Subsequent**
> - Liver biopsy if alcoholic hepatitis suspected
> - Microbiology and cytology of ascites fluid
> - Abdominal ultrasonography
> - Computerized tomography (CT) or magnetic resonance imaging (MRI) if tumour or Budd–Chairi syndrome suspected
> - Mesenteric angiography to identify varices and bleeding sites
> - Autoantibodies, serum caeruloplasmin, serum ferritin, α_1-antitrypsin, α-feto-protein for chronic liver disease

results in a reduction in splanchnic arterial flow. However, its systemic action results in a range of side effects including constriction of the coronary arteries, leading to discontinuation of therapy in 30% of cases. Terlipressin, a new derivative of vasopressin, is replacing vasopressin because its side effects are similar, but milder. These drugs are administered by continuous intravenous infusion. Vasopressin and terlipressin are sometimes used in combination with nitroglycerin, which helps counter the systemic effects and produces some additional reduction in portal pressure. Somatostatin and its long-acting analogue, octreotide, are used as alternatives to vasopressin. They increase splanchnic resistance and reduce blood flow through the varices. Pharmacotherapy aims to achieve short-term control of the bleeding, but about 25% of patients with variceal haemorrhage require further measures (Sutton and Shields, 1995).

Balloon tamponade

If pharmacotherapy fails to stop the bleeding a Sengstaken–Blakemore (*Figure 15.6*) or Minnesota tube can be used to control the haemorrhage mechanically. It will control bleeding in about 80% of cases, but haemorrhage recurs in 20–50% of cases when the balloon is deflated (Neal *et al.*, 1996). Sutton and Shields (1995) emphasize that insertion of these tubes is uncomfortable and should only be attempted if the haemorrhage is continuous. Nursing care of a patient with a Sengstaken–Blakemore tube is discussed on (p. 327).

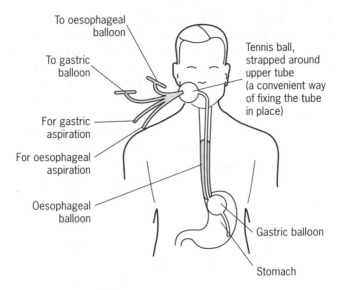

To oesophageal balloon

To gastric balloon

Tennis ball, strapped around upper tube (a convenient way of fixing the tube in place)

For gastric aspiration

For oesophageal aspiration

Oesophageal balloon

Gastric balloon

Stomach

The Sengstaken-Blakemore tube has four channels: one each for gastric aspiration, the gastric balloon, the oesophageal balloon, and oesophageal aspiration

Figure 15.6 Sengstaken–Blakemore tube. (Reproduced from Sutton and Shields (1995) by kind permission of The Medicine Group (Journals) Ltd).

Transjugular intrahepatic portosystemic shunting

TIPSS is a new procedure for controlling variceal haemorrhage and is currently under assessment. Using angiographic techniques, a portosystemic shunt is created between a hepatic vein and a branch of the portal vein and a stent is inserted to keep the channel patent. The procedure can be performed without general anaesthesia, but is associated with complications including shunt stenosis, thrombosis, and recurrence of bleeding. The place of this procedure in the management of portal hypertension and variceal bleeding has yet to be established.

Injection sclerotherapy

Oesophageal varices can be injected with a sclerosing agent (e.g. ethanolamine) during endoscopy. The sclerosant induces thrombosis of the vein. This treatment is currently the main treatment for variceal haemorrhage. Some patients require a second session of treatment. Complications include worsening of the haemorrhage, oesophageal perforation, and oesophageal erosion. A newer technique, endoscopic banding, may produce better results than sclerotherapy, although it is less suitable for patients with acute variceal haemorrhage.

Surgical control

With portal hypertension the risk of haemorrhage can make surgery difficult. The decision to proceed is made if the haemorrhage continues despite transfusion of five or more units of blood. After transfusion of ten or more units the risk of death increases significantly due to the complications of massive transfusion, and surgery is required before this occurs. Surgery can be targeted at the varices or decompression of the portal system. Emergency portocaval shunting success-fully controls the bleeding, but is associated with a high operative mortality (about 30%), which is related to the Child's grading, and a high incidence (15–30%) of postoperative hepatic encephalopathy (Copeland and Shields, 1991; Neal *et al.*, 1996). Sutton and Shields (1995) recommend oesophageal transection (*Figure 15.7*) as a simpler alternative to portocaval shunting. Oesophageal tran-section may be combined with the formation of a narrow-bore H-graft portocaval shunt (*Figure 15.8*) to reduce the risk of postoperative hepatic encephalopathy.

Once bleeding is under control treatment focuses on preventing recurrence. Sclerotherapy is the main treatment, and the recurrence rate is reduced if elec-tive sclerotherapy is combined with the daily oral administration of the beta-adrenoceptor-blocker propanolol, which can help reduce portal pressure. Endoscopic banding requires fewer treatments than sclerotherapy and seems to cause fewer complications. It may become the new treatment of choice. For patients under 60 years of age graded as A or B by the Child's classification Sutton and Shields (1995) recommend narrow-bore H-shunting or distal splenorenal shunting (see *Figure 15.8*). For patients in the Child's C category they suggest TIPSS.

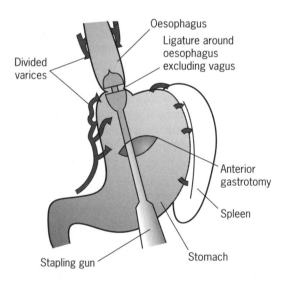

The stapling gun is positioned through the gastrotomy and the lower oesophagus tied into the firing line for transection and re-anastomosis

Figure 15.7 Oesophageal transection. (Reproduced from Sutton and Shields (1995) by kind permission of The Medicine Group (Journals) Ltd).

Narrow-bore H-graft portacaval shunt

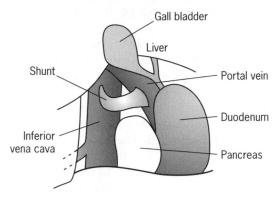

Distal splenorenal shunt

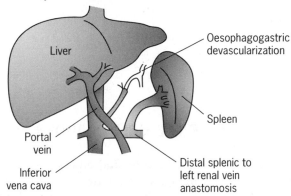

Figure 15.8 Narrow-bore H-graft portacaval shunt and distal splenorenal shunt. (Reproduced from Sutton and Shields (1995) by kind permission of The Medicine Group (Journals) Ltd).

Nursing Management

In acute variceal haemorrhage with haematemesis nursing priorities relate to maintaining a clear airway and monitoring for signs of shock (see Chapter 4). Vital signs are recorded every 30 minutes and suction must be available at the bedside. Intravenous therapy and blood transfusion will need to be maintained. A urinary catheter will be required and all intake and output recorded carefully due to the risk of renal hypoperfusion. The patient is likely to be fasted for theatre. If drug therapy or sclerotherapy or both fail to stop the haemorrhage a Sengstaken–Blakemore tube will be passed. The patient (and family) will be experiencing considerable anxiety and fear. The nurse must try to appear calm and provide clear concise explanations. The patient should not be left un-attended and the nurse must remain alert for indications of sudden circulatory failure. A benzodiazepine sedative may be prescribed to help relieve anxiety and antiemetics may be required to manage nausea and vomiting. The strain of retching and vomiting can cause increased pressure adding to the variceal bleeding.

If balloon tamponade is required the patient will need a careful explanation of the procedure and aftercare. A local anaesthetic spray is applied to the pharynx and the tube is well lubricated and passed down the oesophagus. Encouraging the patient to swallow will help the passage of the tube. At approximately the 40 cm mark the gastric balloon is inflated to hold the tube in place. The oesophageal balloon is filled with a mixture of water and radiopaque dye and continuous low-grade suction is applied. The position of the tube and oesophageal cuff pressure are checked hourly. The tube may be deflated after 12 hours to check for bleeding. It may then be necessary to re-inflate for another 12 hours. Nursing priorities for control of acute variceal haemorrhage relate to the underlying liver disease:

■ Fluid and electrolyte balance.
■ Prevention of hepatic encephalopathy.
■ Nutrition.
■ Managing the underlying condition.

SURGICAL DISORDERS OF THE GALL BLADDER

Surgical problems affecting the gall bladder and biliary tract include congenital cysts, trauma, and benign and malignant tumours, but these are all quite rare. The formation of gall stones is the commonest disease affecting the biliary tract. Bile is produced by the liver and stored in the gall bladder where it is concentrated. Hepatic bile contains about 97% water, the gall bladder absorbs about 90% of the water within four hours. The main constituents of hepatic bile are:

■ Water.
■ Bile acids (salts).
■ Bile pigments (bilirubin, biliverdin).
■ Cholesterol.
■ Proteins.
■ Phospholipids.
■ Electrolytes.

Gall Stones

Cholecystitis (inflammation of the gall bladder) is generally due to the presence of gall stones in the gall bladder (cholelithiasis). Gall stones may also lodge in the bile duct (choledocholithiasis) with resulting inflammation (cholangitis).

Cholesterol is the main component of most gall stones, although only about 6% of stones are pure cholesterol (Keen, 1993). Most gall stones are made up of cholesterol, bile pigment, and some calcium salts. About 15% of gall stones are composed mainly of bile pigments. Gall stones vary in size and shape. Pure cholesterol stones are generally large, round, and pale. Pigment stones are usually small, black, and brittle, and vary in shape from spiky (jackstones) to oval. Mixed stones may be faceted or irregular and when cut open show concentric rings of alternating pigment and cholesterol, often arranged around a pure cholesterol core. Large mixed stones that fill the cavity of the gall bladder and take its shape are called barrel stones. Cholesterol is held in solution in bile in the form of micelles with bile salts and lecithin (a phospholipid). Cholesterol stones are thought to form when there is an increase in the concentration of cholesterol or a decrease in the concentration of bile salts or lecithin. Cholesterol precipitates out of solution resulting in stone formation. Mixed stone formation is probably initiated by the same mechanisms, but excess mucus formation or bacterial infection may also be involved in the formation of these stones. Pigment stones are more common when there is a raised concentration of bile pigments and are often associated with cirrhosis or haemolytic disorders such as sickle cell anaemia and spherocytosis.

Gall stones are twice as common in women as men. They are associated with obesity and advancing age. Cholelithiasis is more common in developed countries, but the incidence is also high in the Far East where cirrhosis due to viral hepatitis is common (Keen, 1993). Cholelithiasis can be asymptomatic or silent when the gall stones produce no pathological effects. However, if the gall stone blocks the exit of the gall bladder or the cystic duct it will cause cholestasis (obstruction or suppression of bile flow) resulting in a chemical acute cholecystitis. Repeated episodes of inflammation can cause fibrosis and thickening of the gall bladder wall and infection may develop, resulting in chronic cholecystitis. Gall stones, particularly small stones, can enter the common bile duct. Common bile duct stones are found in 10–12% of patients requiring a cholecystectomy, and less than 10% of patients with common bile duct stones will remain asymptomatic (Peel, 1991). Common bile duct stones usually produce acute biliary colic with an obstructive jaundice. Back pressure can result in liver damage (biliary cirrhosis). Inflammation and infection of the common bile duct (cholangitis) is common. Gall stones may also be associated with acute and chronic pancreatitis (see below) and carcinoma of the gall bladder. Other complications of cholelithiasis include:

- Perforated cholecystitis. Necrosis of the gall bladder wall results in leakage of bile into the peritoneal cavity and peritonitis or subhepatic abscess may then develop.
- Fistula. A fistula may develop between part of the biliary tract and the other abdominal organs, most often the duodenum.
- Gall stone ileus. Perforation of the gall bladder and fistula formation may result in a gall stone entering and obstructing the bowel.

Acute Cholecystitis and Cholangitis

Acute cholecystitis is usually due to an impacted stone in the gall bladder exit or cystic duct. Generally there is a history of chronic cholecystitis and infected cholecystitis is found in about 75% of cases. The patient will complain of pain, which is sometimes severe. The upper quadrant of the abdomen will be tender and the gall bladder may be palpable. The patient will be pyrexial (38–39°C) with leukocytosis, and toxaemia can develop. A mild obstructive jaundice can develop if the swollen gall bladder presses on the common bile duct. The presence of gall stones in the common bile duct will result in acute cholangitis, which typically presents with pain, fever (with rigors), and jaundice. The urine may appear dark because of the presence of bile pigments, and the stool may be pale or clay coloured due to the reduced amount of bilirubin available in the intestines to colour the faeces. The pain is often severe and may be termed biliary colic. The smooth muscle in the wall of the gall bladder contracts in an attempt to dislodge the stone, causing severe pain in the right subcostal and epigastric regions. The patient appears shocked with pallor, sweating, and extreme restlessness. Vomiting often accompanies this condition. Sometimes the contractions succeed in moving the stone along the duct to be excreted via the intestines.

Investigations for acute cholecystitis

Investigations required for the differential diagnosis of acute cholecystitis are summarized in *Box 15.3*. Liver function tests are essential to assess hepatic involvement. Plain abdominal radiography is probably of limited value, but ultrasound provides a noninvasive and effective imaging if the operator is skilled. Endoscopic retrograde cholangiopancreatography (ERCP) and percutaneous transhepatic cholangiography (PTHC) are more invasive and are considered in more detail below.

Endoscopic retrograde cholangiopancreatography

ERCP of the biliary ducts involves inserting a flexible fibreoptic endoscope down the oesophagus to the duodenum to identify the ampulla of Vater. The ampulla is cannulated and the catheter passed into the common bile duct (or pancreatic duct). Contrast medium is injected and a rapid sequence radiograph taken to visualize the biliary tree. ERCP requires a cooperative patient and it is important that the procedure is fully explained and understood. There is a small risk of complications such as perforation. ERCP is not performed in patients with GI bleeding – blood will be taken for coagulation studies, grouping, and crossmatching before the procedure. The patient will have to lie motionless on an X-ray table for about one hour. A visit to the endoscopy suite before the procedure may help allay fears. Fasting is required before the procedure and premedication (e.g. diazepam) may be prescribed. If stones are seen in the common bile duct a sphincterotomy may be carried out. This means a diathermy wire is inserted through the biopsy channel of the endoscope and the sphincter of Oddi cut to allow the stones to pass. The stones are sometimes removed after

Box 15.3 Investigations in acute cholecystitis (adapted from Peel, 1991).

Full blood count
- Elevated white cell count

Blood culture
- Essential for patients with high fever

Liver function test
- Performed if jaundice is a current or past feature

Amylase
- Raised with associated acute pancreatitis

Plain abdominal radiography
- Only 10% of stones are radiopaque

Ultrasound
- Valuable for stones in the gall bladder, but unreliable in detecting stones in the bile ducts. It can demonstrate dilatation of the duct system

Oral cholecystogram
- Generally replaced by ultrasound. May be useful if dissolution (drug) therapy is considered

Intravenous cholangiography
- This procedure usually demonstrates pathology of the gall bladder and bile ducts. Depends on the ability of the liver to function adequately, so only of value if there is no jaundice

HIDA scanning
- Gives similar information as an oral cystogram, but can also demonstrate bile duct pathology

ERCP
- See text

PTHC
- See text

HIDA, Technetium-99m-labelled scintigraphy iminodiacetic acid sphincterotomy using a basket or balloon catheter. The patient will be drowsy after the ERCP and should be allowed to rest quietly until fully awake. The patient should have nothing to eat and drink for at least one hour. If a sphincterotomy has been performed the fasting should be extended for four hours. Vital signs of temperature, pulse, respirations, and blood pressure should be recorded half-hourly for the first four hours and four-hourly for 24 hours after this procedure because of the risk of bleeding, laryngospasm, hypertension, bradycardia, and respiratory depression. When fully awake, the patient may be offered a wash, mouthwash, and change of clothes. Ensure the patient has voided within eight hours. Any discomfort experienced from a sore throat can be eased by using soothing lozenges and fluids.

Percutaneous transhepatic cholangiography
PTHC is usually attempted when ERCP is not indicated. Initially ultrasound is used to identify dilated bile ducts as PTHC is difficult to carry out unless the ducts are dilated. PTHC requires fasting and laxatives or an enema to clear the bowel. A premedication may be required. An intravenous infusion may be established before the patient goes to the radiography department for intravenous access. The patient lies in a supine position and the skin of the upper right abdominal quadrant is prepared and draped. Local anaesthetic is injected, and under fluoroscopic guidance a long needle is inserted through the skin into the liver. When bile flow is observed a cannula can be passed down the needle into the biliary system. Radiopaque dye is injected and a rapid sequence of films is taken. The procedure takes 30–60 minutes. PTHC is contraindicated in patients with iodine sensitivity, cholangitis, or coagulation disorders. There is a risk of haemorrhage, biliary leakage, infection, and peritonitis. Antibiotic cover is usually given. After the procedure vital signs are monitored until stable and bed rest for six hours is recommended. Often the patient will be prepared for surgery and after PTHC go directly to the operating theatre for appropriate surgery because of the risk of biliary peritonitis.

Treatment
Treatment of cholelithiasis and cholecystitis depends on the severity of the condition. There is some disagreement about the treatment of asymptomatic cholelithiasis. Routine ultrasound examination of the abdomen has increased the diagnosis of silent stones. Some authorities may advise nonsurgical treatment or cholecystectomy in younger patients on the grounds that symptoms will develop later with the risk of complications (Ellis and Calne, 1993). However Neal et al. (1996) suggest that only 1–4% of patients with asymptomatic stones will develop complications and advise that there is little evidence justifying prophylactic treatment. Surgical treatment is normally advised for acute cholecystitis, although nonsurgical approaches may be indicated in a few cases.

Nonsurgical treatment includes drug therapy and lithotripsy. Small non-calcified stones in a functioning gall bladder may be treated by oral administration of bile salts in the form of chenodeoxycholic or ursodeoxycholic acid

(*British National Formulary*, 1996a). The stones should be no more than 1.5 cm in diameter and the patient must not be obese (Peel, 1991). Soloway *et al.* (1980) maintain that chenodeoxycholic acid has been effective in dissolving about 60% of cholesterol gall stones. However, the patient should be reminded that small fragments of the stones may pass through the ducts periodically, causing attacks of biliary colic. Treatment lasts for 6–36 months and patient compliance is poor. Drug therapy is successful in 20–70% of suitable cases, but there is a 50% recurrence at five years. Long-term prophylaxis is required. Gall stones recur in up to 25% of patients within one year of termination of treatment (*British National Formulary*, 1996b).

Extracorporeal shock wave lithotripsy (ESWL) has been used for the non-surgical fragmentation of gall stones in selected patients. Hood *et al.* (1988) describe the use of piezo-ceramic machines to direct shock waves at gall stones located in the gall bladder or common bile duct. Peel (1991) advises that ESWL is only suitable for about 16% of patients: those with three or less radiolucent stones. Approximately 5% of patients have a recurrence at two years and 10% experience complications such as pain and obstruction of the common bile duct by fragments. The fragments may pass spontaneously from the gall bladder, but concurrent administration of bile salts is recommended. Peel also notes that ESWL may remove the gall stone, but the symptoms of cholecystitis may persist.

Nonsurgical treatment can reduce the length of the hospital stay and enable patients to return to normal activities quickly. However, it is important that the nurse ensures that the patient understands the limitations of these treatments and the need to comply with drug therapy and dietary changes.

Surgical treatment
Acute cholecystitis is usually treated by cholecystectomy (i.e. removal of the gall bladder). There are two approaches:

- Immediate cholecystectomy.
- Conservative management with elective cholecystectomy.

Many surgeons regard immediate surgery within 72 hours as the treatment of choice as the risk of recurrence of an acute episode is high if surgery is delayed (Peel, 1991). Other surgeons advocate conservative management (i.e. bed rest, antibiotics, nasogastric drainage, nil orally, and pain control) until the symptoms settle and then an elective cholecystectomy about six weeks later (Ellis and Calne, 1993). Peel (1991) lists the disadvantages of the conservative approach as:

- Prolonged hospitalization and the need for a second admission.
- Longer time away from work.
- Risk of recurrence of an acute episode requiring readmission.
- Possibility that the patient will not attend for treatment until the next acute episode.
- Increased cost to the health service.

Neal *et al.* (1996) describe a compromise approach:

■ If the patient presents within 72 hours of onset of symptoms a laparoscopic cholecystectomy is performed.
■ If the patient presents more than 72 hours after the onset of symptoms, conservative treatment and an elective cholecystectomy is carried out within 4–6 weeks.
■ Deterioration or failure to respond to medical management is managed by cholecystectomy.

Surgical interventions for cholecystitis and cholangitis include:

■ Open cholecystectomy.
■ Laparoscopic cholecystectomy.
■ Operative cholangiography.
■ Cholecystostomy.
■ Choledochostomy.

Open cholecystectomy
A right subcostal incision is made, the cystic duct and artery are ligated, and the gall bladder is removed. The gall bladder space is drained of blood, bile, and serous fluid. An operative cholangiogram can be carried out during this procedure. The cystic duct may be cannulated, or if this is difficult the common bile duct may be used, and contrast media is injected. Fluoroscopy or serial films are used to assess the biliary tree. If the common bile duct has been entered it may be necessary to place a drain in the subhepatic space.

Laparoscopic cholecystectomy
This procedure involves making two small incisions in the abdominal wall and filling the peritoneal cavity with carbon dioxide (CO_2) gas. The surgery is carried out using a laparoscope with an attached video camera. Laparoscopic cholecystectomy is discussed in more detail as an example of minimal access surgery in Chapter 11. An operative cholangiogram can also be carried out during this procedure.

Cholecystostomy
Cholecystostomy provides an alternative when inflammation is too extensive or the patient is too ill for cholecystectomy. The gall bladder is opened and drained and the stones are removed. A drainage tube is placed in the gall bladder and exteriorized for external drainage. Cholecystostomy may be performed as an open or percutaneous procedure.

Choledochostomy
In this operation the common bile duct is incised to remove stones. A T-tube is then inserted into the duct for drainage of bile until the oedema subsides (*Figure*

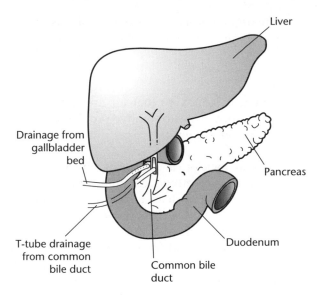

Figure 15.9 Drainage after cholecystectomy and exploration of the common bile duct.

15.9). The T-tube is connected to a drainage bag suspended from the bed just below the patient's body. A T-tube operative cholangiogram may be performed during this procedure to assess the full biliary tract.

Nursing management in acute cholecystitis or cholangitis

A patient presenting with acute cholecystitis will be severely ill and immediate concerns are pain control, antibiotic therapy, monitoring of vital signs, fluid and electrolyte balance, and controlling vomiting. The patient will require regular, adequate analgesia (100 mg pethidine intramuscularly is the usual choice, but nonsteroidal anti-inflammatory drugs (NSAIDs) and antispasmodics may also prove useful. Rest is critical. The pain in cholangitis may be particularly severe (biliary colic) and bile salts in the skin (due to obstructive jaundice) may cause considerable irritation. Skin irritation may be relieved by the appropriate antihistamine and by keeping the skin cool and dry. The patient will initially be nil by mouth and may also have a nasogastric tube in place. Intravenous therapy and careful monitoring of fluid intake and output are usually required. In addition to nasogastric aspiration an antiemetic may be necessary to control vomiting. Vital signs will be monitored hourly until the patient is stable. Pyrexia is common and a broad-spectrum antibiotic such as cefuroxime may be required. The patient will require oral care, and pyrexia will cause sweating and increase the need for washing and changes of bed linen.

Pain and anxiety may interfere with the patient's ability to communicate problems and take in information. In addition the jaundiced patient may experience irritability, lethargy, and depression. The nurse must explain that these feelings are characteristic of the condition and will abate when the obstruction is removed. When adequate analgesia has been established the patient will be better able to understand information and take informed decisions with regard to treatment.

Open cholecystectomy

Preoperative management is similar to that for any upper abdominal laparotomy. There are, however, specific postoperative problems that the nurse should discuss with the patient before surgery:

■ Because the abdominal incision is subcostal, the patient may experience additional discomfort when breathing, coughing, and moving. It is important to emphasize the importance of deep breathing, coughing, and moving to avoid atelectasis and pneumonia. The physiotherapist and nurse should teach the patient how to overcome this problem.

■ The nurse should explain the need for the presence of drainage tubes after operation, for example a wound drain or T-tube for the drainage of bile. Wound drains are likely to be removed within 24–48 hours. The T-tube will drain up to 500 mL in the first 24 hours, but the amount will reduce as the bile duct heals. A T-tube cholangiogram may be performed 7–10 days after the operation to assess patency of the duct before the T-tube is removed. The amount of drainage must be accurately recorded and care taken to avoid traction or accidental removal. The tube should always be handled aseptically and the insertion point regularly inspected for leakage of bile onto the skin.

■ Depending on the patient's age, condition, and the extent of the procedure the patient will be ready for discharge at between 6–10 days. Abdominal sutures are usually removed at 7–10 days. The patient will need to avoid heavy lifting or activities that might strain the wound for 4–6 weeks. Depending on the nature of their employment patients can usually return to work within 4–6 weeks.

Laparoscopic cholecystectomy

Laparoscopic cholecystectomy usually causes minimal postoperative pain and no postoperative ileus. The wounds are small and the patient can be discharged from hospital in 48 hours and may be back to work by the eleventh postoperative day. However, there are some reported complications of laparoscopic cholecystectomy, and these include abdominal wall haematoma, the unanticipated presence of common bile duct stones, and the risk of puncture of bile duct, blood vessels or organs such as the liver or intestines. Meyer (1992) maintains that selected patients with acute cholecystitis and common ductal stones may benefit from laparoscopic surgery. However, he emphasizes that the surgeon must be properly trained and experienced in this procedure. Stillman (1993) reports that patients who have had a laparoscopic cholecystectomy initially appear more restless and uncomfortable than those who have had an open cholecystectomy. It is therefore important that the nurse ensures that the effect of the postoperative medication is evaluated carefully and the dose increased if necessary. The evening after surgery the patient is usually permitted to drink clear liquids; it is important to avoid carbonated fluids as they can cause abdominal discomfort and distension. Patients are allowed to progress to a normal diet when they wish. When the patient is tolerating fluids well, the intravenous fluid therapy can be discontinued. The nurse should encourage the patient to be ambulant the day following surgery and to take a shower on the second day. Some patients complain of pain for up to one week following surgery as the residual amounts of CO_2 used during the operation are absorbed. Oral analgesics and NSAIDs may be used to relieve this problem. The nurse should advise patients to gradually resume normal activities and to see their general practitioner if they have any questions or problems relating to the surgery.

THE PANCREAS

The pancreas (*Figure 15.10*) is a retroperitoneal organ lying in the epigastric and left hypochondriac regions of the abdomen. It is located with its head in the curve of the duodenum. The body lies posterior to the stomach and the tail extends towards the spleen. The major pancreatic duct (of Wirsung) extends along the entire pancreas and enters the duodenum at the ampulla of Vater. The minor pancreatic duct (of Santorini) enters the duodenum at an accessory papilla about 2 cm

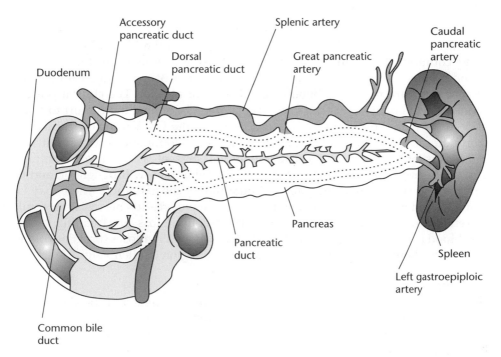

Figure 15.10 The pancreas and spleen.

above the ampulla of Vater. In most individuals the common bile duct and duct of Wirsung both enter the duodenum at the ampulla of Vater. In theory, spasm or blockage at the sphincter of Oddi can cause pancreatic stasis or a reflux of bile into the pancreas resulting in pancreatitis; however, this mechanisms has not been proven in humans. Over 80% of pancreatic tumours are found in the pancreatic head. This can cause compression of the common bile duct and obstruct the flow of bile. The splenic artery provides the arterial supply to the pancreas. Pancreatic veins empty into the splenic and mesenteric veins. The pancreas has exocrine and endocrine functions. The exocrine pancreas produces pancreatic juice, which is carried by the pancreatic duct to the small intestine. The endocrine pancreas consists of the pancreatic islets or islets of Langerhans, which secrete the hormones glucagon and insulin. Diabetes mellitus results from a failure of the beta cells of the islets of Langerhans. Pancreatic or islet cell transplants are being used to treat insulin-dependent diabetes mellitus; however, transplant surgery is beyond the scope of this book and this aspect of pancreatic surgery will not be considered.

The main disorders of the pancreas that may require surgical intervention are:

■ Pancreatitis.
■ Pancreatic cysts.
■ Pancreatic tumours.

Acute Pancreatitis

Pancreatitis is inflammation of the pancreas and may be classed as acute or chronic. Acute pancreatitis is a common condition in the UK and other developed countries, but chronic pancreatitis, although a problem in the USA and France, is less common in the UK. *Box 15.4* lists causes of acute pancreatitis. Over 75% of cases are related to biliary tract disease or alcohol. The clinical presentation of acute pancreatitis can vary from a mild abdominal discomfort to acute abdominal pain with haemorrhage and shock. In the UK acute pancreatitis is a common cause of admission to hospital with acute abdomen, and in about 10% of cases is fatal (Larvin, 1992). The patient will present with nausea, vomiting, and epigastric pain radiating to the back. The abdomen will be tender, and in severe cases rigid with acute pain and guarding of the abdomen. There may be jaundice and abdominal wall staining. In severe pancreatitis necrosis can result in retroperitoneal haemorrhage, with a large volume loss precipitating shock. The blood loss can track through the tissues causing ecchymoses (bruising) of the skin of the flank (Turner's sign) or periumbilical region (Cullen's sign).

Investigations
Blood tests and abdominal imaging are the main investigative procedure when diagnosing acute pancreatitis. Specific tests include:

■ Serum amylase.
■ Serum lipase.

> **Box 15.4** Causes of acute pancreatitis (after Larvin, 1992).
>
> **Major causes**
> - Alcohol
> - Biliary tract stones
>   (About 75% of cases are due to these causes)
>
> **Minor causes**
> - Trauma
> - Obstruction (neoplasia, cysts, parasites)
> - Metabolic (hypercalcaemia, hyperlipoproteinaemia)
> - Renal failure
> - Cushing's syndrome
> - Anorexia nervosa, bulimia
> - Vascular
> - Drugs
> - Infection (viral, bacterial)

- Urine amylase.
- Ultrasonography.
- CT scan of the abdomen.
- ERCP.

Amylase is mainly produced by the pancreas and salivary glands. Serum amylase is elevated in 95% of patients with acute pancreatitis. The normal value is 80–150 Somogyi units dl^{-1}. Levels of 200–500 Somogyi units dl^{-1} are suggestive of alcoholic pancreatitis, while levels higher than 1000 Somogyi units dl^{-1} may indicate a biliary tract cause. However, false-positive and false-negative results are common. A variety of other conditions can cause an elevated serum amylase and Yeo and Cameron (1991) warn that in an acute hospital setting nearly one-third of cases with raised amylase levels may be unrelated to acute pancreatitis.

Lipase is a pancreatic enzyme and serum lipase measurement is used to supplement amylase measurements in the diagnosis of acute pancreatitis. Elevated serum lipase suggests acute pancreatitis or pancreatic duct obstruction. If biliary obstruction is involved then serum bilirubin levels will also be elevated. The amylase:creatinine clearance ratio provides an accurate measure of amylase clearance and can be more sensitive than serum amylase in identifying acute pancreatitis (Vernick, 1996). Ultrasound scanning can be useful in identifying pancreatic changes and the presence of gall stones, but CT scanning may provide more detailed information. A plain abdominal radiograph is often of limited value. With the escape of enzymes into the pancreatic tissue and peritoneal cavity, fatty tissue is broken down into glycerol and fatty acids. The fatty acids combine with calcium to form insoluble calcium compounds. As a result the serum calcium concentration falls and this may be sufficient to provoke heart dysfunction or tetany. A lowered serum calcium concentration is an indicator of a poor prognosis in acute pancreatitis.

ERCP is the radiological examination of the pancreatic ducts and biliary system after injection of contrast medium into the ampulla of Vater. It should not be used within the first five days of acute pancreatitis because it is associated with an increased mortality at this time.

Complications of acute pancreatitis include:

- Hypovolaemic shock and fluid sequestration.
- Respiratory complications.
- Renal failure.
- Duodenal ileus.
- Jaundice.
- Pancreatic abscess formation.
- Pancreatic necrosis.
- Pancreatic fluid collections and pseudocyst.
- Diabetes mellitus.

Treatment

Initial treatment is conservative. Pain relief is a priority. Pethidine analgesia is standard as morphine can cause spasm of the sphincter of Oddi. Intravenous therapy is required to replace electrolyte and fluid losses. Haemorrhage will require blood transfusion, and cortisone may be given to combat severe shock. Antibiotics are prescribed to reduce the risk of abscess formation or a secondary peritonitis, and calcium gluconate may be required if serum calcium concentration falls. Fasting and a nasogastric tube are used to control nausea and vomiting, to reduce pancreatic stimulation, and to treat GI distension due to ileus. Blood gases and chest radiographs are required to monitor for respiratory distress.

Surgery is indicated in acute pancreatitis to:

- Confirm the diagnosis in severe cases not responding to medical management.
- To treat biliary tract obstruction (cholecystectomy).
- To drain an abscess, psuedocyst or fluid collection.

Nursing management

Nursing priorities focus on the key areas of:

- Pain control.
- Observation.
- Fluid balance and nutrition.
- Reducing the risk of complications.

The pain associated with acute pancreatitis can be severe, even excruciating. Pain arises from pancreatic trauma and intestinal distension. Pancreatic enzymes and inflammatory mediators attack tissues causing injury rather like that produced by a 'chemical burn'. Analgesia is always a priority in severe attacks. The pain can add to the shock and cause nausea and vomiting. It may make it difficult to carry out investigations and for the patient to fully understand the choices involved in treatment. Intramuscular pethidine is the usual approach. An intravenous infusion may be required if shock is developing, and alternative approaches to pain control such as patient-controlled analgesia and epidural analgesia have proved valuable. Sedatives and antiemetics may also be prescribed. The nurse must assess the pain rapidly and be alert for verbal and non-verbal indicators of its resurgence. Pain and tenderness should be regularly reassessed. Anxiety, pain, and the need for frequent observations may make it difficult for the patient to sleep.

Observation and monitoring are critical to identify problems and complications early. Pain can interfere with respiratory effort. Sputum retention and inadequate ventilation may promote pulmonary collapse or pneumonia. Pleural effusions are common and usually on the left side; the fluid may contain amylase. Frequent respiratory assessment is essential: blood gases should be monitored and serial chest radiographs may be required. If hypoxia develops, oxygen therapy and pulse oximetry or regular blood gas monitoring are necessary. Breathing exercises and physiotherapy are important. Aspiration pneumonia is a risk because of the vomiting. Shock can rapidly develop and regular observation of vital signs is essential. Blood glucose is monitored 4–6 hourly because there is a risk of diabetes mellitus. Careful recording of fluid intake and output is also important. Renal failure is a common complication. Oral intake is withheld, nasogastric drainage is standard, and catheterization of the urinary bladder is likely. Intravenous therapy, usually crystalloids, is started to replace fluid and electrolytes lost due to vomiting, nasogastric suction, oedema, and third-spacing (extravasation into the peripancreatic spaces). The patient should be offered frequent mouthwashes and oral care.

After the immediate crisis is over the patient will require support and reassurance. If the episode was due to biliary factors preparation may be required for appropriate interventions. If the episode was related to alcohol then education about alcohol and its relationship to pancreatic disease is important. An episode of acute pancreatitis is a major trauma. The patient will be tired and fatigued and is unlikely to be ready to return to work for 4–6 weeks. At discharge an outpatient appointment will be made for review within four weeks and the patient's general practitioner will need a detailed report of the episode.

Pancreatic Tumours

Pancreatic tumours can be classed as benign, primary malignancies, or secondary malignancies (*Box 15.5*). However, many of these pancreatic tumours are quite rare and this section will focus on carcinoma of the pancreas, the

---

Box 15.5 Pancreatic tumours (after Ellis and Calne, 1993).

Benign
- Adenoma
- Cystadenoma
- Zollinger–Ellison (islet non-beta cell tumour)
- Insulinoma (islet beta cell tumour)
- Glucagonoma (islet alpha cell tumour)

Malignant
- Carcinoma
- Cystadenocarcinoma
- Malignant islet cell tumour
- Secondary invasion from stomach or bile duct

---

commonest pancreatic tumour. Pancreatic adenocarcinoma is becoming increasingly common and in the USA is the fourth most common cause of cancer death in men. The condition commonly occurs between the ages of 50 and 70 years and the rate in men is twice that of women. The head of the pancreas is the site for 60% of tumours, while 25% affect the body and 15% the tail (Ellis and Calne, 1993). Tumours of the head of the pancreas commonly result in obstruction of the common bile duct and jaundice is present in about 75% of cases. Only about 10% of cases of carcinoma of the body and tail present with obstructive jaundice and because of this they are often only detected at an advanced stage.

In the early stages the clinical presentation is nonspecific with epigastric pain, weight loss, depression, and backache. Progressive jaundice may develop and thrombophlebitis migrans is seen in about 10% of patients. Sudden onset diabetes mellitus in an elderly patient may suggest pancreatic cancer. Pancreatic tumours are not easily palpated unless they are very large, but a palpable non-tender gall bladder in the presence of jaundice may indicate carcinoma of the head of the pancreas. Investigations are often used to rule out alternatives rather than prove the diagnosis of pancreatic cancer. There is no effective screening available and pancreatic tumours often prove incurable. CT scanning and ultrasonography can be used to identify the tumour, and percutaneous fine-needle aspiration under imaging control is used to confirm the diagnosis by cytology. ERCP can also be used to identify tumours and obtain a specimen for cytology.

Treatment

The prognosis for patients with pancreatic adenocarcinoma is poor. The five-year survival rate is less than 5%. Most patients die within one year and surgical intervention is associated with a 10% mortality. The diffuse nature of early symptoms and difficulty in diagnosing the condition means that tumours usually present at an advanced stage. Vernick (1996) estimates that only 10% of adenocarcinomas of the pancreas are resectable at the time of diagnosis. Palliative surgery is more common than curative surgery. Whipple's procedure, which involves removal of the head of pancreas, duodenum, gall bladder, part of the common bile duct, and part of the stomach may be attempted in a small number of patients. The procedure has a significant mortality rate and can cause considerable complications. If the disease is more widespread than expected on surgical exploration Whipple's procedure may not be attempted and only palliative measures carried out. Palliative procedures aim to alleviate the distressing symptoms associated with severe and unremitting jaundice, which include:

■ Nausea, vomiting, anorexia, and constipation.
■ Skin irritation.
■ Mental irritation and lethargy.

The obstruction may be relieved by anastomosing the jejunum to the gall bladder (cholecystojejunostomy), thereby providing an outlet for the bile other than through the common bile duct to the duodenum. More extensive surgery may be undertaken involving the removal of most of the pancreas, duodenum, and common bile duct. The remaining portion of the pancreas is anastomosed to the jejunum. The obstructive jaundice caused by pancreatic carcinoma can be relieved by intubation using a stent passed through the duodenal papilla at endoscopy or at operation. This provides a short circuit between the distended gall bladder and a loop of jejunum.

The major patient problems associated with pancreatic adenocarcinoma will be anxiety, pain, anorexia, weight loss, and jaundice. The nurse will need considerable skill in supporting the patient and family through the diagnostic process. From the patient's and family's perspective this will be a rapidly developing condition and health professionals will be able to offer only a limited hope of cure. The patient will need to understand the risks and limitations of curative surgery. Palliative care is usually required and the median survival time for patients with unresectable tumours is six months.

THE SPLEEN

The spleen (see *Figure 15.10*) is located in the left upper quadrant of the abdomen (left hypochondriac region) immediately under the diaphragm, and is protected by the eighth to eleventh ribs. The size and weight of the spleen is variable, but a normal spleen weighs 150–200 g. The spleen has a variety of functions, but its main role is to filter blood. The functions of the spleen include:

■ Removal of old or abnormal red blood cells.
■ Removal of abnormal white blood cells and cell debris.
■ Removal of normal and abnormal platelets.

- Storage of platelets.
- Immunological functions (opsonin production, antibody synthesis, protection from infection).

In view of these functions the spleen is therefore a highly vascular organ supplied by the splenic artery, a branch of the coeliac axis. The splenic vein, a major branch of the hepatic portal vein, provides venous drainage.

The two common disorders requiring surgical removal of the spleen (splenectomy) are trauma and splenomegaly. Rupture of the spleen is one of the most common results of non-penetrating injury of the abdomen. Splenomegaly is enlargement of the spleen, but as Ellis and Calne (1993) note, the spleen must be enlarged to about three times its normal size before it can be palpated. Hypersplenism is a condition in which there is splenomegaly and pancytopenia (i.e. a reduction in the cellular elements of blood: red cells, white cells, and platelets). Primary hypersplenism is rare and hypersplenism usually occurs secondary to:

- Disorders of splenic blood flow (i.e. portal hypertension).
- Haemopoietic disorders (e.g. hereditary spherocytosis, thalassaemia major).
- Immune disorders (e.g. idiopathic autoimmune haemolytic anaemia).
- Infiltrative disorders (e.g. myeloid metaplasia, sarcoidosis, Gaucher's disease).
- Infectious disease.
- Neoplasia (e.g. Hodgkin's disease, non-Hodgkin's lymphoma, leukaemias).

Ruptured Spleen

Rupture of the spleen commonly occurs after non-penetrating abdominal trauma, but may be caused by penetrating trauma or be spontaneous or iatrogenic. Carabasi and Kairys (1996) report that iatrogenic injury is responsible for 20% of all splenectomies. The spleen may be damaged during operations on the stomach, pancreas, left kidney or adrenal gland, transverse or descending colon, oesophageal hiatus, and vagal nerve (Sheldon *et al.*, 1991). It is important to note that rupture of the spleen:

- Is commonly associated with other injuries (e.g. liver trauma, kidney trauma, pancreatic trauma, diaphragmatic injury, fractured ribs).
- Can cause a massive internal haemorrhage resulting in rapid death from shock.
- Can develop slowly with progressive blood loss and there may be evidence of peritoneal irritation causing pain in the left shoulder and abdomen. The patient's condition will gradually deteriorate unless steps are taken to remove the damaged spleen.
- May occur as a delayed rupture hours or even several days after the initial trauma.

Splenectomy

Box 15.6 lists indications for splenectomy. Splenectomy is a major procedure and will require a complete preoperative work-up and careful postoperative observation and care. The procedure involves handling the stomach and as there is some risk of injury to the gastric wall a nasogastric tube will usually be passed. Atelectasis is the commonest postoperative complication and observation of respiration is essential. A splenic abscess may develop and is often accompanied by a pleural effusion. Due to the increased risk of pulmonary complications the nurse must encourage breathing and coughing exercises and physiotherapy will be an important part of both pre- and postoperative care. The procedure requires an abdominal incision and appropriate postoperative pain is essential for encouraging adequate ventilation and mobilization. Monitoring for postoperative haemorrhage is an essential nursing priority. The pancreas may also suffer some trauma during splenectomy and the nurse must be alert for signs of pancreatitis, particularly any changes in the type of pain reported.

Splenectomy has a major impact on the composition of the blood and on immune function. Thrombocytosis (an increased platelet count) occurs in up to 75% of patients after splenectomy, and anticoagulant therapy (usually heparin) may be prescribed. Passive exercise, deep vein thrombosis (DVT) prevention, and early mobilization are particularly important for these patients. Removal of the spleen also increases susceptibility to infection, notably encapsulated bacteria such as the pneumococci. Singer (1973) reported that in a series of 2796 splenectomies, 119 (4.2%) of patients suffered a postsplenectomy sepsis and 71 patients (2.5%) died from sepsis. The risk is especially high in patients who have a splenectomy because of a haematological disorder. For high-risk patients some authorities recommend prophylactic antibiotic therapy for up to three years after splenectomy. About 80% of cases of post-splenectomy sepsis occur within the first two years. Pneumococci are the common cause of post-splenectomy sepsis and polyvalent pneumoccal vaccine may be given. The vaccine is given two

---

Box 15.6 Indications for splenectomy (from Eichner, 1979).

Ruptured spleen
Primary splenic tumour
Bleeding oesophagogastric varices associated with splenic vein thrombosis
Splenic cysts or abscess
Hereditary spherocytosis
Idiopathic autoimmune haemolytic anaemia
Hodgkin's disease
Idiopathic thrombocytopenic purpura (ITP)
Thrombotic thrombocytopenic purpura (TTP)
Severe chronic hypersplenism

weeks before splenectomy and prophylactic antibiotics should be continued after immunization (*British National Formulary*, 1996c).

References

British National Formulary (1996a) No. 32, p. 56. British Medical Association and Royal Pharmaceutical Society for Great Britain, London.

British National Formulary (1996b) No. 32, p. 55. British Medical Association and Royal Pharmaceutical Society for Great Britain, London.

British National Formulary (1996c) No 32, p. 507. British Medical Association and Royal Pharmaceutical Society for Great Britain, London

Carabasi RA, Kairys JC (1996) Spleen. In *Surgery*, 3rd edition. Jarrell BE, Carabasi RA (eds). pp. 409–418. Williams and Wilkins, Baltimore.

Copeland G, Shields R (1991) Portal hypertension and oesophageal varices. *Surgery* **98**:2342–2347.

Eichner ER (1979) Splenic function: normal, too much and too little. *Am J Med* **66**:311–320.

Ellis H, Calne R (1993) *Lecture Notes on General Surgery*, 8th edition. Blackwell Scientific Publications, London.

Hood KA, Keighley A, Dowling RH, Dick JA, Mallinson CN (1988) Piezo-ceramic lithotripsy of gallbladder stones: initial experiences of 38 patients. *Lancet* **1**:1322–1324.

Keen CE (1993) Pathogenesis and pathology of gall stones and urinary calculi. *Surgery* **11(2)**:334–336.

Larvin M (1992) Acute pancreatitis. *Surgery* **10(3)**:49–57.

Meyer H (1992) Tighter rules urged on new galbladder surgery. *Am Med News*, June 1, cited in Schade R, Caffano J (1992) Trends in gallbladder disease and its treatment (part 1). *Hosp Med* **28(10)**:77.

Neal DD, Moritz MJ, Jarrell BE (1996) Liver, portal hypertension, and biliary tract. In *Surgery* 3rd edition. Jarrell BE, Carabasi RA (eds). pp. 231–264. Williams and Wilkins, Baltimore.

Peel AG (1991) Cholecystitis and its consequences – the techniques of cholecystectomy. *Surgery* **89**:2122–2130.

Sheldon GF, Croom RD, Meyer AA (1991) The spleen. In *Textbook of Surgery*. Sabiston DC (ed.) pp. 1108–1133. WB Saunders, Philadephia.

Singer R (1973) Postsplenectomy sepsis. In *Perspectives in Pediatric Pathology*. Rosenberg HS, Bolande RP (eds), Vol. 1, pp. 285–311. Medical Publishers Inc., Chicago.

Soloway RD, Balistreri WF, Trotman BW (1980) Gallbladder and biliary tract. In *Recent Advances in Gastroenterology 4*, pp. 251–290, Bouchier IAD (ed.). Churchill Livingstone, Edinburgh.

Stillman A (1993) Laparoscopic cholecystectomy. *Association of Operating Room Nurses J* **57(2)**:429–436.

Sutton R, Shields R (1995) Portal hypertension and oesophagogastric varices. *Surgery* **13(6)**:121–125.

Vernick JJ (1996) Pancreas. In *Surgery*, 3rd edition. Jarrell BE, Carabasi RA (eds). pp. 265–277. Williams and Wilkins, Baltimore.

Yeo CJ, Cameron JL (1991) The pancreas. In *Textbook of Surgery*. Sabiston DC (ed.). pp. 1076–1107. WB Saunders, Philadephia.

Chapter 16

Surgery of the Urinary System

CONTENTS

The urinary system (*Figure 16.1*) consists of the kidneys, the ureters, the bladder, and the urethra. The major function of the kidney is the formation of urine and excretion of waste products. In this chapter the surgical management of patients with disorders of the urinary system and male reproductive organs is discussed. Urological nursing is now a well-developed medical and surgical speciality with its own journals and specialist texts. A single chapter cannot hope to cover all the details of this speciality and in this chapter some of the more common problems that may be encountered on general surgical wards as well as specialist units are considered. Highly specialized topics such as renal dialysis and transplantation are not covered. This chapter will consider:

- Basic anatomy and physiology of the urinary system.
- Common investigations of the urinary tract.
- Urinary tract infection (UTI).
- Urinary calculi.
- Retention of urine and prostatic disease.
- Urethral strictures.
- Surgical problems of the male reproductive organs.

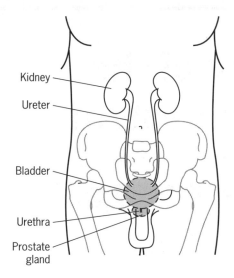

Figure 16.1 The urinary system.

ANATOMY AND PHYSIOLOGY

The paired kidneys occupy a superior–posterior position in the abdominal cavity and are found embedded in fatty tissue (the perinephric and paranephric fat) on either side of the vertebral column. The right kidney lies 2–8 cm lower than the left kidney. The kidneys are extraperitoneal, that is they lie outside the peritoneal membrane that encloses most of the abdominal contents. In size the kidneys are 9–15 cm long, 4–5 cm in width, and about 3 cm thick, and weigh approximately 150 g in men and 135 g in women. The superior–posterior aspect of each kidney is in contact with the diaphragm and each kidney is capped by an adrenal (suprarenal) gland. The kidneys are surrounded by a fascia that anchors them to surrounding structures, and the perinephric (within the fascia) and paranephric (outside the fascia) fatty pads help cushion and protect them. The fascia tends to limit the spread of kidney infections, but infection may track from a renal abscess between the layers of the fascia into the pelvis. The kidneys have limited mobility to accommodate changes of position as the body moves from supine to upright positions, but occasionally a condition called 'floating kidney' or nephroptosis occurs. If the supporting fascia is damaged the kidneys may be displaced causing traction and even torsion of the renal vessels and nerves. Nephroptosis frequently occurs among lorry drivers, motorcyclists, and horse riders. The condition can be serious particularly in malnourished patients who have little fatty tissue protecting the kidney.

Figure 16.2 shows the general features of the bean-shaped kidney. The prominent indentation where the renal vessels and ureter enter the kidney is called the hilus. The kidney is covered by a tight fibrous capsule, the renal

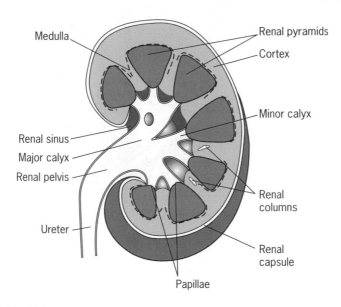

Figure 16.2 The kidney.

capsule, which provides a further barrier to infection. The capsule folds inwards at the hilus to form a cavity called the renal sinus. The renal artery and vein branch extensively within the sinus to supply the renal segments. The renal pelvis is the funnel-shaped distension of the ureter, which is continuous with the major calyces of the kidney.

In section the kidney can be separated into the outer cortex and the inner medulla. The cortex is primarily made up of the renal corpuscles (glomeruli and Bowman's capsules) and proximal and distal convoluted tubules. The medulla consists of 9–18 renal pyramids with the tips or papillae of the pyramids projecting into the renal sinus. The renal columns are fingers of cortex extending between the pyramids. The basic functional unit of the kidney is the renal lobe formed by the renal pyramid and adjacent cortex. The papilla of the pyramid projects into a minor calyx and the minor calyces fuse to form the major calyces. The major calyces join to form the renal pelvis. The kidney has an extensive vascular supply. The renal artery is a direct branch of the abdominal aorta and divides into segmental branches, which in turn form interlobar, arcuate, and interlobular arteries (*Figure 16.3*). The kidney is innervated by sympathetic nerves arising from the twelfth thoracic to second lumbar vertebrae. Renal pain is referred to and experienced in the lumbar area, inguinal regions, and the anterior aspects of the upper thigh.

At the histological level the nephron is the functional unit of the kidney. The basic structure of a nephron is shown in *Figure 16.4*. Blood flow through the capillary tuft of the glomerulus forms an ultrafiltrate of plasma. As the filtrate passes through the proximal convoluted tubule, the loop of Henle, the distal

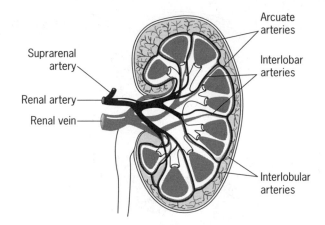

Figure 16.3 Renal blood supply.

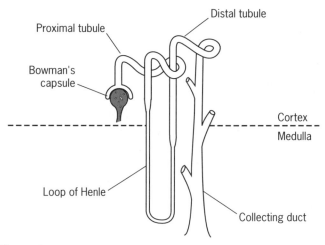

Figure 16.4 The nephron.

convoluted tubule, and the collecting duct, the processes of selective reabsorption and secretion alter its composition. The collecting duct carries the urine to the renal pelvis and into the ureter. From the ureter urine flows to the bladder for storage until it can be conveniently excreted via the urethra.

The ureters are thin muscular tubes approximately 30 cm long and connect the kidney to the urinary bladder. The ureter arises from the renal pelvis and descends retroperitoneally to enter the posterior–inferior aspect of the bladder. The wall of the ureter contains a thick layer of circular and longitudinal muscle, which helps move urine into the bladder. The muscle is involuntary muscle with peristaltic waves occurring about six times a minute. The diameter of the ureter varies down the length of the ureter. It is particularly constricted at the ureteropelvic junction where it crosses the iliac vessels and at the junction with the bladder (Pansky and House, 1964). Urinary calculi commonly lodge at these areas of constriction. The anatomy of the urinary bladder, urethra, and male reproductive organs are considered in more detail below.

The kidneys regulate extracellular fluid volume and composition and are critical for the maintenance of the body's internal environment. The central role of the kidneys in fluid and electrolyte homeostasis means that kidney disease can have severe effects and if untreated may quickly become life-threatening. The five major functions of the kidney are:

- Excretion of inorganic compounds (e.g. sodium, potassium, calcium, magnesium, hydrogen, and bicarbonate ions).
- Excretion of organic waste products (e.g. urea, creatinine).
- Regulation of blood pressure (by the formation and release of renin, which is part of the renin–angiotensin–aldosterone mechanism, and by regulating fluid volume).
- Regulation of red cell volume (by release of erythropoietin).
- Vitamin D activation (the kidney converts vitamin D into its active form).

INVESTIGATIONS OF THE URINARY TRACT

Investigation of urinary tract dysfunction may require a range of clinical tests, including radiography and imaging, biochemical tests, biopsy, and histopathology. As with all investigations there may be some discomfort, and sensitivity about the genitourinary system may increase anxiety for the patients. It is important that the surgical nurse fully explains the procedure, what is involved, and why it is required. The nurse must be able to answer any questions confidently to reduce the patient's anxiety. Informed consent requires that the reasons for specific preparations for investigations are clearly understood by patients and that time is given for patients to ask questions. Some investigative procedures are invasive and consent for the relevant procedure must be given in writing by the patient after the doctor's initial explanation. If the patient's bladder, ureters, and bowel need to be empty for the investigation, it is important the nurse clearly explains that food and fluids need to be withheld. It is equally important that patients know when they can resume eating and drinking, and the date when the results of the investigation will be available to them.

Urine Tests

Urinalysis
Routine urinalysis is an important measure for screening for systemic as well as urological disease. It is carried out when the patient is admitted and may be repeated if there is a change in the urine. The surgical nurse should inspect a

sample of urine, noting its colour and smell. Concentrated urine may be dark and pungent, but any foul smell is likely to indicate infection. Urine is normally clear to amber in colour; the presence of blood, pus, or sediment will require further investigation. *Box 16.1* lists changes in the macroscopic appearance of urine and the possible causes. Routine urinalysis is generally carried out using reagent strips. There is a wide range of strips available and these can be used to test for

---

Box 16.1 **The varying macroscopic appearances of urine with causes listed below (adapted from Sweny and Varghese, 1988).**

Straw to dark yellow
- Normal

Milky
- Urate crystals forming in acid urine
- Insoluble phosphates in alkaline urine
- Pus, UTI
- Spermatozoa
- Chyluria

Smoky pink
- Haematuria less than 0.5 mL L^{-1}

Foamy
- Proteinuria

Blue–green
- Pseudomonas UTI
- Bilirubin

Pink–red
- Blood, haemoglobin, myoglobin (brown on standing)
- Porphyrins (on standing)
- Anthocyanins (beetroot)
- Drugs

Orange
- Excess urobilinogen
- Drugs

Yellow
- Conjugated bile

Sediment
- UTI
- Acute tubular necrosis
- Nephrotic syndrome

an increasing number of substances. *Box 16.2* lists the normal findings for routine urinalysis.

If a urinary infection is suspected the urine can be examined microscopically and a specimen sent for culture and sensitivity testing. The nurse must ensure that:

- An aseptic technique is used to avoid contamination of the specimen.
- The specimen is transported to the laboratory in a firmly capped sterile bottle.
- The specimen is labelled clearly and correctly.
- The specimen is sent to the laboratory immediately and not left standing around as this may alter the bacterial count.

To collect a midstream specimen of urine (MSU) the patient's genitalia must be clean. In the male patient, the prepuce is retracted and the glans washed. In the female patient, the vulva is washed with soap and water, patients usually prefer to do this themselves. The patient is then asked to start urinating. The initial flow is discarded and the specimen is collected into a sterile container before the flow stops. The specimen is transferred to a sterile specimen container labelled 'midstream specimen of urine'. If the patient is catheterized, the nurse should withdraw the urine from the clean catheter specimen port with a sterile needle and syringe and label the specimen as a 'catheter specimen of urine'.

Biochemical analysis of the urine may be requested and often a 24-hour urine collection is needed to assess kidney function or to measure for particular metabolites, for example creatinine. For a 24-hour urine collection, the patient is asked to empty the bladder immediately before the collection of urine is scheduled to begin. This urine is then discarded, but all urine passed over the following 24 hours is then collected in a special container. Depending on the analysis, the collection bottle may contain a preservative.

Box 16.2 **Routine urinalysis with normal findings and values in parentheses.**

- pH (4.5–8.0)
- Specific gravity (1.005–1.035)
- Protein (Negative)
- Glucose (Negative)
- Ketones (Negative)
- Bilirubin (Negative)
- Urobillinogen (up to 1.0 Ehrlich unit)
- Haemoglobin (Negative)
- Red blood cells (RBC) (Negative)
- White blood cells (WBC) (Negative)
- Nitrites (bacteria) (Negative)

A creatinine clearance test is used as a measure of glomerular filtration rate (GFR) and is a common test of renal function. The test requires a 24-hour urine collection and a blood sample for serum creatinine. No special diet is required, but it is essential that all the urine is collected. The patient needs to be aware that even one missed specimen means that the collection has to be started again. The patient may also need reminding to urinate before defaecation and not to discard toilet paper into the urine collector. The normal values are 97–137 mL min^{-1} for males and 88–128 mL min^{-1} for females. Ageing causes a decrease in GFR of about 6.5 mL min^{-1} per decade (Pagana and Pagana, 1990).

Blood Tests

A wide range of blood tests can be used when investigating urinary tract function. The tests used will vary depending on the suspected disease state and may include haematology and blood chemistry tests. Blood urea nitrogen is an indicator of kidney function, and an elevated concentration may indicate renal disease. Serum creatinine is used to assess GFR and screen for renal damage. An elevated level indicates serious renal damage. Serum uric acid is primarily used to confirm a diagnosis of gout, but an increased concentration may indicate renal dysfunction. Electrolyte regulation is a function of the kidney and serum sodium, phosphate, and potassium, and the anion gap can all be used to assess renal disease. Serum calcium may be raised in certain metabolic conditions predisposing to calculi formation. Specific enzymes may also be assessed. An elevation in the levels of serum acid phosphatase and prostate-specific antigen are indicators of prostatic disease. Blood will also be screened for anaemia and indications of infection (e.g. white cell count).

Imaging of the Kidneys, Ureter, and Bladder

Radiography and more recently magnetic resonance imaging (MRI) are critical tools in urological investigations. *Box 16.3* lists some of the more common procedures used in urological radiography. In addition therapeutic interventions (e.g. dilation of stenosis) may be carried out using radiographic imaging to guide the surgeon. Plain radiography of the kidneys, ureters, and bladder (KUB) is useful for checking the position of structures and detecting calculi (90% of calculi are radiopaque and can be visualized in an abdominal radiograph), but more extensive investigation usually requires the use of a radiopaque contrast medium.

Intravenous urography
Intravenous urography (IVU) is used to provide more detailed anatomical assessment of the urinary tract. It can be used to:

- Assess the position, size, and shape of the kidneys.
- Visualize the renal pelvis, calyces, and ureters.
- Assess upper urinary tract drainage.

> ### Box 16.3 Procedures used in urological radiography (adapted from Sweny and Varghese, 1988).
>
> - Plain radiography of kidney, ureter, and bladder (KUB)
> - Intravenous urogram (IVU)
> - Antegrade and retrograde pyelograms
> - Renal angiography
> - Digital subtraction angiography (DSA)
> - Computed tomography (CT)
> - Ultrasound
> - Micturating cystourethrogram
> - Isotope renography

- Assess bladder shape and emptying.
- Identify filling defects and masses in the renal pelvis and bladder.

A radiopaque contrast medium that is excreted only by glomerular filtration (e.g. Omnipaque or Niopam) is administered intravenously and radiographs are obtained before injection and then at timed intervals after injection to allow visualization of the body of the kidney (nephrogram), the collecting system (pyelogram), the ureters, and the bladder. An aperient may be required before the urogram to reduce bowel and gas shadows, which can interfere with detailed visualization of the urinary tract. IVU carries a slight risk of causing an allergic reaction to the contrast medium, but this is less than 1% when modern low osmolality contrast media are used (McCahy *et al.*, 1995). In cases of renal pain or upper urinary tract obstruction, IVU can demonstrate the presence of stones and dilation above the obstruction. Renal or bladder masses may be evident, but masses or filling defects are likely to require additional radiographic investigations or cystoscopy.

Although the non-ionic contrast media such as Omnipaque or Niopam seldom give rise to allergic reactions, patients should be asked about any known sensitivity. As urine or faeces can obscure the structures being visualized an aperient might be required the night before and a phosphate enema on the day of the procedure. Fluids will be restricted and the patient limited to a light breakfast. Patients will be encouraged to empty their bladder immediately before the investigation.

Pyelography

Retrograde pyelography involves an injection of contrast medium directly into the ureter to help visualize the collecting system and ureter. It is mainly used to investigate ureteric obstruction or provide additional information on upper tract filling defects identified by IVU. Antegrade pyelography in which the contrast is injected directly into the renal pelvis is less commonly used, but may be necessary if retrograde pyelography is contraindicated. Pyelography is not commonly used in modern urological investigation.

Renal angiography
The renal arteries may be catheterized via the femoral artery and the arterial supply to the kidneys visualized using a contrast medium. Renal angiography can be used to investigate the renal vasculature and to identify neovascularization due to renal tumours and may be used in some therapeutic interventions.

Digital subtraction angiography
This is a computerized method of visualizing major blood vessels using an intra-arterial injection.

The patient should avoid eating and drinking for four hours before going to the X-ray department for angiography. The patient will also need to remove all clothing, jewellery, and prostheses, and wear a gown. The groin area will need to be clean as an injection will be given at this site before the catheter is inserted. The patient is likely to be in the X-ray department for 4–6 hours and will need to be transported home afterwards. If the patient is having angiography as an out-patient, written instructions must be made available. After the procedure, the patient may eat and drink, and after a rest can be driven home. The patient should be warned that the groin area will be tender and possibly bruised for a few days. If bleeding should occur, firm pressure should be applied over the puncture site until the bleeding stops. If bleeding persists, the general practitioner or Accident and Emergency Department should be contacted at once.

Computed tomography
Computed tomography is widely used to provide more detailed visualization of masses and calcification identified by radiography. It is very sensitive and can help in staging as well as identifying renal, ureteric, and bladder tumours. It is not very effective in identifying carcinoma of the prostate, but may allow assessment of lymph node involvement.

Magnetic resonance imaging
Magnetic resonance imaging is becoming increasingly important in the investigation of the urinary tract and associated structures. It seems likely that it may replace CT in the evaluation of bladder cancer (McCahy et al., 1995) and it is effective in assessing larger renal masses. MRI has the advantage of not requiring contrast media. However, CT is still more efficient for assessing renal masses of less than 3 cm diameter (McCahy et al., 1995). MRI is also very effective in assessing and staging prostate tumours and in visualizing the scrotal contents.

Ultrasonography
Ultrasound scanning provides a non-invasive painless method for visulizing soft tissues. It can be used to assess size and shape of structures and scanning of the kidney is used to evaluate cysts, tumours, obstruction, hydronephrosis, and

urinary calculi. It can also be used to detect non-radiopaque stones. Ultrasound is about 95% effective in identifying benign cysts and in differentiating renal tumours from abscesses or cysts (Booth, 1983). Ultrasonography of the bladder can be used to identify tumours as small as 3 mm, but is of limited value in staging the disease. It can also be used to assess postmicturition bladder volume and prostate size and volume, and to visualize prostate carcinoma, although it may miss about 20% of prostate tumours (McCahy *et al.*, 1995). Colour-coded doppler ultrasound, a development of ultrasonography may be more accurate for identifying malignancy. Ultrasound is probably the ideal method for imaging scrotal masses and other testicular problems.

Cystoscopy

A flexible fibreoptic cystoscope can be passed via the urethra to allow direct visualization of the bladder. Modern cystoscopes are thin and highly flexible, which means that although the procedure is uncomfortable it is relatively painless and does not require a general anaesthetic. Operative procedures involving the bladder and prostate may be carried out by cystoscopy; however, a more rigid cystoscope and a general anaesthetic may be necessary. Flexible ureteroscopes are also available that allow the ureters and renal pelvis to be visualized and samples taken for cytology.

The nurse must ensure that patients understand that they will be awake during the procedure, which may entail some discomfort, but will not last long. They can expect to be told the result of the examination straight away, although biopsy results may not be immediately available. No special preparation is required and the patient can eat and drink as normal. The patient is asked to change into a gown and empty the bladder. The urethral area is cleaned, and local anaesthetic and lubricant are applied. The flexible cystoscope is inserted into the urethra and into the bladder. Men may be asked by the doctor to try to pass urine allowing the cystoscope to pass through the bladder sphincter more easily. Once the cystoscope is in the bladder, the whole of the lining may be visualized. Saline may be inserted via the cystoscope and this can be passed out once the examination is over. Specimens (biopsies) may be taken from the bladder lining without causing pain. Fine catheters may be passed into the ureters to take radiographs of the kidneys if necessary (retrograde ureterogram). The nurse should explain that after cystoscopy, some patients experience a burning pain on passing urine and there may be a little bleeding. The patient is encouraged to drink three litres of fluid daily and these side effects will usually stop within 24 hours. Should problems of burning or bleeding persist, the patient is asked to contact their general practitioner as soon as possible.

Biopsy

Needle biopsies can be obtained from the kidney, ureter, bladder, and prostate to help with the diagnosis of a mass or a suspicious lesion. Bladder and ureteric biopsies are obtained during endoscopy. Prostatic biopsies can also be obtained using the transrectal route. Renal biospy may be indicated in:

- Nephrotic syndrome.
- Nephritic syndrome.
- Unexplained haematuria.
- Asymptomatic proteinuria.
- Acute renal failure (unexplained).

A renal biospy is usually carried out using radiography or ultrasound to guide the procedure. The left kidney is preferred as this avoids the risk of liver trauma (Sweny and Varghese, 1988). Bleeding is a common and serious complication, and coagulation and clotting studies must be assessed beforehand. It is important that patients understand the procedure and are cooperative and able to hold their breath for about 30 seconds. The nurse needs to emphasize the importance of not moving during the procedure and sedation may be helpful. The patient should be encouraged to stop breathing each time the needle is advanced to avoid trauma to the kidney and adjacent organs. Blood pressure should be recorded before the procedure and quarter-hourly blood pressure, pulse, and respirations should be monitored for about four hours after the procedure and then 4-hourly if satisfactory. It is essential that haemorrhage is detected as early as possible. The wound site should be checked and urine assessed for haematuria. Bed rest is essential after renal biopsy.

URINARY TRACT INFECTIONS (UTIs)

The presence of micro-organisms in the urinary tract is referred to as a UTI. UTIs can be bacterial, viral, or parasitic in origin (*Box 16.4*), but bacterial UTI is the main problem in surgical practice. UTI is of particular relevance to surgery for three main reasons:

- Pathological changes due to UTI may require surgical intervention.
- UTI increases the risk of postoperative complications after surgery of the urinary tract.
- UTIs are associated with other urological problems such as prostatic obstruction, urinary calculi, and bladder tumours.

UTIs are generally considered to be an ascending infection, most usually due to faecal organisms: *Escherichia coli* is responsible for 80% of UTIs (Farrar and Chinegwundoh, 1994). The periurethral area in men and the introitus in women may become colonized by opportunistic pathogens, which gain access to the urethra and ascend, infecting the urethra, bladder, and eventually the kidney. UTI is more common in women, probably due to the shorter urethra. Bacteriuria is the presence of bacteria in urine after contamination from the vagina or

Box 16.4 Causes of urinary tract infections.

Bacterial
- Enterobacteria (*Escherichia coli, Proteus mirabilis*)
- *Pseudomonas aeruginosa*
- *Streptococcus faecalis*
- Coagulase-positive staphylococcus
- *Chlamydia*
- *Mycobacterium tuberculosis*

Viral
- Herpes zoster

Fungal
- *Candida albicans*

Parasitic
- Schistosomiasis
- Hydatid disease
- Filariasis
- Onchocerciasis
- Amoebiasis

prepuce has been ruled out. Farrar and Chinegwundoh (1994) define significant bacteriuria as urine that produces a colony count greater than 10^5 mL^{-1} on culture. Bacteriuria can be symptomatic or asymptomatic, and symptoms may include pyuria (pus in the urine), pyrexia, dysuria, and cystitis.

Cystitis is inflammation of the bladder and may be of bacterial or non-bacterial origin. The clinical manifestations of cystitis include urinary frequency, urgency, dysuria, and cloudy and foul-smelling urine. Pyelonephritis is infection or inflammation of the renal pelvis and presents with similar symptoms as cystitis, but also causes fever, chills, and flank pain.

Upper UTIs can lead to surgical complications, including perinephric abscess and pyonephrosis.

Factors that increase the risk of UTI include:

- Vesicoureteric reflux (primary or acquired defect of the bladder–ureter junction).
- Urinary tract obstruction and stasis (e.g. calculi, tumours, pregnancy).
- Urinary tract fistula.
- Sexual trauma.
- Catheterization or instrumentation of the urinary tract.

Steps to reduce the risk from catheterization are reviewed in Chapter 4.

SURGERY OF THE KIDNEYS AND URETERS

In the adult a variety of conditions affecting the kidneys and ureters may require surgical intervention. Renal cysts may require aspiration under ultrasound control. Renal infections, renal abcesses, and perinephric abscesses are serious conditions requiring excision and drainage, but are relatively uncommon. Renal trauma or cancer are the two main causes of nephrectomy (i.e. removal of the kidney) in general surgery. However, urinary calculi are the most common reason for surgical treatment of the kidney and ureters and are considered in some detail below.

URINARY CALCULI

The treatment of urinary calculi (urolithiasis) is one of the most rapidly advancing areas of modern surgery. New approaches developed in the early 1980s now allow 95% of urinary tract calculi to be removed using minimally invasive techniques (Whitfield, 1989) making open surgery for removal of urinary calculi the exception rather than the rule. Urinary calculi affect about 2% of the population in Britain. About 40% of stones pass spontaneously. Men are twice as likely to be affected as women. Urinary calculi are generally radiopaque and Keen (1993) identifies the main types of calculi as:

- Calcium oxalate stones. About 33% of calculi are composed entirely of calcium oxalate.
- Calcium oxalate and calcium phosphate stones. About 33% are composed of a mixture of calcium oxalate and calcium phosphate (as apatite).
- Triple phosphate and struvite stones. About 15% of stones are of this type. They include the so-called staghorn calculus, which forms a cast of the renal pelvis and calyces.
- Uric acid stones. These are radiolucent and account for about 6% of urinary calculi.
- Cystine stones. These account for 2–3% of urinary calculi.
- Brushite stones (calcium hydrogen phosphate dihydrate) stones, which account for another 2% of stones, often in combination with oxalate or apatite.
- Uncommon urinary stones, which include combinations of free fatty acids (urostealiths), cholesterol, and xanthine.

The exact causes of calculi formation remain uncertain, but several factors predispose to stone formation. Conditions that promote urinary stasis, concentration of constituents, and, in particular, an alkaline pH, contribute to calculi formation. Hypercalciuria, usually without an accompanying hypercalcaemia, is found in about 60% of patients with calcium oxalate stones (Keen, 1993). Other conditions promoting stone formation include UTI, metabolic disease, and renal tubular acidosis (Paulson, 1991). Bladder stones are more common in hot, dry regions. Triple phosphate stones are most often associated with urinary infection. Urea-splitting bacteria increase urinary pH by converting urea to ammonia and cause precipitation of calcium ammonium phosphate. These uric acid stones are often very large. Cystinuria, an autosomal recessive inherited metabolic condition, is associated with the formation of cystine stones. Keen (1993) notes that excessive ingestion of magnesium trisilicate is associated with the formation of silicon dioxide stones.

Urinary calculi can vary greatly in size, shape, and composition. They can be found at any level in the urinary tract, but commonly originate from the renal pelvis. Small stones can pass into the ureters where they may cause pain (ureteric colic) and haematuria. Obstruction can lead to hydroureter and hydronephrosis. In the urinary bladder stones can grow, becoming quite large. Infection (pyelonephritis and pyonephrosis) is a potential complication (Ellis and Calne, 1993). Pain is the main presenting symptom, although some stones are asymptomatic. Ureteric colic has been described as 'the dreadful agony.' It is often accompanied by vomiting and sweating. Small mobile stones are more likely to cause pain than larger immobile calculi (Whitfield, 1989).

Investigations

Urine is tested for the presence of blood, and KUB abdominal radiography will reveal the majority of stones. IVU will be carried out to explore the renal anatomy and the risk of hydronephrosis. A urine specimen is required for culture and sensitivity testing. Serum uric acid and calcium estimation are also recommended, and a more detailed investigation of renal function (urea, electrolytes, and creatinine) may be required if the stones are large or bilateral (Whitfield, 1989). Any stones that are passed should be sent for chemical analysis.

Treatment

Treatment depends on the patient, the presenting symptoms, and the results of the investigations. Whitfield suggests that treatment will depend on:

■ The patient's symptoms.
■ The patient's age.
■ The size and position of the calculi.
■ Renal function.
■ The presence of infection.
■ The patient's general health.

Small asymptomatic calculi can generally be left alone, but the patient requires regular reassessment. Most ureteric stones of less than 5 mm in diameter will pass spontaneously in the urine within 48 hours of the acute attack. The nurse's role is to encourage the patient to maintain adequate hydration and reassure the patient that oral analgesia will be available in the event of further pain. Patients are advised to call their general practitioner in the event of nausea, vomiting, fever, or intractable pain. There is little evidence that encouraging a high fluid load and diuresis will help pass the stone more quickly or easily. Any stone causing obstruction, intractable pain, renal disease, or UTI must be removed. Symptom control is critical until removal can be arranged. Ureteric stones can cause acute renal colic: the patient complains of severe intermittent pain and commonly presents with tachycardia, nausea, and vomiting. If a UTI is also present the patient may be pyrexial. Bed rest and analgesia are required, and the pain may be severe enough to require an intramuscular narcotic such as pethidine or diamorphine (Whitfield, 1989). An antiemetic such as prochlor-perazine intramuscularly may be prescribed to control the vomiting.

Open surgery is generally only required for large staghorn calculi within the renal calyces or if there is a pre-existing disorder of the collecting system that can be corrected at the time of stone removal. The majority of stones can be treated by minimally invasive techniques such as percutaneous nephrolithotomy (PCNL) and ureteroscopy or noninvasively by extracorporeal shock wave lithotripsy (ESWL). Approximately 75–80% of patients with urinary calculi can be treated by ESWL and nearly all by a combination of lithotripsy with PCNL (Paulson, 1991). Stones can also be removed using endoscopic methods (ureteroscopy). Temporary relief of obstruction can be produced by flush back and stenting or insertion of a nephrostomy tube. ESWL is, however, the general treatment of choice.

Extracorporeal shock wave lithotripsy

ESWL is based on the principle that shock waves generated in a fluid medium can be focused through the body to shatter the stone. The original lithotripter used an electrohydraulic system to generate shock waves. The patient had to be placed in a fluid bath and positioned so that the calculus was sited at the focus point. Electromagnetic lithotripters are more compact and the patient is positioned on a water cushion (Dawson and Whitfield, 1994). The most modern lithotripters use ultrasound imaging to locate the stones and piezoelectric crystals to generate the shock waves, eliminating the need for a water tank. With piezoelectric systems and depending on the patient's age and condition, ESWL can be performed without anaesthetic or analgesia on an outpatient basis. Analgesia is usually required with electrohydraulic or electromagnetic systems. Dawson and Whitfield (1994) suggest a diclofenac (100 mg) suppository and note that about 10% of patients may require addition analgesia such as pethidine. It can take up to 2000 individual shocks to reduce a large calculus to particles small enough to be excreted, and the procedure can take 30–90 minutes. ESWL can also be used to break up larger calculi for removal by PCNL. ESWL is costly to establish and may be limited to specialist regional centres.

Although ESWL is not necessarily painful, the patient will require careful explanations and reassurance. An anxiolytic premedication (e.g. diazepam or temazepam) may be prescribed. The nurse must emphasize the importance of the patient not moving during the lengthy procedure. Reassurance is a critical nursing role during this treatment. The patient should be accompanied by a known nurse who stays throughout the procedure. Background music may help alleviate stress and boredom. Vital signs are monitored during the procedure. The patient will usually stay in the unit until urine is passed and oral frusemide may be given after the procedure to encourage diuresis. Antibiotics and analgesia may also be prescribed as a prophylactic measure. Most patients can return home with no ill effects, but some may experience pain, dysuria, haematuria, and occasionally ureteric obstruction, and require hospitalization until the symptoms settle. Discharge advice should be given verbally and as an information leaflet. The patient is advised to drink three litres of fluid daily. Some blood and sediment will be noticed when passing urine. It is also important to emphasize that the patient must attend for a follow-up assessment when check radiographs will be taken. There may be some discomfort and analgesics can be taken. Patients should notify their general practitioner in the event of pain, nausea, pyrexia, clots in the urine, or decreased urinary output.

Ureteroscopy
Technical advances and miniaturization mean that modern ureteroscopes are much less traumatic, allowing for a better range of endoscopic procedures. Stones can be removed from the upper ureter using a ureteroscope and from the lower ureter using a cystoscope. Stones are fragmented using an ultrasonic probe, laser lithotripsy, or lithoclast, and then removed with a wire endoscopic stone basket (Dawson and Whitfield, 1994). As the procedure may take some time a general anaesthetic is usually used.

Percutaneous renal surgery
If ESWL is not available or appropriate, stones in the kidney can be removed using percutaneous renal surgery. The procedure is carried out using a general anaesthetic and requires the usual preparation for surgery under a general anaesthetic. A premedication is usual and the nurse must ensure that the patient understands that a catheter and intravenous infusion will probably be in place postoperatively. The patient is placed in a prone position and a needle inserted through the skin between the iliac crest and the subcostal region. The needle follows a posterior–lateral direction to enter the renal pelvis or calyces. Ultrasound or radiological imaging is used to ensure correct placement. A wire is threaded through the needle and this is used to guide a series of dilators forming a direct tract into the kidney. A plastic sheath (Amplatz sheath) is placed in the tract. *Figure 16.5* shows a percutaneous nephroscope positioned to fragment a stone using ultrasound. Stones can also be fragmented using an electrohydraulic probe, or if small, removed using forceps. When the nephroscope is removed a drain is inserted to allow drainage of blood, urine, and fragments.

On return to the ward, the nurse must ensure that the infusion rate and urinary drainage are satisfactory. The patient's vital signs are monitored regularly. As soon as the patient is tolerating fluids, the infusion and catheter are removed. Normal diet is resumed, and if the dressing is comfortable,

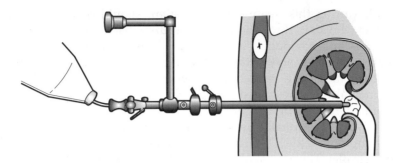

Figure 16.5 Percutaneous nephroscope positioned to fragment a stone. (Reproduced with kind permission from Sabiston DC (1991) *Textbook of Surgery*, 14th edn. WB Saunders, Philadelphia.)

mobilization is encouraged. After 48 hours a nephrostogram is carried out to ensure normal drainage of the collecting system, and if this is satisfactory the nephrostomy drain can be removed. The patient can expect to be discharged on the fourth day. Advice must be given to drink at least three litres of fluid daily and to return for check-up in six weeks (Latham and Marden, 1986).

Temporary relief of obstruction

Temporary measures may be adopted to relieve ureteric obstruction due to urinary calculi (Morrison *et al.*, 1994). In flush back and stenting the stone a small stone in the upper ureter can be flushed back into the renal pelvis and a small tube or stent inserted to prevent the stone re-entering the ureter. A nephrostomy tube can be inserted when flush back fails. Under radiographic guidance a small catheter is inserted into the collecting system of the kidney, sutured in place, and connected to a closed drainage system. These methods are occasionally used to provide short-term relief of obstruction until the patient can be scheduled for removal of the calculi.

SURGICAL DISORDERS OF THE BLADDER

The urinary bladder is shown in *Figure 16.6*. It is situated immediately behind the pubic symphysis and superior pubic rami. The fundus of the bladder is extraperitoneal, the base lies on the pelvic floor. The bladder is highly distensible, accommodating up to 500 ml of urine, but the trigone, the portion at the base of the bladder where the ureters enter and the urethra exits is less distensible. The detrusor muscle forms the walls of the bladder and contraction of the detrusor muscle is responsible for bladder emptying. The bladder is lined by a transitional epithelium. The peristaltic action of the ureters forces urine into the bladder. Males become aware of bladder distension when the bladder contains 100–150 ml of urine; the awareness becomes urgent at 350–400 mL, and painful

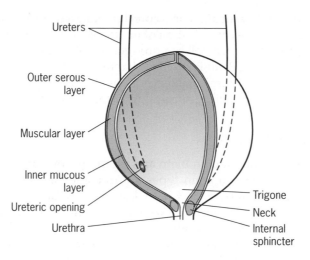

Figure 16.6 The urinary bladder.

when it contains over 400 mL. Involuntary micturition will occur when the bladder contains about 500 mL of urine in the healthy male, but may occur at a much lower volume in the elderly or those with bladder disease. The bladder innervation is illustrated schematically in *Figure 16.7*.

Surgical problems of the bladder include bladder cancer, bladder trauma, fistulas, bladder stones, and neurogenic bladder. Bladder trauma is usually associated with pelvic trauma, and repair will often be carried out during general surgery. Bladder fistulas are usually traumatic, inflammatory, neoplastic, or iatrogenic. A vesicoenteric fistula is a tract between the bladder and the gut and is

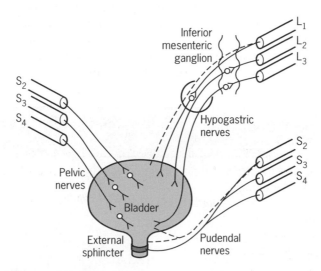

Figure 16.7 Innervation of the bladder.

usually secondary to diverticulitis or colorectal malignancy. A vesicovaginal fistula is commonly seen as a complication of unattended childbirth or secondary to gynaecological procedures. Calculi can produce irritable bladder symptoms, and the treatment of urinary calculi is discussed above (p. 361). Neurogenic bladder dysfunction is treatable by surgical interventions (MacDonagh and Swami, 1995), but the major condition requiring surgical intervention is bladder carcinoma.

Bladder Tumours

Bladder cancer is a worldwide problem and represents one of the most common urological tumours. The two main types are transitional cell carcinoma (TCC) and squamous cell carcinoma (SCC). In Europe and the USA about 90% of bladder tumours are TCC, while SCC accounts for only 6–8%, and about 2% are adenocarcinomas. TCC of the bladder is the fifth most common cancer in men and the tenth most common in women although the incidence in women is rising (Woodhouse, 1992a). In developed countries bladder cancer tends to be a disease affecting middle-aged to elderly people and is associated with certain occupations (*Box 16.5*). There is a higher incidence in smokers, and this might be one reason for the increasing incidence in females. In Africa the picture is quite different. SCC is the most common bladder tumour, affecting many men and women at a much younger age, and is usually associated with parasitic infection due to *Schistosoma haematobium* (Elem, 1991). This section will concentrate on TCC of the bladder. It is, however, worth noting that the same condition can arise in the ureters and kidney.

Woodhouse (1992a) suggests that TCC can be divided into two categories: superficial, accounting for about 70%; and invasive. Superficial TCC is limited to the epithelium, but can progress into the invasive form affecting the bladder muscle. Haematuria is the main presenting symptom and occurs in approximately 70% of cases. Otherwise superficial TCC may be asymptomatic. With the more invasive forms of TCC bladder irritability results in dysuria, urgency, and frequency. Symptoms may be mistaken for UTI or not reported due to embarrassment, and patients may present for treatment at an advanced stage.

Box 16.5 **Bladder cancer and associated occupations (adapted from Woodhouse, 1992a).**

- Known exposure to carcinogens associated with transitional cell carcinoma
- Coal gas manufacturing
- Rubber manufacturing and destruction
- Cable manufacturing
- Dye manufacturing
- Rodent extermination
- Sewage work

Investigations include urinalysis, cytological examination of the urine, IVU, and cystoscopy. Cytology of the urine may identify cancer cells, although cancer cell-free urine does not rule out bladder cancer, and IVU is performed to exclude renal causes of haematuria, for example renal pelvic carcinoma. On cystoscopy a benign condition – transitional cell papilloma – may be identified. Papillomas of the bladder wall may predispose to malignancy. A biopsy of the papilloma can be taken and at the same time it can be treated by diathermy. Recurrence is common and it must be emphasized to the patient that regular check cystoscopy is essential to ensure early treatment of any recurrence. Cystoscopy and biopsy are the key investigations for staging bladder cancer. Woodhouse (1992a) emphasizes that staging must be exact because it forms the basis for decisions on the type of treatment. If the tumour is classified as superficial, further investigations may not be necessary as distant spread is rare before there is invasion of the bladder muscles. Patients with invasive tumours, however, need further investigations such as pelvic CT to identify local spread and chest radiography, bone scan, and liver function tests to check for distant metastases. The TNM method of staging is in common use, but other staging systems may also be used. *Box 16.6* illustrates the staging of cancer using the TNM system.

Box 16.6 **TNM staging of bladder cancer.**

T (tumour)
T_x: Primary tumour cannot be assessed
T_0: No evidence of primary tumour
Tis: Carcinoma *in situ*
Ta: Noninvasive papillary carcinoma
T_1: Tumour invades submucosa or lamina propria
T_2: Tumour invades superficial muscle
T_{3a}: Tumour invades deep muscle
T_{3b}: Tumour invades perivesicular fat
T_4: Tumour invades adjacent organs

N (regional lymph nodes)
N_x: Regional lymph nodes cannot be assessed
N_0: No regional lymph node involvement
N_1: Metastases in single node less than 2 cm
N_2: Metastases in single node larger than 2 cm and less than 5 cm or multiple nodes less than 5 cm
N_3: Metastases in nodes larger than 5 cm

M (distant metastases)
M_x: Distant metastes cannot be assessed
M_0: No distant metastases
M_1: Distant metastases

Treatment of superficial TCC

Management of superficial TCC is based on regular cystoscopy and local treatment with transurethral resection of the tumour (TURT). On cystoscopy tumours can be cauterized or resected depending on their size. A general anaesthetic is usually needed for cautery or resection, and newer approaches based on laser treatment and photodynamic therapy are being developed. General care will be as for cystoscopy. Woodhouse (1992a) suggests four main outcomes for cystoscopy and cautery or resection:

- No recurrence (30%).
- Single recurrence (20%).
- Low-activity multiple recurrences of less than five tumours per episode with mean time to recurrence two years (25%).
- High-activity multiple recurrences with episodes recurring within 15 months, often with multiple tumours on each recurrence (25%).

Patients cannot be considered in the no recurrence group until they have been clear for six years. Cystoscopy and treatment will depend on the individual's pattern of recurrence and radical treatment is required in 20–30% of cases. Radical treatment is necessary if the disease shows progression of grade or stage or if the symptoms are unacceptable, causing discomfort and lifestyle alterations. Cystectomy (i.e. removal of the bladder) is the main form of radical treatment. Moore *et al.* (1993) describe the use of intravesical chemotherapy for treating recurrent superficial TCC. Locally acting cytotoxic drugs are instilled and have few systemic side effects. However, local effects may include frequency, urgency, dysuria, and an occasional reduction in bladder capacity (*British National Formulary*, 1996). Intravesical bacille Calmette–Guérin (BCG) has also been used to treat some types of invasive bladder cancers.

The patient may be treated as a day case. Before the procedure an IVU may be required to ensure that there is no obstruction of the renal tract, and urine is cultured to exclude UTI. The nurse must explain the procedure and answer any questions the patient may have. The main agents and their use are listed in *Box 16.7*. It must be emphasized that the catheter is inserted in order to instil the drug and will be removed as soon as this has been completed. The drug is given slowly and the patient is asked to try to retain the fluid for two hours, alternating position on the bed from side to side. During this time, the nurse should listen to the patient for fears that may exist about for example loss of control of micturition or of having to have the bladder removed. Before discharge, the patient should be advised about aftercare and possible side effects. The patient should be warned about the possibility of dysuria (burning sensation on micturition), urgency, frequency, and haematuria, and advised to drink at least two litres of fluid a day and to report any fever. A nonsteroidal anti-inflammatory drug (NSAID) may be prescribed to control any pain or discomfort.

Box 16.7 The main cytotoxic agents used in bladder instillations and their uses (*British National Formulary*, 1996).

Doxorubicin
Used for recurrent superficial bladder tumours and some papillary tumours. Solution 50 mg in 50 mL sterile sodium chloride 0.9% instilled monthly.

Epirubicin
Used for papillary tumours. Solution 50 mg in 50 mL sterile sodium chloride 0.9% instilled weekly for 8 weeks.

Mitomycin
Used for recurrent superficial bladder tumours. Solution 10–40 mg in 20–40 mL sterile water instilled weekly or 3 times weekly for a total of 20 doses.

Thiopeta
Used for recurrent superficial bladder tumours. Solution 15–60 mg in 60 mL sterile water instilled weekly for 4 weeks, then after a break of 2 weeks, at intervals of 1–2 weeks for a further 4 doses.

Treatment of invasive carcinoma of the bladder

Once bladder cancer has become invasive penetrating the lamina propria and into the muscle the condition becomes much more serious. Deep or invasive TCC is an aggressive condition with a mortality of 50–70% and requires radical treatment. Other invasive types of bladder carcinoma, namely squamous cell carcinoma and adenocarcinoma, also have a poor prognosis and usually require radical cystectomy. Surgery is likely to be used in combination with chemotherapy or radiotherapy. As invasive bladder cancer tends to present at a later stage surgical treatment alone is seldom sufficient as there is usually both local and distant spread. However, the condition most often presents in elderly patients who may be too frail to tolerate combined treatment by surgery, chemotherapy, and radiotherapy. Surgical treatment may be by TURT or partial or complete cystectomy. Cystectomy also requires some type of reconstruction or urinary diversion.

If invasion is limited and the muscle is not affected, cystoscopic resection (TURT) is possible. Partial cystectomy in which only the affected area is removed may also be considered. Intravesical therapy with mitomycin or BCG may also be effective. Careful follow-up with three-monthly check cystoscopy is essential, and more radical treatment is required for any recurrence. For very localized deeper tumours, a partial or segmental cystectomy may occasionally be considered, but recurrence in the residual bladder is high and some authorities do not recommend this approach (Paulson, 1991). Total or radical cystectomy is advised for cases where there is clear muscle involvement and is the mainstay of treatment for patients under 65 years of age (Woodhouse, 1992b). Radical cystectomy in men can involve removal of the bladder, prostate, seminal vesicles, and some adjacent tissue. In women, the bladder, uterus, fallopian tubes, anterior vagina, and urethra may be removed (Paulson, 1991). However, Woodhouse (1992b) emphasizes that surgery alone is seldom sufficient.

Systemic chemotherapy and external beam radiotherapy are used in combination with surgery or may be used alone if surgery is not an option. Radiotherapy may be used before or after surgery and in combination with chemotherapy. Chemotherapy may be intravesicular or systemic. Systemic treatment with a combination of cytotoxic drugs may be used as a pre- or postoperative therapy. Examples of intravenous cytotoxic regimens include M-VAC (methotrexate, vinblastine, doxorubicin, and cisplastin) and CISCA (cisplastin, cyclophosphamide, and doxorubicin). Radiotherapy or chemotherapy may be used as purely palliative measures.

Removal of the bladder requires the formation of a urinary diversion. In an ileal conduit diversion a section of the ileum is isolated, keeping the blood supply intact, an anastomosis is formed with the ureters, and a stoma is formed on the abdominal wall (*Figure 16.8*). Paulson (1991) describes an alternative procedure, the orthotopic bladder, which can be used if the urethra can be preserved (*Figure 16.9*), although Woodhouse (1992b) observes that the female urethral sphincter is seldom strong enough to keep this type of reservoir continent. Woodhouse (1992b) also suggests that for some patients an exteriorized ileal conduit can be avoided. Instead the ileal reservoir can be approached by submucosal tunnelling to form a catheterizable stoma.

Nursing care for patients treated with cystectomy and urinary diversion

Preoperative care
As with all cancers the patient may require a great deal of information and support when considering the options for treatment. The nature of the surgery will mean that the patient has to make some major psychological adjustments. The procedures can have a serious impact on body image and sexuality. Stoma

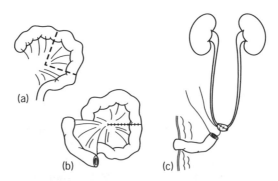

Figure 16.8 Ileal conduit urinary diversion.

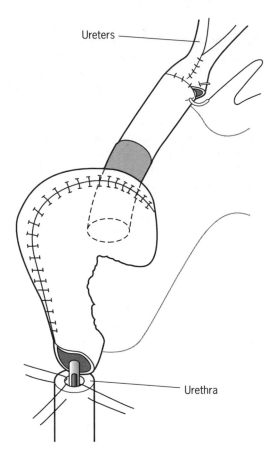

Ureters

Urethra

Figure 16.9 The orthotopic bladder. (Reproduced with kind permission from Sabiston DC (1991) *Textbook of Surgery*, 14th edn. WB Saunders, Philadelphia.)

formation will affect self-image, and male impotence is a consequence of radical cystectomy. The cancer patient will also be concerned about possible pain and whether the operation will actually cure the condition. The surgical nurse will need to be prepared to discuss and reinforce the information provided by the surgeon. The patient may find it useful to meet someone who has a urinary stoma and to plan the placement of their own stoma with the surgeon. The patient can be encouraged to handle samples of stoma pouches, which are odour- and waterproof.

Preoperative preparation will include bowel preparation. A low-residue or fluid-only diet will be required and enema or colonic washouts will be used to clear the bowel before surgery. Local antibiotics may be prescribed in the form of suppositories and systemic antibiotics may be used to 'sterilize' the bowel. Prophylactic antibiotic therapy will start before surgery and is continued in the postoperative period.

Postoperative care

On return from theatre the patient will require general postoperative care. A nasogastric tube will be in place for aspiration of gastric contents and intravenous therapy will be in progress. A midline incision and surgical drain will impede movement. In addition there will be aspects of care specific to the procedure. The stoma will be sited as agreed and will have a moist red appearance. The colour of the stoma is monitored to ensure it is receiving an adequate blood supply and oxygenation. Two drains will protrude from the stoma. These are fine catheters that have been placed in the junction between the ureter and ileal reservoir to support the anastomosis and ensure urinary drainage. It is important to ensure that urine is draining from both ureters. A collecting bag with a valve to prevent backflow of urine will cover the stoma. The bag should be emptied frequently to reduce the risk of ascending infection. Intravenous therapy can be discontinued and the nasogastric tube removed when bowel sounds have returned and the patient is accepting oral fluids, usually within 24–48 hours. The incisional drain can be removed when drainage reduces, usually 4–5 days after surgery. The ureteric drains are retained until postoperative swelling subsides. They can usually be removed 7–10 days after surgery, although some surgeons may leave them in for two weeks.

An important aspect of nursing care will be preparing the patient for discharge and helping them to come to terms with the stoma. It may be useful to involve a stoma care specialist. The patient is taught how to clean and protect the stoma and surrounding skin. They will need practice in changing the bag and shaping replacement flanges. Patients will react to a stoma in different ways. Some may be eager to take an active part from an early stage, others may be reluctant to look at or touch the stoma. Family members may also require help in adjusting to the stoma and learning about stoma care. It should be emphasized that with good care and correct fitting of appliances the stoma should not be socially embarrassing. The patient needs to take about two litres of fluid a day and to observe the urine for signs of infection (i.e. cloudiness or unpleasant odour).

After radical cystectomy, the patient may wish to discuss sexual function. In men, the bladder, prostate, and seminal vesicles will have been removed, but if a nerve-sparing type of operation has been performed, an erection may be possible. In women, the uterus, ovarian tubes, ovaries, and urethra may have been removed, but sexual function and orgasm are usually preserved. Invasive bladder cancer is a life-threatening condition, and treatment may have a profound effect on body image and sexuality, so it is important that the patient and family are fully aware of the implications of treatment and have ample opportunity to discuss this and ask questions both before and after the operation.

After about 14 days the patient will be ready for discharge. An outpatient follow-up will be arranged for 6–8 weeks later and the patient is advised to contact his own doctor if problems develop. After bladder cancer there is a need for continuous surveillance and, in addition, the urinary diversion will need to be periodically assessed.

Retention of Urine

Retention of urine is a common complaint in surgical urology. Although urinary retention can affect men and women of all ages, it predominantly occurs in elderly men, and this discussion will consider causes of lower urinary tract obstruction in men. The problem may present as acute or chronic retention of urine. *Box 16.8* lists the causes of urinary retention. Acute retention is usually painful with complete obstruction of urine output; chronic retention is often painless and may be accompanied by overflow incontinence. Acute retention presents as a sudden painful distension of the bladder, which is easily confirmed by gentle palpation. The patient is likely to be acutely distressed and may be pale and shocked because of the severe pain. Lawrence (1990) identified eight factors that can precipitate acute retention as follows:

- Surgery.
- Drugs (e.g. diuretics, anticholinesterases, antidepressants, and sympathomimetics).

Box 16.8 **Common causes of urinary retention (adapted from Lawrence, 1990).**

Urethral
- Meatal stenosis
- Stricture
- Phimosis
- Benign prostatic hypertrophy

Bladder
- Clot retention
- Detrusor failure

Neurological
- Neurological disease (e.g. multiple sclerosis)
- Spinal cord trauma
- Surgical trauma
- Diabetic neuropathy

Precipitating factors
- Surgery
- Alcohol
- Drugs
- Cerebrovascular thrombosis or haemorrhage
- Prolonged immobility
- Acute UTI

- Alcohol.
- Cerebral thrombosis or haemorrhage.
- Constipation.
- Haemorrhoids or other painful perianal conditions.
- Prolonged bed rest.
- Acute UTI.

In chronic retention, the bladder gradually distends. The patient complains of little or no pain, but has dribbling incontinence of urine. Chronic retention can develop into a compete obstruction. Palpation will reveal an enlarged bladder, although this will not be as marked as in acute retention. In chronic retention the build-up of urea and other metabolites may contribute to confusion in the elderly patient.

It is important that the nurse provides psychological support and information during the initial stages of treatment and investigation. Severe pain, severe infection, and impaired renal function require urgent intervention – usually immediate catheterization of the urinary bladder. In chronic retention without pain, immediate catheterization may not be required and treatment can be guided by the results of diagnostic investigations. Immediate catheterization is the most appropriate pain control method in acute retention. Traditionally a urethral catheter has been used to achieve rapid decompression of the bladder in the emergency situation. Suprapubic catheters were only used when the urethral route proved problematic. However, modern approaches to suprapubic catheterization allow a Foley balloon catheter to be inserted without the need for skin sutures or additional fixation, and suprapubic catheters are often preferred, particularly if catheterization is required for more than a few days.

Specific investigations for retention of urine include:

- Catheter specimen of urine for culture and sensivity.
- Haemoglobin estimation, blood grouping, and crossmatching.
- Blood test for renal function.
- Serum acid phosphatase levels (raised level can indicate malignancy of prostate and secondary bone deposits).
- IVU or ultrasound.
- KUB, radiographs of the chest, lumbar spine, and pelvis (a bone scan may be carried out if necessary to detect evidence of secondary deposits or other conditions).
- Rectal examination for prostate enlargement.

The nurse should support the patient during the rectal examination to diagnose whether the enlargement of the gland is benign or malignant. A benign enlargement feels smooth, but with a malignant enlargement, an irregular hard mass can be felt. It is important to explain to the patient that this examination may be repeated after catheterization and before operation as the prostate may appear larger than it really is if it is being pushed downwards by an enlarged bladder. If the findings of a digital rectal examination and transrectal ultrasound suggest that a patient has a high likelihood of prostate cancer, a transrectal biopsy under ultrasound guidance can be performed (Andriole and Winfield, 1993). The patient is given antibiotic cover to prevent infection in the blood stream. This procedure may be carried out on a patient as a day case and it should be carefully explained to the patient that over the following few days any flu-like symptoms such as a high temperature or backache, must be reported to the general practitioner immediately. Also the patient must be advised that he may pass blood in his urine, semen, or stools after this procedure for as long as a week, but if this persists, it should be reported.

THE PROSTATE

The prostate (*Figure 16.10*) is one of the accessory glands of the male. It is a fibromuscular gland that secretes a fluid that contributes to the seminal fluid of the ejaculate. The prostate lies at the base of the bladder surrounding the urethra (the prostatic urethra) as it enters the bladder. The prostate is subdivided into five lobes: left and right lateral lobes, left and right posterior lobes, and the median lobe. The median lobe, which surrounds the prostatic urethra, is the most prone to benign prostatic hypertrophy, while the posterior lobes are more prone to malignant transformation. An enlarged prostate can be readily palpated on digital rectal examination. The prostate is supplied by the inferior vesical and internal pudendal arteries, and venous drainage is via well-developed venous plexuses, which empty into the internal iliac veins.

The prostate may be damaged during pelvic trauma, and infections of the prostate causing acute or chronic prostatitis are not uncommon urological infections, but the two main diseases of the prostate are benign prostatic hypertrophy and carcinoma of the prostate.

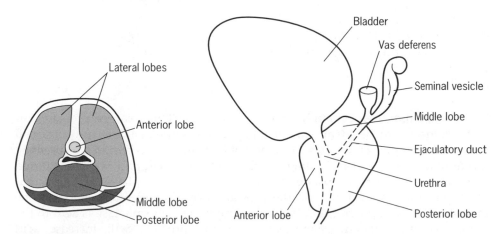

Figure 16.10 The prostate.

Benign Prostatic Hypertrophy

Benign prostatic hypertrophy is the commonest cause of bladder obstruction in men. The prostate gland remains fairly constant in size until middle age, when benign hypertrophy may develop. Hypertrophy is observed in the median and posterior lobes. In benign hypertrophy the smooth muscle mass of the prostate increases from 25% to 40% of the prostate mass (Rosario and Chapple, 1995). The normal ageing process will also contribute to an increase in prostatic connective tissue, but the cause of hypertrophy is poorly understood. Some degree of hypertrophy is common from 45 years of age, but this is usually asymptomatic. By the age of 80 years about 80% of men will suffer from benign prostatic hypertrophy, although only about 10% of cases require surgical intervention. Prostatic enlargement can cause mechanical obstruction of the bladder and problems associated with urinary stasis. In the early stages the patient will complain of reduced force and size of the urinary stream, and as the condition progresses increased frequency, dysuria, and possibly nocturia. A hesitant intermittent stream with terminal dribbling may also occur in the later stages. Terminal dribbling may be due to residual urine in the bladder or in the elongated prostatic urethra. Pressure from the enlarged gland and straining to urinate may cause congestion and rupture of the venous plexus resulting in haematuria. Haematuria can be a frightening symptom for the patient. Urinary stasis will also predispose to infection and increase the risk of urinary calculi. Prostatic enlargement can sometimes compromise sexual function. Back pressure on the ureter may cause a progressive bilateral hydronephrosis with eventual renal failure (Weinerth, 1991). Progressive renal failure and uraemia may result in drowsiness, headache, and intellectual impairment. Ellis and Calne (1993) recommend palpation for bladder enlargement and a check on blood urea when assessing elderly men for sudden behavioural changes.

Special investigations for benign prostatic hypertrophy include:

- Rectal examination.
- Haemoglobin estimation.
- Serum acid phosphatase and urea levels.
- MSU.
- IVU.

Rectal examination in benign hypertrophy will reveal an enlarged prostate, but distinct lobes can be identified. In malignant enlargement, the prostate will present as a single craggy mass. Haemoglobin estimation is required as uraemia can inhibit erythropoeisis, leading to anaemia. Serum acid phosphatase is raised in about 50% of cases of prostate cancer. A raised acid phosphatase suggests that the tumour has spread beyond the prostatic capsule and often denotes bone metastasis. It is important that blood for serum acid phosphatase is sent to the laboratory immediately. Manipulation of the prostate will increase acid phosphatase levels so the sample should not be taken within 48 hours of rectal examination of the prostate. Blood urea is checked to rule out uraemia. The MSU is required to check for urinary infection, although infection is more common in prostatic disease after catheterization or instrumentation of the urinary tract. IVU is used to assess renal function, bladder enlargement, and incomplete emptying of the bladder.

Prostatectomy

Conservative medical management of benign prostatic hypertrophy causing bladder obstruction is seldom effective, although treatment with low-dose oestrogens may produce some reduction in prostatic mass. Surgical treatment is the method of choice. In acute retention an emergency prostatectomy may be required, but usually catheterization and decompression of the bladder is sufficient and the operation can be scheduled as an elective procedure. Four approaches can be used for prostatectomy:

- Suprapubic prostatectomy.
- Perineal prostatectomy.
- Retropubic prostatectomy.
- Endoscopic transurethral prostatectomy.

The first three involve open surgery and are generally only used if the prostate is very large or unless there is some coexisting intravesical pathology such as a large tumour that requires removal at the same time. With improvements in endoscopy the transurethral prostatectomy has become the method of choice (Ellis and Calne, 1993). Milne (1988) describes transurethal resection of the prostate gland (TURP). General or spinal anaesthesia may be used. The patient is placed in the lithotomy position and the bladder is checked with a cystoscope. A resectoscope sheath is inserted into the viewing telescope, and a wire loop attached to a diathermy machine is used to cut away small fragments of prostatic tissue, which are later evacuated from the bladder. A tissue specimen will be sent for histopathology. Cautery is used to control bleeding. The surgeon's view is kept clear of blood by continuous irrigation using an optically appropriate solution, usually isotonic glycine, which does not easily conduct current and is not as readily absorbed into the blood stream as other isotonic fluids. Once the operation has been completed, the resectoscope is removed and a large-bore irrigation catheter is inserted. The catheter allows continuous irrigation of the bladder to prevent the formation of blood clots. Using this approach the mortality associated with TURP is less than 1% and complications are minimal. The patient is usually in hospital for one week or less.

Nursing care

Before prostatectomy the patient will have experienced prostatic symptoms including dysuria, poor stream, frequency or urgency, nocturia, and dribbling incontinence. These symptoms are disconcerting and cause embarrassment and distress to a previously continent patient. It is important that the patient is placed in a bed close to the toilets or bathroom. The nurse should discretely ensure that the patient has sufficient change of pyjamas. The patient may require time to rest and recover from acute or chronic retention of urine before undergoing surgery. Details of investigative procedures and of the operation should be carefully explained and time allowed for questioning. A patient requiring prostatectomy is often in the older age group and may have difficulty with hearing, vision, and mobility.

UTI due to stasis is a major risk, especially if the patient is catheterized. To avoid the potential problem of UTI via the catheter, the patient should be encouraged to drink freely. Recording of fluid intake and output will help monitor fluid status. The patient's urinary meatus must be kept clean and the patient should be advised to ensure his prepuce or foreskin is not retracted to avoid paraphimosis. Informed consent is necessary. The patient must have a clear understanding of the consequences of TURP. Prostatectomy invariably results in retrograde ejaculation (i.e. the ejaculate flows into the bladder rather than into the urethra). It may be necessary to emphasize to the man that although he will not be sterile or impotent it is unlikely that he can father children by normal intercourse. Sensitivity is required, and the nurse should not assume that the elderly patient is sexually inactive or that loss of the ability to father children normally will not be a concern.

TURP is an invasive procedure requiring the usual rigorous preoperative assessment and preparation. As patients are often elderly, spinal anaesthesia may be required but, as Lympany (1993) points out, a full assessment is required so that a general anaesthetic can be given if necessary. A small-scale study of preoperative information-giving and TURP indicated that use of a preoperative information booklet could improve patients' understanding (Brewster, 1992). Postoperatively the patient may experience problems with anxiety, pain, sleep disturbance, immobility, and nutrition. Of particular concern are the risks of haemorrhage, anaemia, infection, and fluid and electrolyte imbalance.

Anxiety

The patient will be concerned about the success of the surgery and his prognosis in recovery. Despite preoperative information about benign hypertrophy, the patient may still have a fear of cancer. Surgery involving the genito-urinary system can be particularly stressful, and the presence of a urinary catheter may cause additional embarrassment. The patient should be reminded about retrograde ejaculation, but reassured that 'dry ejaculation' need not interfere with his or his partner's sexual satisfaction. Sexual intercourse can be resumed about two weeks after the operation provided the patient is comfortable and confident. Visible haematuria due to bleeding from the prostatic bed may further increase anxiety. Feelings of control and a reduction of anxiety can be encouraged by involving the patient in his own care. Morrison et al. (1994) suggest that the patient is encouraged to:

■ Make entries on his own fluid balance chart.
■ Drink at least three litres in 24 hours.

- Record the colour and amount of urine.
- Take responsibility for personal hygiene including regular catheter care.
- Take regular gentle exercise.

Pain

After prostatectomy pain may be experienced from the site of surgery due to the presence of a urinary catheter or because of blockage of the catheter by blood clots. Pain should be monitored and postoperative analgesia used as prescribed. Ensuring patency of the bladder irrigation system will be an effective contribution to pain control.

Haemorrhage and anaemia

Haemorrhage is a serious potential complication of prostatectomy. Initial postoperative care will include careful observation and monitoring of vital signs for indications of shock. Urinary drainage must be monitored: haematuria is to be expected, but any indication of increased blood loss needs to be reported. Oral anticoagulants will have been discontinued as part of the preoperative preparation and patients requiring anticoagulant therapy will be treated with heparin until oral anticoagulants can be resumed. Intraoperative and postoperative blood loss can be substantial and the patient may require postoperative transfusion to avoid anaemia.

Nutrition and fluid balance

The patient may be reluctant to eat due to postoperative nausea, and immobility may reduce appetite in the immediate postoperative period. A normal diet can be quickly resumed, but the patient should be encouraged to eat fruit and vegetables to avoid constipation and straining. Fluid and electrolyte imbalance can be a particular problem after prostatectomy. Glycine used as irrigating fluid during TURP can cause a transient hyponatraemia postoperatively. The patient needs to be observed for any rise in pulse rate, hypotension, hypothermia, signs of pulmonary oedema, or confusion. Intravenous therapy and bladder drainage or irrigation are likely in the postoperative period. Fluid intake and output must be carefully monitored and recorded.

Postoperative infection

The presence of a urinary catheter increases the risk of a postoperative UTI. Asepsis must be maintained when handling any part of the irrigation or drainage system. Patient hygiene, particularly handwashing and meatal care, should be encouraged. The foreskin should cover the glans as sustained retraction can cause paraphimosis. The need to drink and maintain an adequate urinary output must also be emphasized. It will help if the catheter is comfortably positioned and secured. The patient can be encouraged to observe the colour and smell of the urine and report any abnormalities. Because of the risk of UTI prostatectomy is often carried out under antibiotic prophylaxis followed by a course of antibiotics in the postoperative period.

Bladder irrigation and catheter care

After prostatic surgery continuous bladder irrigation may be used to prevent the formation and retention of blood clots. A three-way catheter is used: the irrigation fluid flows into the catheter via the inlet channel and drainage is via a separate outlet channel. The third channel is for inflation of the retention balloon. Irrigation fluid, usually saline, flows in under gravity and flow is controlled by a normal intravenous-style clamp. Usually two three-litre bags of saline are set up using a Y-connector as in *Figure 16.11*. It is important that input and output is closely monitored. The bags are usually numbered and the amount given is recorded on a special fluid balance chart. The volume of drainage is also monitored, and urine volume can be calculated by subtracting the volume of irrigation fluid given from the volume of drainage. The patient's abdomen should be observed: distension could indicate bladder obstruction. Drainage is observed for volume and colour, and any sudden drop in volume may indicate

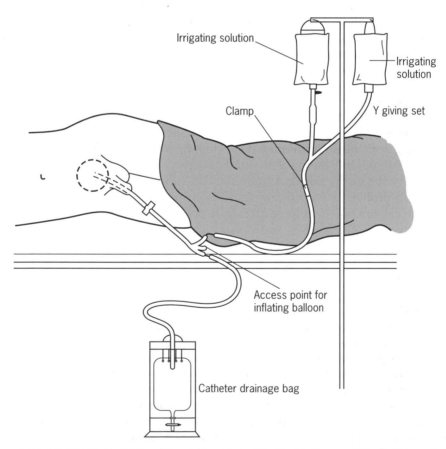

Figure 16.11 Bladder irrigation. (Reproduced from *The Royal Marsden Hospital Manual of Clinical Nursing Procedures* with kind permission of Blackwell Science Ltd.)

obstruction. Clot retention is a common problem, especially in the first 24 hours. Bladder irrigation can usually be discontinued the day after surgery provided the patient can maintain an adequate fluid intake.

The urinary catheter may stay in place another day or two. It is normally removed by the third postoperative day. Adequate urine output is essential and it is also important that the patient has defaecated because constipation and straining can result in further bleeding from the prostatic bed. After removal of the catheter the patient may still experience some urgency and frequency. The nurse can reassure the patient that a normal pattern of micturition will become established over the next few weeks. Pelvic floor exercise should be taught (i.e. where the patient is encouraged to tighten his perineal muscles as if holding back the flow of urine, to maintain the hold for 3–5 seconds while breathing normally, and then to relax). This exercise is repeated up to five times, doing ten sets of five repetitions daily until continence recovers. It can be combined with trying to stop urinating midstream. The nurse must emphasize that the urinal is used once only and then replaced with a clean one to avoid the possibility of infection.

Sleep and mobility
Pain, regular monitoring of vital signs, management of bladder irrigation, and intravenous therapy may contribute to sleep disturbance, particularly during the first postoperative night. Pain, intravenous therapy, and the presence of a urinary catheter and irrigation will also severely limit mobility. Early discontinuation of irrigation will encourage mobilization, although some patients may be embarrassed by the need to carry around the urine drainage bag.

Discharge planning
It is important that the nurse gives the patient discharge advice in writing, leaving time before the actual time of discharge for the patient to take in the information and ask questions. The patient needs to understand that the prostatic bed may take several weeks to heal. He may pass blood in his urine for a few weeks, and urgency and frequency will still be a problem. It is important that a generous fluid intake is maintained and constipation is avoided. Secondary haemorrhage of the prostatic bed sometimes occurs around the fourteenth postoperative day and patients are advised to remain off work for three weeks and during that time not to lift, play golf, or cycle. Driving can be resumed twenty days postoperatively, and sexual activity twenty-eight days postoperatively. The patient should be reassured that he will not need to be seen in the hospital outpatients department after discharge home because he should have no more difficulty passing urine. However, in some cases the prostatic tissue may regenerate, so the operation may have to be repeated in ten years' time. Also the urethra may narrow over the years and cause the urine stream to start flowing slowly again. If the patient thinks that the problem is recurring he should be advised to consult his general practitioner.

Prostate Carcinoma

Adenocarcinoma of the prostate is the fourth most common cause of cancer-associated death in the UK and the second most common cause in the USA (Kirby, 1991). It is rare below the age of 50 years, but affects about 15% of men over the age of 50. It has been suggested that as many as 90% of men over the age of 90 years will have histological evidence of prostate malignancy. Prostate cancer is an incidental finding in about 10% of TURP specimens. The cause of prostate carcinoma is unknown, but genetic, environmental, social, and dietary factors may influence development. Genetic influence is suggested by the findings in the UK and USA that prostatic cancer is twice as common in Afro-Caribbeans as Caucasians, and that the incidence is low in Japanese and Chinese people. Prostatic cancer is positively associated with a high-fat diet and there is a suggestion that phyto-oestrogens found in plants such as soya may be protective. The incidence is also high in married men and those who have had many sexual partners (Kirby, 1991). Environmental influences are suggested by the higher rates associated with some industries.

The growth is usually an infiltrating hard adenocarcinoma situated beneath the prostatic capsule. In over 70% of cases the cancer arises in the posterior lobes and the hard enlarged mass can be palpated on rectal examination. Some authorities have suggested regular screening for men over the age of 55 years: in the early stages the tumour may be identified as a single hard nodule in one lobe. At this stage it is often asymptomatic. However, as screening would involve yearly rectal examination for all men over 55 years of age the costs would be high. Untreated the single nodule will expand, crossing to the other lobe, and eventually the lobular structure is obliterated and the cancer presents as a single large mass. There may be invasion of the bladder, urethra, seminal vesicles, iliac nodes, pelvis and spine, with secondary deposits appearing in the liver and lungs.

The clinical presentation of prostate cancer is generally the same as for benign prostatic hypertrophy. However, weight loss, back and pelvic pain, anaemia, and lymphadenopathy are additional findings that suggest cancer rather than benign prostatic hypertrophy. Initial investigations are also the same as for benign prostatic hypertrophy. As discussed above, serum acid phosphatase will be raised in about 50% of cases of prostate cancer. Additionally blood can be tested for prostate-specific antigen (PSA). Approximately 80% of patients with prostate cancer have elevated values of PSA. However, approximately 20% of patients with benign hypertrophy also have elevated PSA, so the test is not sufficiently accurate to be used as a sole screening method. Screening using digital rectal examination and PSA testing would identify the majority of prostate cancers. PSA levels are lower in the earlier stages of the disease and increase as the condition progresses. PSA estimation therefore provides a useful tool for assessing progress and the effectiveness of treatment. If prostate cancer is suspected transrectal fine-needle biopsy is essential to confirm the diagnosis. Laparoscopic pelvic lymph node dissection has been used for staging the condition, but transrectal prostatic ultrasonography is proving useful for identifying and staging the condition. However, about 20% of prostate cancers are iso-echoic and will therefore be missed by transrectal ultrasonography (McCahy *et al.*, 1995). Additional radiographic investigations to identify possible secondaries will be required.

Treatment of prostatic cancer depends on the stage of the disease and presenting symptoms. Histopathological confirmation of malignancy is essential and staging is required to classify the patient as having prostate-confined or disseminated cancer. In organ-confined prostatic cancer the patient will have a negative bone scan, normal acid phosphatase, PSA levels less than 20 µg ml^{-1}, and no evidence of lymphatic metastases. However, as prostatic cancer is often asymptomatic many patients only present for investigation when the disease has reached a more advanced stage. Kirby (1991) suggests that prostate-confined cancer can be treated by:

■ Conservative or deferred therapy.
■ Radical radiotherapy.
■ Radical prostatectomy and internal iliac lymphadenectomy.

Conservative management (observation only) may be suggested for older (70 years plus) asymptomatic patients with small localized well-differentiated tumours. George (1988) reported that only 10% of 120 patients (mean age 74 years) managed conservatively developed metastases and prolonged survival of many patients, with death being due to conditions other than prostatic cancer. If conservative management is suggested, the patient will need to be advised that there is a 50% chance of death within two years of the appearance of metastases (Kirby, 1991).

Radical radiotherapy of the prostate is usually by external beam irradiation. If the patient is generally fit and well radiotherapy can be delivered on an out-patient basis. It is non-invasive and has the advantage of including the external and internal lymph nodes. There are still debates about the relative value of radiotherapy versus radical prostatectomy for organ-confined prostate cancer, but studies suggest survival rates may be broadly equivalent (Weinerth, 1991). Side effects of prostate radiotherapy include rectal irritation, which can result in diarrhoea and rectal bleeding, bladder irritation and dysuria, and erectile impotence (in 30–40%).

Radical prostatectomy and internal iliac lymphadenectomy is usually performed as open surgery using the retropubic approach. Andriole and Winfield (1993) describe a nerve-sparing prostatectomy, which allows preservation of the cavernosal nerves regulating penile erection. This operation is particularly suitable for men with low PSA levels and small tumours. The patient should be advised that complications of this operation include urinary leakage, but this is usually temporary and can be relieved by the correct use of pelvic floor exercise.

Cure is not an option for disseminated prostatic cancer, but limited remission can be achieved. Endocrine manipulation is the mainstay of therapy. A large percentage of prostatic tumours are androgen-dependent and anti-androgen therapy will produce symptomatic relief in about 75% of patients with disseminated prostatic cancer (Ellis and Calne, 1993). Oestrogen therapy (stilboestrol, fosfestrol tetrasodium, polyestradiol phosphate) will provide symptom relief, but side effects include gynaecomastia, testicular atrophy, and fluid retention. In patients with cardiovascular disease whose condition would be worsened by additional fluid retention, bilateral subcapsular orchidectomy may be necessary. However, orchidectomy has major psychological disadvantages and chemical alternatives may be considered. These include luteinizing hormone releasing hormone (LHRH) or androgen antagonists (e.g. buserelin, goserelin, leuprorelin, and cyproterone acetate).

In the more advanced cases of prostatic carcinoma, radiotherapy may be necessary to relieve the pain of bony deposits. Chemotherapy appears to be ineffective in disseminated prostatic cancer. TURP may be considered if the patient has urinary obstruction.

The available treatments for disseminated prostatic cancer are essentially palliative: 50% of patients will be dead within two years of the appearance of metastases. The patient will be treated mainly at home with hospital admissions for assessment and symptom control. Quality of life can be maintained, but in the final stages of the disease the nurse's role will be to help the family and patient deal with the impending death with dignity.

URETHRA

Urethral Strictures

A urethral stricture is an abnormal narrowing of the urethral lumen. Strictures are generally caused by trauma, inflammation, or malignancy, or are sometimes a side effect of radiotherapy. Once strictures occur they can present the patients with problems for the rest of their lives. Urethral stricture seldom occurs in females of any age (the adult female urethra is only approximately 3.75 cm long) and is rare in children, but common in adult males. This discussion will be limited to the anatomy and management of urethral stricture in men. The male urethra is divided into prostatic, membranous, bulbar, and penile segments (*Figure 16.12*). The membranous urethra is the shortest, narrowest segment (1–2 cm long) and has relatively thin walls. The membranous urethra is more prone to trauma from catheterization and instrumentation than the other segments. Mundy (1992) emphasizes that while any part of the urethra may be affected, the aetiology varies depending upon the area involved:

- Bladder neck strictures usually occur because of scarring following TURP or catheterization.
- Membranous urethral strictures are due to catheterization, TURP, or pelvic trauma.

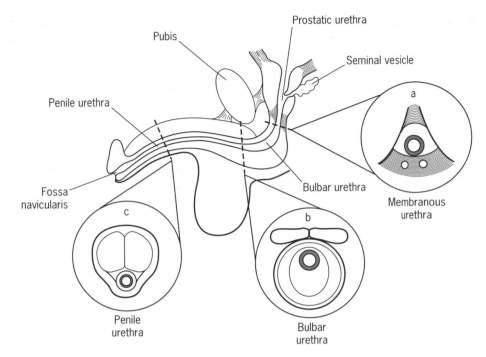

Figure 16.12 The male urethra. (Reproduced from Woo H, Chapple CR (1995) Urethral strictures. *Surgery* **13(2)**:38 by kind permission of The Medicine Group (Journals) Ltd.)

- Bulbar urethral strictures are caused by catheterization or instrumentation or infection (e.g. nonspecific urethritis, gonorrhoea).
- Penile urethral strictures are caused by instrumentation or ischaemia and are more common in the elderly.

Symptoms of stricture include poor flow, frequency, dysuria, and haematuria. These symptoms do not usually become evident until the narrowing is sufficient to markedly reduce flow. Chronic retention of urine may also occur, with incomplete emptying of the bladder and dribbling incontinence. Investigation includes a careful physical examination, urine culture, contrast urethrography, flow rate assessment, and urethroscopy. Woo and Chapple (1995) identify the main surgical approaches to treatment as:

- Regeneration procedures.
- Excision and re-anastomosis.
- Substitution.

Urethral dilatation and urethrotomy are regeneration procedures; they remove the urethral stenosis and allow the urethral epithelium to regenerate, hopefully without adhesion. They are relatively simple procedures and are the most widely used form of surgical treatment. In urethral dilatation the urethra is stretched by a series of bougies. The procedure can be carried out in the outpatient department, but will tend to control rather than cure the problem. Urethrotomy is usually performed endoscopically. The surgeon divides the stricture under direct vision. Intermittent self-dilatation using a self-lubricating catheter can reduce the need for repeated urethral dilatation or urethrotomy (Woo and Chapple, 1995).

Recurrence after regeneration procedures is about 50%, and if repeated treatment fails, excision and re-anastomosis or substitution procedures or both may be required. In patients unable to cope with repeated self-dilatation or unsuitable for more extensive surgery a urethral stent can be inserted. Surgical removal of the stricture is called urethroplasty. Small strictures can be excised with primary re-anastomosis. Longer strictures may require more extensive two-stage procedures.

Nursing Management

Preparation for urethral procedures or surgery is similar to that for any invasive procedure. One area of particular importance is preparing the patient for dealing with intermittent self-catheterization. Morrison *et al.* (1994) suggest that the primary nurse may find the following points helpful when helping the patient adjust to this procedure:

- No-one needs to know the patient is using the procedure.
- The treatment although not appealing will reduce the risk of future readmission.
- Infection risk can be reduced by careful meatal and hand hygiene and maintaining adequate fluid intake.
- Initially dilatation will be daily, but it can later be reduced to once weekly.
- Dilatation does not need any major adjustment of lifestyle.

The patient may also seek reassurance that the procedure will not have any adverse effects on sexual function.

THE TESTIS

The male reproductive organs are shown in *Figure 16.13*. The male urethra and prostate have been discussed above. In this section the surgical problems affecting the scrotum, testes, and penis are considered. The scrotum contains the testes, the epididymides, and the lower part of the spermatic cords. It is a thin-walled pouch of pigmented skin with a thin sheet of involuntary muscle known as the dartos muscle dividing it into two cavities. Each compartment contains a testis, epididymis, and the testicular portion of the spermatic cord. The scrotum is continuous with the abdominal wall, and the testis descends into the scrotum during development.

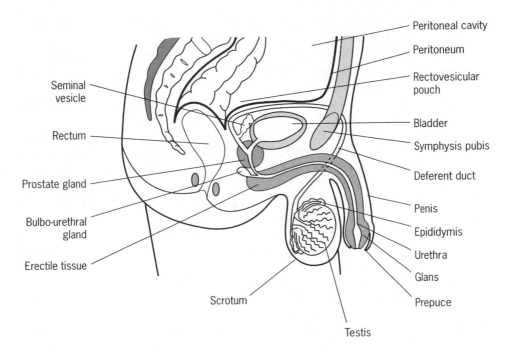

Figure 16.13 The male reproductive organs.

Each testis (*Figure 16.14*) has three coverings known as tunicae. The tunica vaginalis is the outer covering and is formed from a portion of peritoneum, which descends into the scrotum. Like the peritoneum it is a folded serous membrane with a parietal and visceral layer. Hydrocele is a condition that arises in the tunica vaginalis. The tunica albuginea lies under the visceral layer of the vaginalis and ingrowths of this form septa, which divide the glandular structure

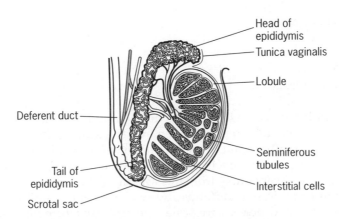

Figure 16.14 The testis.

of the testes into lobules. The tunica vasculosa is a network of capillaries that lines the tunica albuginea.

The lobules of the testes are composed of germinal epithelial cells, which form the convoluted seminiferous tubules. These become the epididymis, which continues as the ductus deferens enclosed within the spermatic cord. The seminiferous tubules produce the spermatozoa, which are conveyed through the epididymides to the deferens duct. The addition of fluid from the seminal vesicles results in the formation of semen. Cells that lie between the tubules secrete the hormone testosterone, which influences the development and function of the male reproductive organs. The testicular artery provides the main blood supply to the testes, but there is also an extensive collateral supply. Venous return is via the testicular veins. Each testicular vein is formed from the 8–10 veins of the pampiniform plexus found at the inferior end of the spermatic cord. Varicocoele is a condition affecting the pampiniform plexus.

The penis is composed of three columns of vascular erectile tissue. The central column, the corpus spongiosum, contains the penile urethra and on either side are the corpora cavernosa. The erectile tissue is surrounded by a dense connective tissue that helps produce erection when the penis is engorged with blood. Externally the main features are the urinary meatus, glans penis, frenulum, and prepuce. In this section the surgical treatment of scrotal and testicular swellings and penile conditions requiring circumcision are considered.

Swellings of the Scrotum and Testis

Scrotal swelling is probably the main feature of problems of the scrotum or testis presenting for surgical investigation. Scrotal swellings can be of scrotal or abdominal origin. If on examination the fingers can meet above the swelling the problem is probably of scrotal origin. If the fingers cannot identify the top edge then it is likely to be a herniation of abdominal origin (an inguinoscrotal hernia). Scrotal swellings fall into five main categories:

- Epididymal cysts.
- Infection.
- Hydrocele.
- Varicocele.
- Testicular neoplasia.

Cysts of the epididymis usually develop during adult life and if large and producing symptoms may require surgical removal (Ellis and Calne, 1993). Cysts are often bilateral and multiple and transillumination of the scrotum demonstrates a translucent swelling similar to a hydrocele. However, with epididymal cysts the testis can be palpated separately from the swelling. Acute and chronic infections of the testis can result in scrotal lumps and swelling, for example orchitis due to mumps. However, hydrocele, varicocele, and testicular tumours are the main causes of scrotal swelling presenting for surgical treatment.

Hydrocele

Hydrocele is an excessive collection of fluid in the tunica vaginalis, the membranous sac surrounding the testis. In primary or idiopathic hydrocoele the scrotum will be large and tense, but there is no underlying disease of the testis. In secondary hydrocoele the volume of exudate is smaller and not under tension, but the condition is associated with inflammation or neoplasia of the testis or epididymis (Ellis and Calne, 1993). Infantile hydrocoele is a common form of hydrocele, but only adult forms of the condition will be considered here. Hydrocele is usually unilateral and although there may be extensive scrotal swelling pain is not a common feature. However, the size and weight of the swollen scrotum may cause discomfort, anxiety, and acute embarrassment.

The hydrocele should be transilluminated to locate the position of the testis and the fluid removed by means of a trocar and cannula under local anaesthetic. Once the fluid has been removed, the testis is palpated to exclude malignancy or infection. Blood-stained fluid may be an indication of the presence of malignancy in which case, further investigations including ultrasonography may be indicated. A primary hydrocele may require intermittent tapping, in which case the patient may prefer to have the hydrocele sac excised surgically. This operation can cause the patient considerable discomfort. An ice pack applied carefully to the scrotum will reduce some of the oedema and bruising and afford some relief. The patient should be advised to wear a scrotal support while the discomfort persists.

Varicocele

The veins of the pampiniform plexus of the spermatic cord can become varicose leading to the condition of varicocele. This most often affects the left side. The cause is unknown and in most cases is not associated with any other pathology. Occasionally varicocele may develop due to blockage of the testicular vein by a tumour. Varicoceles are often asymptomatic although the patient may sometimes complain of dragging or an aching feeling in the scrotum. The condition does not usually require treatment, but discomfort or subfertility may be an indication for division and ligation of the varicosities.

Testicular Cancer

Although it represents only 1–2% of all cancers in men, testicular cancer is the most common cause of cancer in men aged 20–40 years. In 3–5% of cases the testicular tumours are bilateral. However, with medical progress over the last 20 years the condition is treatable and has a cure rate of more than 90%. Indeed the high cure rate even for advanced cancer of the testis has led some authorities to suggest that screening for testicular cancer is not indicated. However, others believe that regular physical examination and testicular self-examination could significantly reduce the number of deaths from cancer of the testis. Testicular tumours can be classed by cells of origin into germinal cell and non-germinal cell tumours:

■ Non-germinal cell tumours (i.e. interstitial cell tumours, Leydig cell tumours, or androblastomas) are relatively rare, accounting for less than 3% of testicular tumours.
■ Germinal cell tumours account for 97% of testicular tumours. The two main types are seminoma and teratoma, but embryonal carcinoma and chorio-carcinoma also occur.

Embryonal carcinoma is occasionally seen in younger men, but is the main testicular tumour in children. Choriocarcinoma is a rare, but very invasive form of teratoma with a poorer prognosis. Seminomas account for over 50% of testicular tumours and arise from the cells of the seminiferous tubules. Seminoma usually occurs in men of 30–40 years of age and is characterized by slow growth and late invasion (Weinerth, 1991). Spread is via the testicular lymphatics. Seminomas are solid tumours and may be characterized by cells varying from well-differentiated spermatocytes to poorly-differentiated round cells. They may be described as typical, anaplastic, or spermocytic seminoma. Teratomas are thought to arise from more primitive germinal cells and tend to present as more cystic tumours. Teratomas are associated with a younger age group (i.e. 20–30-year-olds) and more rapid blood-borne spread to the lungs and liver. Although testicular tumours spread locally, spread through the capsule is rare.

Testicular tumours usually present as a painless lump in the testis. If the lesion has metastasized, there may be back and abdominal pain, weight loss, and general weakness. Unfortunately tumours may go unnoticed by the patient until a dull aching type of pain develops. Suspicion of testicular tumour requires early surgical exploration and high inguinal orchidectomy if the diagnosis is confirmed. Other specific investigations may include:

■ Abdominal and scrotal ultrasound.
■ Abdominal and chest radiography and CT for secondary deposits.
■ Blood tests for tumour markers (i.e. alphafetoprotein (αFP) and beta-human chorionic gonadotrophin (β-HCG)).

Treatment

Orchidectomy with adjuvant radiotherapy or chemotherapy is the treatment of choice. If there is no lymph node involvement five-year survival rates of 100% have been reported. Radiotherapy is seldom used for non-seminoma testicular cancer, but seminomas are radiosensitive. After orchidectomy for seminoma low-dose radiotherapy is used to treat the lymph nodes. The remaining testis will be affected by scattering of the beam and there will be some transient reduction in sperm count, but fertility should not be permanently affected. Adjuvant combination chemotherapy is used after surgery for metastatic non-seminoma and to treat advanced metastatic seminoma (Horwich and Hendry, 1993).

Preoperative and postoperative care for the patient undergoing orchidectomy is similar to that for any major surgery. Pain relief, preventing wound infection, and reassurance and information are key aspects of nursing care after orchidectomy. It is important to emphasize that it is now a very treatable condition with a good prognosis. The nurse must be able to discuss issues concerning sexuality with the patient if he wishes. Men will worry about the effects of surgery, radiotherapy, and chemotherapy on sperm function. They may fear infertility or worry about whether the effects on spermatogenesis will increase the risk of genetic malformation. The patient may have had the opportunity to bank sperm before starting treatment and will need to be reassured about the true effects of his treatment. The effects will depend on the severity of the disease and the dose of radiotherapy or type of chemotherapy required. Obviously the patient requiring bilateral orchidectomy will be infertile and may need significant support and counselling. If the patient is concerned about the deformity or shape of the scrotum when a testis has been removed, a prosthetic testis can be inserted. It is important that the nurse emphasizes the importance of close follow-up after this condition. Although testicular cancer is very treatable one-third of patients will relapse within 18 months of orchidectomy. Relapse is usually successfully treated by further chemotherapy.

THE PENIS

The anatomy of the penis is shown in *Figure 16.15*. In the adult the main problems of the penis presenting for surgical treatment are phimosis and paraphimosis. Cancer of the penis is a rare condition in the UK, but a common problem in Africa

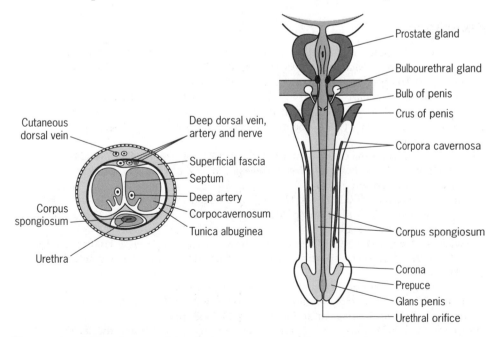

Figure 16.15 The anatomy of the penis.

and Asia. Problems with erection and impotence are beyond the scope of this chapter. In phimosis there is a marked narrowing of the foreskin or prepuce, which becomes too contracted to allow retraction over the glans penis. It can develop due to chronic balanitis (i.e. inflammation of the foreskin and glans) or after trauma due to forcible retraction of the foreskin. Paraphimosis is a condition in which the foreskin is retracted over the glans and cannot be drawn back into position. It interferes with venous return resulting in swelling and pain. Anti-biotics can be used to treat any infection and the partner of a sexually active patient may also require treatment. Circumcision, the surgical removal of the prepuce, is the treatment of choice, although occasionally a dorsal slit may provide relief from these conditions.

Circumcision can be performed as day surgery. Postoperative care is directed towards patient education and the promotion of wound healing. The importance of good personal hygiene, daily washing of the area with soap and water must be emphasized. In the immediate postoperative period the patient can be instructed to protect the wound from chafing by covering it with a non-adhesive dressing. There will be some postoperative oedema, which might cause a degree of dysuria. Erection may prove painful and a local anaesthetic gel can be used to provide relief. Sexual intercourse should be avoided until the wound has healed. If urine leaks onto the wound there is a risk of infection and delayed healing. This can be managed by increasing the frequency of washing and dressing changes, but sometimes short-term catheterization is needed to control the problem.

References

Andriole GL, Winfield HN (1993) New Options in Urology. *Patient Care* **27(2)**:12–27.

Booth JA (ed.) (1983) *Handbook of Investigations*, pp. 129–131. Harper & Row, London.

Brewster J (1992) Operations explained. *Nurs Times* **88(39)**:50–52.

British National Formulary (1996) No. 32, p. 503. British Medical Association & Royal Pharmaceutical Society for Great Britain, London.

Dawson C, Whitfield HN (1994) The management of urinary stone disease part 1. *Surgery* **12(4)**: 73–76.

Elem B (1991) Carcinoma of the urinary bladder in Africa. *Surgery* **96**:2284–2287.

Ellis H, Calne R (1993) *Lecture Notes on General Surgery*, 8th edition. Blackwell Scientific Publications, London.

Farrar DJ, Chinegwundoh FI (1994) Urinary tract infections. *Surgery* **12(5)**:104–110.

George NJR (1988) Natural history of localized prostatic cancer managed by conservative therapy. *Lancet* **i**:494–497.

Horwich A, Hendry WF (1993) Treatment of testicular cancer. *Surgery* **11(10)**:505–510.

Keen CE (1993) Pathogenesis and pathology of gallstones and urinary calculi. *Surgery* **11(2)**:334–336.

Kirby RS (1991) Cancer of the prostate. *Surgery* **96**:2302–2307.

Latham E, Marden W (1986) Percutaneous lithotripsy. *Nurs Times* **92(25)**:65–66.

Lawrence WT (1990) Urinary retention. *Surgery* **77**:1838–1843.

Lympany A (1993) Care of a patient undergoing spinal anaesthesia. *Br J Nurs* **2(19)**:962–972.

MacDonagh RP, Swami SK (1995) Neurological bladder dysfunction. *Surgery* **13(8)**:169–174.

McCahy PJ, Murthy LNS, Neal DE (1995) The role of radiology in urology. *Surgery* **13(3)**:49–57.

Milne C (1988) Improving micturition. *Nurs Stand* **3(6)**:22–23.

Moore S, Newton M, Grant EG, Keetch DW (1993) Treating bladder cancer. *Am J Nurs* **93(5)**:32–39.

Morrison M, Shandrau T, Smithers F (1994) The urinary system. In *Nursing Practice: Hospital and Home The Adult*. Alexander MF, Fawcett JN, Runciman PJ (eds). pp. 291–323. Churchill Livingstone, Edinburgh.

Mundy AR (1992) Urethral strictures. *Surgery* **10(2)**:35–40.

Pagana KD, Pagana TJ (1990) *Diagnostic Testing and Nursing Implications*, pp. 230–232. Mosby, St Louis.

Pansky B, House EL (1964) *Review of Gross Anatomy. A Dynamic Approach*, p. 308. Macmillan, New York.

Paulson DF (1991) The urinary system. In *Textbook of Surgery*, 14th edn. Sabiston DC (ed.). pp. 1433–1456. WB Saunders, Philadephia.

Rosario DJ, Chapple CR (1995) Lower urinary tract obstruction. *Surgery* **13(3)**:57–63.

Sweny P, Varghese Z (1988) *Renal Disease Clinical Tests*, pp. 146–149. Wolfe Medical Publications, London.

Weinerth JL (1991) The male genital system. In *Textbook of Surgery*, 14th edn. Sabiston DC (ed.). pp. 1457–1478. WB Saunders, Philadephia.

Whitfield HN (1989) Urinary calculi. *Surgery* **72**:1713–1719.

Woo H, Chapple C (1995) Urethral strictures. *Surgery* **13(2)**:37–43.

Woodhouse CRJ (1992a) Superficial transitional cell carcinoma of the bladder. *Surgery* **10(6)**:133–138.

Woodhouse CRJ (1992b) Carcinoma *in situ* and invasive bladder cancer. *Surgery* **10(6)**:139–143.

Chapter 17

Hernias, Amputations and Other Conditions in General Surgery

CONTENTS

- ❏ Hernias
- ❏ The Skin and its Appendages
- ❏ Lower Extremity Peripheral Vascular Disease
- ❏ Varicose Veins
- ❏ Chest Drains

This chapter covers some conditions and problems commonly encountered in general surgery. Hernias are one of the most commonly presenting surgical conditions and are considered in some detail. Minor skin problems such as cysts are also very common and usually dealt with by the general surgeon. Two conditions affecting the vascular system, amputation due to peripheral vascular disease and varicose veins, are also considered. However, more specialized or complex topics such as cardiac surgery and revascularization procedures are not covered and the reader is directed to specialist texts. Finally the topic of chest drains is introduced as these may be encountered on the general surgical ward and their safe and effective management is an important nursing topic.

HERNIAS

A hernia is an abnormal protrusion of a visceral organ or tissue through a defect in its coverings, usually a weakness in surrounding muscular wall. The abdominal wall and diaphragm are the principal sites for hernias. Hernias may be treated conservatively or by elective surgical reduction. They can be large and unsightly and cause the patients psychological as well as physical distress. Untreated abdominal hernias cause intestinal obstruction or strangulation if the blood supply to the herniated loop of bowel is impaired.

Strangulated hernia often results in perforation or gangrene. The main types of hernia in adults are:

- Diaphragmatic: traumatic, acquired hiatal.
- Abdominal wall: indirect or direct inguinal, femoral, umbilical, epigastric, ventral, incisional.

Hernias occur for a variety of reasons. Congenital defects in the muscular wall are common, as in indirect inguinal hernia. Ageing can result in a loss of tissue strength and elasticity predisposing to hernia formation, as in direct inguinal hernia. Trauma can be a cause, as in incisional hernia, and this risk is increased by wound infection. Increased abdominal pressure can contribute to the actual occurrence of a hernia when a weakness of the abdominal wall is present. Causes of increased intra-abdominal pressure associated with herniation include:

- Obesity.
- Heavy lifting.
- Abdominal distension (e.g. ascites or intra-abdominal tumour).
- Pregnancy.
- Constipation.
- Respiratory effort (coughing, asthma, chronic obstructive airways disease).

Hernias affect both men and women. Groin hernias are the most common, accounting for 75–80% of all hernias. Incisional hernias account for approximately 8–10% and umbilical hernias for 3–8%. Less common types of hernia include peristomal, perineal, lumbar, obturator, spigelian, gluteal, and sciatic hernias.

A hernia (*Figure 17.1*) may be described as complete if the hernia sac and contents pass through the defect in the abdominal wall, or incomplete if the

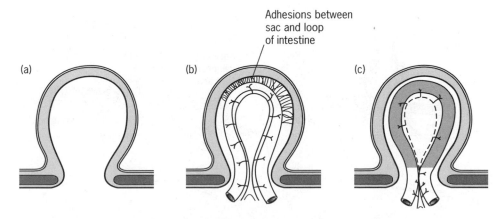

Figure 17.1 Hernias. (a) Reducible. (b) Irreducible. (c) Strangulated.

defect is present, but the hernia sac and contents do not protrude all the way through the defect. A hernia is described as reducible if the contents can be pushed back into the abdomen and irreducible if this is not possible. An irreducible hernia is described as incarcerated when the gut cannot be returned as a result of inflammation or adhesions, but its blood supply is not obstructed. If the loop of bowel is twisted or kinked the hernia is obstructed and in a strangulated hernia disruption of the blood supply has resulted in ischaemia of the herniated tissue. Richter's hernia occurs when one side of the bowel wall rather than a whole loop is caught in the hernia.

Hiatus Hernia and Reflux Oesophagitis

Traumatic diaphragmatic hernias are relatively rare, but may occur after penetrating or crush injuries to the chest. Acquired hiatus hernias will be the main type of diaphragmatic hernia encountered in general surgery. The oesophagus and stomach meet at the gastro-oesophageal junction. Normally the oesophagus passes through the diaphragm (at the oesophageal hiatus) and the last 2–4 cm of the oesophagus lies within the abdominal cavity. Although there is no anatomical sphincter the muscle of the oesophageal hiatus normally encircles the oesophagus tightly. In hiatus hernia the opening becomes enlarged and as a result, the upper part of the stomach moves up into the thorax. *Figure 17.2* illustrates the two main types of hiatus hernia:

■ Type I (axial or sliding) hiatus hernia is the commonest, accounting for about 90% of acquired hiatus hernias.
■ Type II (rolling or paraoesophageal hiatus hernia) accounts for about 10%.

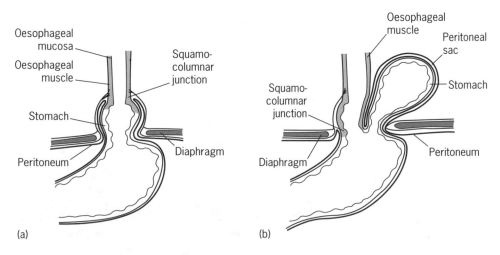

Figure 17.2 Hiatus hernia. (a) Type I. (b) Type II.

Hiatus hernias are thought to result from a progressive weakening of the muscles of the oesophageal hiatus. They tend to develop from middle age onwards and are four times more common in women than men. Obesity is often a contributing factor.

Hiatus hernia is often asymptomatic, but may present with symptoms related to reflux, oesophagitis, and mechanical effects of the hernia. Herniation into the thorax may result in dyspnoea, cough, hiccups, and palpitations. These effects may be seen with both type I and type II hiatus hernias. Type I hiatus hernia may present with heartburn and regurgitation due to reflux of stomach contents into the distal oesophagus. The burning pain may be aggravated when the patient lies down. Reflux can produce oesophagitis with dysphagia, acute or occult haemorrhage, and the risk of oesophageal strictures developing. Type II hiatus hernia is not usually associated with reflux and oesophagitis, but the patient may experience a sense of fullness after eating. Type II hernias may get progressively larger and there is a risk of haemorrhage, obstruction, and strangulation. They are more likely to need surgical treatment than type I hiatus hernias.

Gastro-oesophageal reflux
Reflux of stomach acids into the distal oesophagus can produce oesophagitis. Reflux occurs because the cardiac sphincter becomes incompetent. The symptoms of reflux include heartburn, substernal pain, and dysphagia. Four factors may contribute to dysphagia in acid reflux:

■ Direct chemical injury with oedema and inflammation.
■ Secondary muscle spasm due to chemical irritation.
■ Fibrosis and stricture formation.
■ Mechanical effects of a large hiatus hernia on oesophageal peristalsis.

Oesophageal bleeding may cause a chronic anaemia. Blood loss is usually slow and stools will test positive for occult blood, but occasionally frank blood loss is evident. Heartburn and substernal pain are common, but some patients may present with pain that radiates to the neck, shoulders, and arms, which may be mistaken for angina pectoris. Reflux oesophagitis may also result from repeated vomiting, long-term nasogastric intubation, some types of gastric surgery, and a histological abnormality (Barrett's oesophagus) where the oesophagus contains ectopic acid-secreting gastric-like mucosa (Ellis and Calne, 1993a).

Investigations
A barium swallow is usually carried out to make a diagnosis of hiatus hernia, to identify reflux, and to detect any associated strictures. The patient will be examined in a head-down position to demonstrate any herniation of the stomach into the thoracic cavity. If the barium swallow is inconclusive then a gastro-oesophageal reflux scan may be required. Barium swallow is usually contraindicated in patients with intestinal obstruction. Endoscopic examination of the

oesophagus (oesophagoscopy) can be used to identify oesophagitis or stricture and a biopsy may be required to exclude carcinoma.

Treatment
The medical treatment of hiatus hernia depends on the degree of oesophagitis and the type of hernia. Type II hernias may become very large and there is the risk of strangulation so surgical intervention is the treatment of choice. A conservative approach is common for type I hiatus hernia. The patient is advised to lose weight, to take small frequent meals, to avoid bending, and to sleep propped up in bed. Drug therapy may include antacids and H_2-receptor blockers (ranitidine or cimetidine) to reduce acid secretion. Surgical treatment may be indicated in severe cases if a stricture has developed or if conservative treatment fails. An abdominal or thoracic approach can be used to reduce the hernia. Hernia repair is usually supplemented by anti-reflux surgery designed to improve sphincter tone. Anti-reflux procedures involve returning the distal oesophagus to its intra-abdominal position and plicating or wrapping it with the stomach. Three procedures, which vary in technical approach, are commonly used:

- Belsey Mark IV operation.
- Nissen fundoplication.
- Hill repair.

These procedures appear to produce similar results (Skinner, 1991). Side effects include an inability to belch or vomit, which can result in gaseous distension, dysphagia if the stomach is wrapped too tightly around the oesophagus, and trauma to the stomach or oesophagus from poorly placed sutures.

Nursing management
Nursing care is initially targeted at symptom control and helping the patient understand the condition and necessary changes in lifestyle. Reflux can be painful and distressing. The pain may mimic angina and until a differential diagnosis is confirmed the patient may be very anxious. If the condition is chronic, anaemia and dysphagia may occur. Raising the foot of the bed or sleeping propped up may provide sufficient relief. Nutritional advice is important: small, more frequent meals may help, and weight loss is a priority for the obese patient. If surgery is required general pre- and postoperative care is similar to that required for any gastrointestinal (GI) surgery. Specific points of postoperative care include:

- Observation of respirations (the surgery includes manipulation of thoracic structures).
- Care of an underwater seal chest drain (if a thoracic approach was used).
- Careful monitoring and recording of nasogastric aspirate.

Fluid balance will be monitored and as bowel sounds return oral fluids may be slowly reintroduced. Initially the patient may only tolerate a soft diet, but should be managing a normal diet before discharge. The patient will be advised about diet, weight loss, to avoid smoking, and to avoid heavy lifting.

Abdominal Hernias

The common sites for abdominal wall hernias are shown in *Figure 17.3*. The anatomical basis is similar for all of them (i.e. a weakness in the muscle wall allows the protrusion of peritoneum with or without visceral organs through the defect). Inguinal and femoral hernias are the most common and will be considered in more detail below. Hernias are usually treated by surgical reduction, and depending on the type of hernia and condition of the patient may be suitable for day surgery.

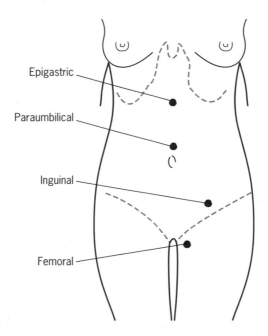

Figure 17.3 Common sites for abdominal hernias.

Umbilical hernia

In adults umbilical hernias are much more common in women than men, probably due to the effects of pregnancy. Umbilical hernia often presents as a painful lump, but may be undected in very obese patients. The hernia occurs due to weakening of the umbilical scar and is associated with ageing, obesity, chronic cough, ascites, pregnancy, large ovarian cysts, ambulatory peritoneal dialysis, or other factors which increase intra-abdominal pressure (Duncan and Rogers, 1991). Surgical repair is recommended and treatment is relatively straight-forward if the patient presents at an early stage. However, many elderly patients present at a late stage and complications and morbidity are more common in this group. The hernia tends to have a narrow neck, and strangulation and obstruction are frequent complications. Surgery is carried out under general anaesthesia with muscle relaxation. Most umbilical hernias contain omentum, but some may contain small intestine or transverse colon. Adhesions are common. The hernia is reduced with division of any adhesions and resection of ischaemic omentum. The defect is closed using a simple transverse repair of the fascial defect.

Epigastric and incisional hernias

Epigastric hernias occur more commonly in men than women (ratio 3 : 1) and consist of one or more small protrusions through defects in the linea alba above the umbilicus. About one in five epigastric hernias prove to be multiple at the time of repair. They can be closed by a simple repair, but recurrence is quite common (i.e. approximately 10%). Ellis and Calne (1993b) note that although epigastric hernias usually only contain extraperitoneal fat, they can be surprisingly painful.

Incisional hernias are the most common type of ventral hernia. Predisposing factors include wound infection, haematoma, obesity, poor surgical technique, malnutrition, advanced age, jaundice, uraemia, coughing, or abdominal distension. In the acute situation the wound may burst open with exposure of the abdominal contents. As the neck of the hernia is wide, strangulation is a rare complication. If the patient is obese, support and advice about following a diet should be provided. A corset dressing may be worn postoperatively to support the repair.

Inguinal and femoral hernias

Groin hernias are the commonest type of hernia presenting in general surgery. It has been estimated that 3% of the adult male population will require surgery for an inguinal hernia, and strangulated groin hernias are an important cause of preventable mortality (Devlin, 1993). Burkitt *et al.* (1990) observed that repair of inguinal hernia accounted for 12% of UK operating time. According to Devlin (1993) inguinal hernia occurs more commonly in men than women (ratio 12 : 1), but femoral hernias are more common in women than men (ratio 4 : 1). However, inguinal and femoral hernias occur with equal frequency in women. Direct inguinal and femoral hernias are considered to be acquired conditions while indirect inguinal hernia is a congenital condition. To understand inguinal and femoral hernias it is necessary to have a clear idea of the anatomy of the groin region.

The abdominal wall in the groin and other regions is made up of layers of tissues from the deepest layer, the peritoneum to the most superficial, the skin (*Box 17.1*). The position of the inguinal canal is shown in *Figure 17.4*. The inguinal canal is about 4 cm long and extends through the abdominal wall from the internal or deep inguinal ring to the external or superficial internal inguinal ring. The inguinal canal (*Figure 17.5*) contains the spermatic cord or round ligament of the uterus. The spermatic cord includes nerves, blood vessels, vas deferens, and

> **Box 17.1** **The layers of the abdominal wall (abbreviated from Nyhus et al., 1991).**
>
> - Skin
> - Fat
> - Fascia (Scarpa's)
> - Aponeurosis and muscle (external oblique)
> - Inguinal canal, muscle (internal oblique), spermatic cord
> - Aponeurosis and muscle (transversus abdominis)
> - Fascia (transversalis)
> - Preperitoneal fat
> - Peritoneum

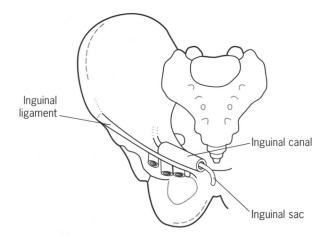

Figure 17.4 The position of the inguinal canal.

the processus vaginalis. The inguinal ligament forms the floor (inferior wall) of the canal and the falx inguinalis forms the roof or superior wall. The falx inguinalis is the free edge of the aponeurosis (tendon sheet attaching muscle to bone) of the transversus abdominis muscle. The anterior wall is formed by the external oblique aponeurosis and fibres of the internal oblique muscle. The posterior wall of the inguinal canal is formed by the transversalis fascia and the interfoveolar ligament.

Indirect inguinal hernias pass through the internal inguinal ring into the canal and exit the abdomen via the external ring. If large enough the hernia will descend into the scrotum. There is a high risk of strangulation because the hernia is passing through the muscular inguinal canal.

A true congenital indirect inguinal usually presents during the first year of life. *In utero*, the processus vaginalis descends through the inguinal canal into the

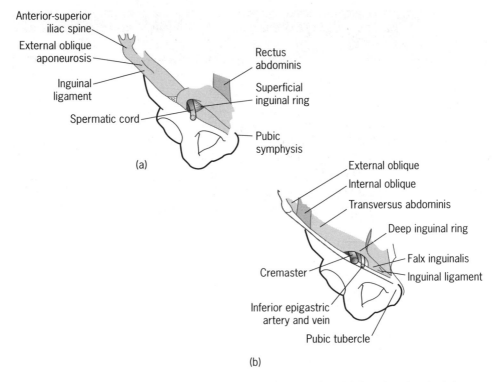

Anterior-superior
iliac spine

External oblique
aponeurosis

Inguinal
ligament

Spermatic cord

Rectus
abdominis

Superficial
inguinal ring

Pubic
symphysis

(a)

External oblique

Internal oblique

Transversus abdominis

Deep inguinal ring

Falx inguinalis

Inguinal ligament

Cremaster

Inferior epigastric
artery and vein

Pubic tubercle

(b)

Figure 17.5 The inguinal canal. (a) The superficial inguinal ring. (b) The deep inguinal ring.

scrotum with the descending testes. The processus vaginalis may persist forming an extension of the parietal peritoneum (i.e. a hernial sac).

In adults inguinal hernias are considered to be acquired as they usually present from middle-age onwards. Direct inguinal hernias do not enter the inguinal canal and seldom enter the scrotum, so the risk of strangulation is much lower than that of an indirect inguinal hernia. They are a direct herniation through the inguinal triangle and exit the abdominal wall through the external inguinal ring. The inguinal triangle is made up of the lateral edge of the rectus sheath medially (the linea semilunaris), the inferior epigastric artery laterally, and the inguinal ligament inferior–laterally. Direct inguinal hernias are always acquired, but there may be a genetic predisposition to weakness of the abdominal wall in the region of the inguinal triangle.

Femoral hernias, unlike inguinal hernias, lie inferior to the inguinal ligament in the area of the femoral triangle. The inguinal ligament forms the superior border of the femoral triangle, the sartorius muscle represents the lateral border, and the adductor longus muscle, the medial border (*Figure 17.6a*). The triangle can be divided into muscular and vascular compartments. The vascular compartment contains the femoral artery and vein and the femoral ring or canal (*Figure 17.6b*). The femoral canal contains fat and lymphatics and a lymph node.

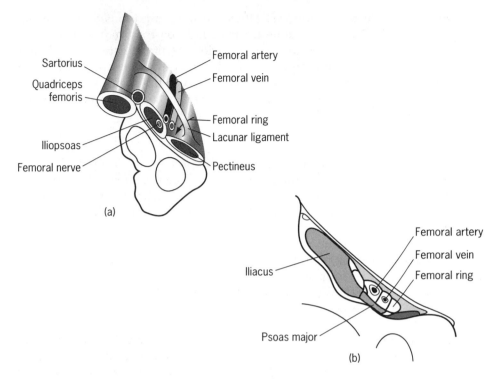

Figure 17.6 (a) Muscle of the femoral triangle. (b) Muscular and vascular compartments.

It is bounded by the inguinal ligament, the femoral vein, the lacunar ligament, and the pectineal ligament, which is a thickening of the periosteum of the superior ramus of the pubic bone. Femoral hernias pass down this canal and because of the tight, ligamentous boundaries there is a high risk of strangulation, incarceration, and bowel necrosis. Femoral hernias are acquired, usually occur in middle age, and are rarely seen in children. They are more common in women than men and may be associated with physical exertion or pregnancy.

Clinical presentation

An inguinal hernia usually presents as the sudden appearance of a lump in the groin. The lump may appear intermittently, be associated with exertion, and may be painful. It can extend into the scrotum (i.e. a complete hernia) and may be unilateral or bilateral. Ellis and Calne (1993b) report that 60% of inguinal hernias appear on the right side, 20% on the left, and 20% are bilateral. Indirect inguinal hernias can usually be differentiated from direct inguinal hernias by the history and physical examination. The direct hernia tends to appear on standing, but reduces or disappears when the patient lies down. The hernia will usually enlarge when the patient coughs because abdominal pressure is easily transmitted through the wide neck. Patients often make their own diagnosis of hernia using the colloquial term 'rupture'. However, it is important to realise that although patients may have a name for the condition they may not have full understanding of the causes and complications. Unfortunately some older patients cope with the condition for a considerable time unaware of the risk of complications. They tend to seek medical advice when the hernia becomes more swollen, tender, or painful. By this time adhesions may have occurred, the hernia is irreducible, and there is a higher risk of strangulation.

Treatment

Surgical intervention is the treatment of choice for groin hernias. However, conservative treatment can be attempted and may be used for elderly patients who represent a poor surgical risk. Conservative treatment involves the use of a truss to support the hernia but drawbacks of this treatment include:

■ Risk of strangulation.
■ Truss has to be worn at all times.
■ Truss needs frequent adjustment.
■ A large hernia can significantly interfere with lifestyle.
■ Local pain or tenderness may develop.

Herniorraphy or repair of a hernia is usually carried out as an elective procedure, but patients who present with complications such as obstruction, incarceration, or strangulation require emergency surgery. These can be life-threatening conditions and the patient may present with the signs of intestinal obstruction (i.e. vomiting, severe abdominal pain, abdominal distension, and constipation). Devlin (1993) identifies the priorities of treatment in this case as:

■ Resuscitate – restore circulating fluid volume, treat concurrent problems (e.g. heart failure) and prepare for surgery.
■ Reduce contents – return only live viable bowel to the peritoneum.
■ Repair – repair the fascial–aponeurotic defect to prevent recurrence.

In an elective repair the main principles are to return the contents of the sac to the peritoneal cavity, to ligate the neck of the sac, and to repair the abdominal wall defect. A variety of different procedures are in use including Shoudice, Bassini, and Stoppa repairs and McVay's method. In some types of repair the abdominal wall defect is reinforced using a polypropylene mesh. Recurrence rates after surgery vary depending on the type of hernia and repair technique, but may be 3–5% of cases. Laparoscopic repair of inguinal hernia is becoming more common and may be offered as day surgery. Sailors et al. (1993) presents a study of successful operations performed from 1991–1992 for inguinal hernia using a standardized laparoscopic technique. Herniorraphy may be performed under local or general anaesthesia and procedures such as the Shoudice repair, which do not require invasion of the main peritoneal cavity, may be suitable for day surgery (Devlin, 1993).

Nursing care
It is important to realise that although groin hernias are common and may be familiar to the nurse and patient they are not without risks. There is a significant mortality in the elderly, particularly with strangulated hernia. Devlin (1993) reported that the 30-day mortality for elective hernia surgery was 0.3% and there was an operation-specific mortality rate of 6% for strangulated hernias. The mortality rate of hernia repairs also rises with age, being 0.1% for patients under 60 years of age, but 3.3% for patients over 80 years of age (Ziffren and Hartford, 1972). Hernias, and particularly groin hernias, represent an important and costly public health problem and nurses need to be knowledgeable about them to help with both prevention and treatment.

When assessing a patient admitted for elective herniorraphy it is important to determine whether the patient has an upper respiratory infection, chronic cough, or sneezing due to allergy. This is particularly critical with the older patient. If any of these problems are identified, it may be necessary to postpone the operation as coughing or sneezing postoperatively could seriously weaken the wound. The physiotherapist will be involved in showing the patient appropriate chest exercises for before and after the operation, and patients are shown how to support the potential wound site should they cough or sneeze. Obesity is a significant risk factor and the overweight patient should be encouraged to lose weight in preparation for an elective hernia repair. Suppositories should be offered to the patient the evening before surgery and the nurse should explain that discomfort can result postoperatively if the bowel is full. The groin area may require skin preparation.

Postoperative care is similar to that required after abdominal surgery. The nurse must be alert for particular problems including sepsis, haemorrhage, scrotal complications, and neurological complications. Scrotal complications include scrotal bruising, hydrocele, and genital oedema. There may be damage to the vas deferens or ischaemic orchitis, which can result in testicular atrophy. A scrotal support may be applied if there is any tendency for the scrotum to swell after repair of an inguinal hernia. Neurological complications include persistent pain, nerve entrapment, and paraesthesia. It is important that both the patient and nurse are aware that a hernia repair may prove more complex than anticipated and involve extensive handling of tissues. Postoperative pain may be much greater than anticipated and it may take longer than expected for bowel function to return. The length of time in surgery and the operation notes will help the surgical nurse anticipate postoperative needs. A hernia repair should not be dismissed as routine or minor surgery.

Day surgery
The suitability, safety, and efficiency of the day care approach to inguinal hernia repair has long been discussed (Farquharson, 1955). Day surgery is becoming increasingly common, reducing waiting lists and allowing otherwise healthy individuals to rapidly resume their normal activities. Careful assessment and discharge planning is essential, and this is often carried out by the nurse in a

preadmission clinic. After the operation the nurse must ensure that every effort is made to get the patient back home before the effect of the local anaesthetic has worn off. Patients should be advised to have 3–4 days in bed, but can get up to go to the toilet. Their general practitioners are asked to visit them, and they usually return to hospital for removal of the sutures nine days after surgery. Age is not a bar to day surgery, but a careful assessment of the patient and home circumstances is important.

Discharge planning and patient education

The nurse should ensure that the following issues have been discussed with the patient and family whether the patient stays in hospital for a few days or goes home directly after surgery:

■ Pain and scrotal swelling may be present after operation for 48 hours. Use of a scrotal support and prescribed medication may be helpful and any severe pain must be reported immediately.
■ Pain or difficulty with urinating must be reported.
■ Constipation or straining during defaecation should be avoided. Ensuring a good fluid intake (at least two litres a day) and a diet containing plenty of fruit and fibre will help. Coughs, colds, or any other problem that may increase intra-abdominal pressure should be avoided if possible.
■ The wound should be kept clean and any drainage from the incision reported.
■ Although frequent gentle activity is encouraged, the patient needs to rest for about seven days after the operation and only resume normal activities gradually. Heavy lifting or other strenuous activities should be avoided for six weeks, and information about correct lifting techniques should be provided.

THE SKIN AND ITS APPENDAGES

Surgical problems affecting the skin and its appendages (i.e. hair, nails, and sebaceous and sweat glands) are common. *Box 17.2* lists skin conditions that may require surgical intervention. Many of these will be managed by specialists in dermatology or plastic surgery, but some of the more common conditions are dealt with in general surgery. Sebaceous cysts, ganglia, pilonidal sinuses, and lipomas are frequently encountered conditions and are briefly discussed in this section.

Sebaceous Cysts

Sebaceous cysts are retention cysts that develop when a sebaceous gland becomes obstructed. They are most common on the scalp, face, vulva, and scrotum, but may be found in any area with sebaceous glands. They do not occur on the palms of the hands or soles of the feet. Infection, ulceration, and calcification are

Box 17.2 Surgical skin conditions (adapted from Ellis and Calne, 1993).

Benign conditions

Cysts
- Epidermal inclusion cysts
- Sebaceous cysts
- Dermoid cysts
- Ganglia

Vascular birthmarks
- Haemangiomas (strawberry birthmarks)
- Capillary haemangiomas (port-wine stains)
- Cavernous haemangiomas (venous)

Vascular tumours
- Pyogenic granuloma
- Telangiectasia (spider naevi)

Lipomas

Nervous tissue tumours
- Neurilemmomas
- Neurofibromas

Other
- Keloid scars
- Hidradenitis suppurativa
- Seborrhoeic dermatitis

Premalignant conditions
- Actinic keratosis
- Bowen's disease
- Keratoacanthoma

Naevi (moles)

Malignant conditions
- Malignant melanoma
- Basal cell carcinoma
- Squamous cell carcinoma

potential complications. Removal is by simple excision and may be performed under local anaesthesia in a general practitioner's minor surgery clinic or in a day surgery unit. Large or adherent cysts may require a general anaesthetic.

Ganglia

Ganglia are common surgical lumps that usually occur on the wrists, along the flexor aspect of the fingers, or on the dorsum of the foot overlying the joints. They are thin-walled cysts with a synovial lining. They may be treated by excision for cosmetic reasons or because of discomfort. Recurrence is common, especially if there is inadequate resection of the base or stalk.

Pilonidal Sinus

This is a common minor condition that typically affects young male Caucasians. It usually develops before the age of 30 and is rare after 40 years of age. Although it mainly affects men with dense dark hair, women are increasingly affected. Edwards (1992) suggests that this may be because women wear tight trousers. The male to female ratio reported in the literature varies from 3 : 1 to 7 : 1. Pilonidal sinus generally affects the sacrococcygeal region, but has been reported between the fingers in barbers, and more rarely involving the umbilicus, perineum, axilla, sole of the foot, anal canal, or clitoris or an amputation stump. There has even been a report of a periareolar pilonidal sinus in a hairdresser (Gannon et al., 1988).

Pilonidal sinus is probably an acquired condition, although in rare cases there may be a congenital origin. The hair follicles in the natal cleft distend and an abscess forms, which may contain loose hairs (*Figure 17.7*). Usually it is the patient's own hair that appears in the sinus, but there have been reports of pilonidal sinuses containing hair of a different colour from the patient's hair, animal hair, wool, and grass (Akwari, 1991). The sinus may initially be asymptomatic, but infection will develop and the patient usually presents with local discomfort, discharge, and occasionally bleeding. Usually the problem is very localized with minimal cellulitis, and systemic reactions are uncommon. Pilonidal sinus tends to be a recurrent problem even after treatment. Although generally described as a minor condition, large recurrent sinuses may require extensive resection.

Treatment

Treatment of pilonidal sinus varies widely and may range from conservative management to Z-plasty plus rhomboid flap. Asymptomatic pilonidal sinus should simply be monitored. Simple incision and drainage may prove sufficient for an acute pilonidal sinus, but often the entire sinus tract is excised. Wide excision is probably needed for chronic pilonidal disease and the wound may be sutured or allowed to heal by granulation. Pilonidal sinuses are commonly infected with aerobic (e.g. *Staphylococcus aureus*) and anaerobic bacteria

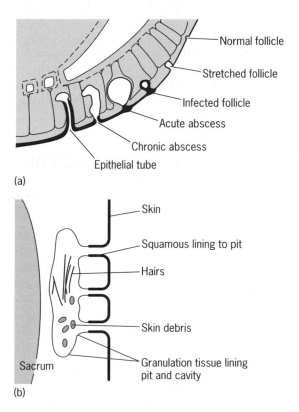

(a)

(b)

Figure 17.7 Pilonidal sinus. (Reproduced with kind permission from Sabiston DC (1991) *Textbook of Surgery*, 14th edn. WB Saunders, Philadelphia; and Edwards MM (1992) *Surgery* **10(12)**:283 by kind permission of The Medicine Group (Journals) Ltd.)

(particularly *Bacteroides*) and antibiotic therapy is usually recommended. Edwards (1992) recommends metronidazole for anaerobes and cephalosporin for aerobes in the absence of specific sensitivities. Acute pilonidal sinus may be treated as day surgery with follow-up as an outpatient. More extensive surgery may require 2–3 days hospitalization and regular attendance as an outpatient until healing is complete.

The nurse has an important role in educating the patient to cope with treatment and reduce recurrence. After incision and drainage the hairs around the incision are usually shaved weekly until the wound has healed. It is important that the area is kept clean. The patient can be taught about local cleansing and care of the wound, which will need frequent dressing changes. For the first few days patients may be required to lie on their abdomen or side. Oral analgesics are usually sufficient for pain control. The patient may be discharged within 24 hours to continue recovery at home and can usually return to work within 1–2 days.

Lipomas

Lipomas are soft lobulated fatty tumours that can be found in many areas of the body, but are most common on the back, shoulders, neck, and thigh. They are extremely common, affecting both sexes, but women may present more often for treatment due to cosmetic concerns. Treatment is by simple excision and may be carried out in minor surgery clinics or as day surgery.

LOWER EXTREMITY PERIPHERAL VASCULAR DISEASE

Atherosclerosis is a disease affecting large and small muscular and elastic arteries. It is the cause of about 50% of deaths in developed countries. Sheehan and Shepherd (1994) reported that in England and Wales in 1991 more than 240,000 people died from atherosclerosis and its consequences. Complications of atherosclerosis include:

- Ischaemic heart disease and coronary thrombosis.
- Cerebral thrombosis.
- Ischaemic bowel disease.
- Peripheral vascular disease.
- Renal failure.

In atherosclerosis atherosclerotic plaques accumulate on the blood vessel wall; this can gradually cause occlusion and reduce blood flow through the vessel. Atherosclerotic lesions may start as fatty streaks, which are discrete subintimal lesions of the vessel wall made up of cholesterol, smooth muscle cells, and macrophages. Fatty streaks do not impede haemodynamic function, but can develop into larger fibrous plaques (*Figure 17.8*), which include extracellular matrix components. Fibrous plaques can obstruct blood flow. Complex plaques develop in advanced disease. These are large obstructive lesions that may show intimal ulceration, calcification, fissuring, or intraplaque haemorrhage. In addition to blocking blood flow complex plaques can result in secondary

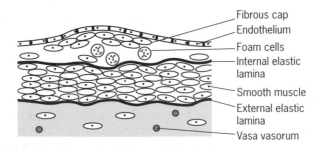

Figure 17.8 Fibrous plaque. (Reproduced from Sheehan and Shepherd (1994) by kind permission of The Medicine Group (Journals) Ltd.)

thrombosis or pieces can break loose causing acute blockage of a disal artery (i.e. embolism). Certain anatomical sites, usually where arteries branch or bifurcate, are particularly prone to plaque formation (*Figure 17.9*). The theories of atherogenesis are beyond the scope of this section, but the four major risk factors are:

- Hyperlipidaemia.
- Hypertension.
- Smoking.
- Diabetes mellitus.

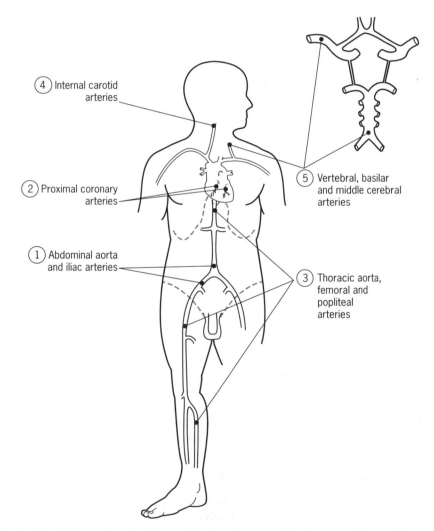

Figure 17.9 Common sites for atherosclerotic occlusion. (Reproduced with permission of Dimitri Karetnikov from Rubin and Farber (1988) *Pathology*, 1st edn, JB Lippincott, Philadelphia).

In addition other factors such as being overweight and lack of exercise may contribute to the risk. Atherosclerosis can affect central and peripheral arteries, but in this section only peripheral vascular disease of the lower extremity will be considered.

If occlusion progresses slowly a collateral circulation can develop and the condition may be asymptomatic at rest. However, intermittent claudication is likely. Claudication is characteristic of peripheral vascular disease. The patient will complain of aching or cramping pain and fatigue in the leg(s) after walking a certain distance. Claudication is usually consistent and reproducible; that is, it occurs consistently once a certain distance has been covered. It is also rapidly relieved by a few minutes' rest. Ischaemic rest pain indicates a more severely compromised arterial supply and is characterized by intense burning pain across the foot, which is made worse by elevation, but may be relieved when the foot is dependent. This condition is very disabling and painful. The risk of ischaemic damage may require surgical intervention. If ischaemia continues there is the risk of ischaemic necrosis and gangrene. Initially necrosis will affect the most distal areas of the toes or occur between the toes, producing non-healing ulcers. Surgical debridement or amputation is often required. Arterial insufficiency also produces other symptoms (i.e. loss of hair, changes in the nails, skin pallor on elevation of the leg, and dependent erythema). If the condition is not adequately treated ischaemia will result in progressive loss of more and more tissue, perhaps culminating in a below-knee amputation. Acute occlusion or embolism is a critical problem because there is no collateral circulation and acute limb ischaemia can result in irreversible muscle damage after about six hours (Campbell, 1990).

Atherosclerosis is the most important cause of lower limb ischaemia, but other diseases can impair arterial blood flow including:

■ Embolism.
■ Thrombosis.
■ Diabetes mellitus.
■ Raynaud's disease.
■ Buerger's disease.
■ Blood vessel trauma.

Embolism is the commonest cause of acute limb ischaemia, but acute thrombosis of vessels already obstructed by chronic atherosclerosis is also common.

Arterial Supply to the Lower Limb

Before considering investigations and treatment for peripheral vascular disease of the legs it is useful to review the arterial supply. The femoral and obturator arteries provide the main arterial supply to the leg with some contribution from the gluteal vessels (*Figure 17.10*). Common sites for occlusion include the superficial and deep femoral, popliteal, and tibial arteries.

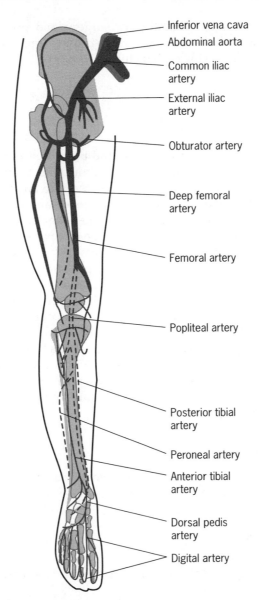

Figure 17.10 Arterial supply to the leg.

Investigations

A variety of invasive and noninvasive diagnostic procedures can be used when assessing peripheral vascular disease. It is important that the nurse understands the significance of the investigations, so that a clear comprehensive explanation can be offered to the patient. The extent of investigation will depend on the patient's history, condition, suitability for surgery, and prognosis. A range of blood investigations, urinalysis, chest radiography, and electrocardiography (ECG) will be required. Specific tests include:

■ Doppler studies.
■ Arteriography.
■ Magnetic resonance imaging (MRI).

The Doppler probe emits a narrow ultrasound beam that can be used to assess the velocity of moving red blood cells. The ultrasound beam is reflected back from moving red cells and the signal is converted into an audible output. This device allows mapping of the arterial flow of the leg and when combined with sphygmomanometry allows measurement of the systolic arterial pressure at the ankle at rest and after exercise. This can then be compared with the pressure at the brachial artery. Normally when an individual is lying down the pressure at the ankle is slightly higher than the brachial pressure. Doppler studies allow identification of arterial obstruction or reduced flow.

MRI is another noninvasive technique that allows an assessment of the arterial tree. Cullimore (1993) points out that MRI can clearly demonstrate blood vessels because the blood in the vessels appears as black on the image and therefore a picture similar to that produced by an arteriogram can be obtained.

Arteriography is the most useful technique for precisely identifying the site and extent of blockage. However, the procedure is invasive and associated with complications. It is only necessary if the patient is going to be treated with a revascularization procedure.

Surgical Treatment

Claudication, ischaemic rest pain, and ischaemic necrosis are all indications for surgical intervention. If the patient is suitable, a revascularization procedure can be attempted, for example:

■ Femoropopliteal bypass.
■ Femorotibial artery bypass.
■ Profundoplasty (repair of the origin of the deep femoral artery).

These procedures are usually carried out in specialized vascular surgery units.

Percutaneous transluminal angioplasty (PTA) offers an alternative to bypass surgery. A catheter with an inflatable balloon is guided under fluoroscopic imaging to the area of occlusion. The balloon is inflated to fracture the plaque and stretch the blood vessel wall. This procedure is useful for localized plaque formation, but is less successful for diffuse atherosclerotic disease. It is also associated with a significant risk of embolism or thrombosis. If the patient is not a candidate for a revascularization operation, amputation is considered. Even if revascularization can be attempted, amputation will occasionally have a better outcome than an extensive revascularization procedure. Amputation may involve removal of a single toe, all the toes, or the foot, or a below-knee or above-knee amputation. Below-knee amputation is preferred as it offers the maximum scope for rehabilitation. The indications for amputation are:

- Unreconstructable vascular disease.
- Poor potential for ambulation even after revascularization.
- Spreading or systemic sepsis.

Nursing Management

Peripheral vascular disease

Peripheral vascular disease has an impact on most aspects of living and nursing priorities include assessment, education, and symptom management. A comprehensive physical and psychosocial assessment is required to establish the extent of the disease and its impact on the patient and family's lifestyle. Claudication and ischaemic rest pain can be major disabling factors and aspects of lifestyle such as diet and exercise may affect the disease process. During physical examination the nurse should pay particular attention to the legs, assessing skin colour, temperature, and condition, and noting any absence of hair and the size of the patient's legs. If only one leg is involved, muscle atrophy may make it noticeably thinner. Often the leg veins are very inconspicuous when compared with normal veins. Temperature differences between the legs or areas of the leg can be identified by palpation with the back of the hand. Any sign of gangrene of the toes or toe tips must be recorded. If pressure is applied to the toes and released there should be a return of colour within three seconds after the pressure is released. Ulcers or lesions should be assessed and their size, location, appearance, and the degree of pain they cause should be documented. The pulses in both legs should be palpated, starting with the dorsalis pedis and working up the leg to include the posterior and anterior tibial, popliteal, and femoral arteries. If it is difficult to palpate the pulses, a hand-held Doppler unit may be useful. The nurse can test the patient's limb for light touch, discrimination, and position.

Another problem that may be experienced by the patient with arterial occlusion is a feeling of tingling, pins and needles, or a crawling sensation in the affected limbs. This is because blood becomes diverted from arterioles supplying the peripheral nerves to arterioles supplying the muscles, and the peripheral nerves become ischaemic. Patients may complain that their limbs are cold and pale. Light touch discrimination can be tested by asking patients to close their eyes while the nurse lightly touches the toes of the affected limb. They are then asked what they can feel. Position can be tested by asking patients to bend their big toe up towards their face and in the opposite direction.

Patient education is an important part of nursing care in this condition. Priorities for patient education include:

- Maintaining a safe environment.
- Coping with pain.
- Minimizing risk factors.

Risk factors

Some risk factors (e.g. cigarette smoking, diet, diabetes mellitus) can be controlled or even eliminated, and it is important that the nurse can explain to patients why these risk factors are dangerous.

Cigarette smoking

Nicotine stimulates the sympathetic nervous system, causing vasoconstriction, particularly in the extremities. As a result, the heart has to work harder to pump blood through the narrowed vessels, and this causes the heart rate and blood pressure to increase. Carbon monoxide in cigarette smoke reduces the capacity of the red blood cells to carry oxygen. Nicotine also increases the risk of thrombosis by increasing the tendency for platelets to stick to each other. Patients must be encouraged to stop smoking or at least reduce the number of cigarettes they smoke.

Diet

Many people with atherosclerosis affecting the lower limbs avoid exercise because it causes pain. If they do not reduce the fat content of their diet they may become overweight and have increased blood lipid levels. Obesity increases demands on the heart and hyperlipidaemia is an important risk factor for atherosclerosis. An adequate fluid intake should also be encouraged as dehydration can increase the risk of thrombosis. The patient will need advice from the dietician, and nurses must reinforce the importance of maintaining an appropriate diet in vascular disease. In chronic peripheral vascular disease the peripheral tissues may be devitalized and ensuring an adequate intake of nutrients, particularly vitamins and trace elements, may be beneficial and help with healing.

Diabetes mellitus

Diabetes mellitus accelerates the process of atherosclerosis, which tends to involve the smaller and more distal arteries. Also microvascular disease, which is associated with diabetes mellitus, means that the patient with diabetes mellitus has a higher risk of losing a limb. Maintaining good diabetic control and adhering to the appropriate diet are critical.

Pain

Claudication and ischaemic rest pain can have a major impact on quality of life, limiting exercise, and sleep. Rest relieves the pain of claudication, but exercise and mobility are important to avoid muscle atrophy, improve peripheral perfusion, and encourage the development of a collateral circulation. The patient may require regular analgesia, and sometimes even opiate analgesia. It is important to encourage adequate use of analgesia and regular appropriate exercise. Some patients with peripheral vascular disease also suffer from arterial spasm; these patients can be advised to keep warm and to occasionally place the limb in a dependent position.

Safe environment

The ischaemic limb suffers from a loss of sensation and poor tissue vitality. It is particularly at risk from injury, infection, heat, and cold. Foot care is important in peripheral vascular disease, and especially for patients with diabetes mellitus. Foot care such as cutting toenails or treating corns should be carried out by the chiropodist. Even a small cut can prove difficult to heal and may result in serious infection. Shoes should be comfortable and well fitting. If a foot injury occurs and the skin is broken, the nurse must emphasize that adhesive tape should not be used. Instead the area can be bandaged, and if the injury does not show signs of healing within 72 hours, the patient should consult his general practitioner. The patient needs to be careful with hot water bottles, electric blankets, open fires, and hot baths due to the reduced sensation in the affected limb. The patient may also suffer from poor sight and can injure the legs by knocking into furniture without being aware of the extent of the tissue injury. Cold may also be damaging, but the patient needs to wear loose layers rather than constrictive clothing (particularly underwear or socks) that may impede the circulation. Due to the poor circulation leg-crossing should be avoided and frequent position changes are recommended. If the skin is very fragile a bed cradle may help keep covers away from the foot. Hygiene and careful skin care is important to reduce the risk of infection.

Below-knee amputation

As with any surgery preoperative assessment and planning is as critical as immediate postoperative care. The patient undergoing this operation may have suffered intractable pain both day and night for a long time and will probably be tired and physically depleted. A clear priority is counselling and support to prepare the patient for the loss of a limb. However, the amputation may actually be welcomed by the patient. The limb will have been causing pain, it will be discoloured, and it will be unsightly, perhaps even infected and necrotic. Nonetheless the nurse needs to expect a grief response to the permanent alteration in body image. As Brunner and Suddarth (1992) point out, coping will be facilitated by skilled professional help and adequate support systems. The patient may benefit from a visit by another amputee or be reassured by visiting the local limb fitting centre if a prosthesis is likely to be helpful. Preoperative care is generally similar to that for any major surgery, but the nurse and physiotherapist need to prepare the patient for the initial alteration in mobility after the amputation. Specific aspects of postoperative care include pain control, mobilization, wound care, promoting independence, and adapting to the amputation.

Pain control

Pain in the wound site must be assessed carefully by means of a pain chart, and the appropriate prescribed medication given. Amputees sometimes experience phantom sensations, complaining of pain in the part of the limb that has been amputated. Phantom pain can persist for months after the surgery. It is important that the nurse explains this phenomenon to allay the patient's anxiety. Phantom pain is a central pain syndrome and the physiological and psychological mechanisms behind it are poorly understood. Effective postoperative analgesia may help reduce its occurrence. It is important that the nurse realises it is a real pain that can have a major impact on the patient's quality of life. Transcutaneous and electrical nerve stimulation may prove useful, and distraction techniques and activity may help. In extreme cases of chronic phantom pain nerve stimulators have been implanted or nerve ablation therapies tried. Phantom pain is less common in lower limb amputations due to occlusive arterial disease.

Stump care
The wound site is commonly covered by a soft padding and a stump bandage (*Figure 17.11*). A wound drain may be in place. The bandage is designed to protect and compress the stump to reduce oedema and prepare the stump for a prosthesis. Exudate will tend to accumulate at the stump, which should be checked for excessive bleeding, drainage, or infection. The usual postoperative

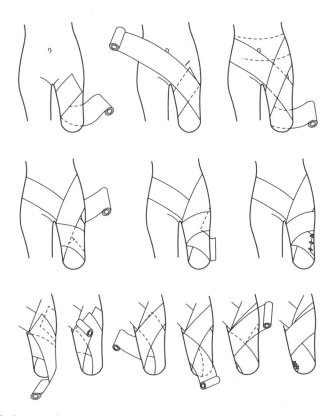

Figure 17.11 A stump bandage.

observations are required due to the risk of haemorrhage and infection. If excessive haemorrhage occurs a pressure dressing can be applied and medical staff alerted. If haemorrhage is uncontrollable a tourniquet may be applied, but this should be used only as a last resort. The historical practice of keeping a tourniquet at the foot of the bed is not required and can create anxiety in the patient. The stump bandage may be replaced by a special elasticated stump dressing or 'sock.' There is a danger of flexion contracture of the stump so the nurse should encourage the patient to move as much as possible and to lie in the prone position for periods during the day to stretch the flexor muscles.

Mobilization
The patient can usually get out of bed after the first postoperative day and will require a wheelchair to help with mobilization. Some amputees will not be candidates for a prosthesis and it is important that these patients are taught wheelchair management so that they can move easily from bed to chair. Patients will find their balance affected and will need to practice standing and walking under nursing and physiotherapy supervision. Clothing may need to be adapted so that it does not impede movement.

Promoting independence
To encourage independence patients must be actively involved in postoperative care. Patients can be taught to care for their stump, to learn to use the wheelchair, and to take responsibility for hygiene and excretory activities. After the immediate postoperative period rehabilitation becomes the nursing priority. The patient will follow a planned rehabilitation coordinated by the physiotherapist, and if appropriate, the limb fitting services. The occupational therapist may carry out a home visit to assess the patient in the home environment and to advise on any necessary adaptations in preparation for discharge. Modifications may need to be made in the home such as hand rails or ramps.

Adapting to the amputation
The realization that the limb has gone may shock the patient regardless of how much time there has been to prepare for the amputation. It is important that the nurse is prepared to listen and discuss further care options with the patient. Referral to an amputee support group may be required.

VARICOSE VEINS

Although varicose veins may occur in any part of the venous system the condition most frequently affects the superficial veins of the legs. Varicosities are long, dilated, tortuous, and unsightly veins. The condition results from valvular incompetence affecting the deep, superficial, or perforating veins of the legs (*Figure 17.12*). The most common sites for varicose veins are the long and short saphenous veins and their tributaries. These veins are superficial, lying outside

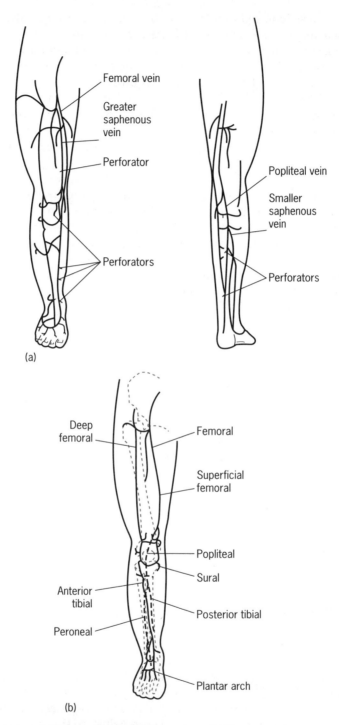

(a)

(b)

Figure 17.12 Veins of the legs. (a) Superficial system. (b) Deep system.

the deep fascia that surrounds the leg muscles. The superficial veins are large muscular veins with relatively thick walls located just under the skin. The deep veins, which are less muscular and have thinner walls, lie within the muscles and are supported and protected by the surrounding muscles and fascia. The thin deep veins act as pumps or bellows. As the surrounding muscle relaxes and contracts it pushes blood up the veins. Veins have strong bicuspid valves that prevent backflow of blood. Deep veins have more valves than superficial veins. Perforating veins connect the deep and superficial veins.

The valves of the leg veins can resist quite high pressures. During muscle contraction blood moves up the veins in short sections (*Figure 17.13a*). However, if a valve becomes incompetent it effectively creates a much longer column of blood (*Figure 17.13b*) and allows retrograde filling. This increases pressure on the distal valve, which may in turn fail. The condition tends to get progressively worse as more valves are put under excessive pressure and fail.

Varicose veins can be classified as primary or secondary. Primary varicose veins involve the superficial venous system with failure of the valves allowing reflux of blood at the saphenofemoral venous junction. Secondary varicose veins are associated with deep vein involvement or venous hypertension due to pregnancy. Gage and Gage (1987) describe Trendelenburg's test to differentiate between incompetence of the great or small saphenous veins and the saphenofemoral junction from incompetence in the deep perforating veins. The patient is asked to lie flat and elevate the leg. A tourniquet is applied to the thigh and the patient is asked to stand up.

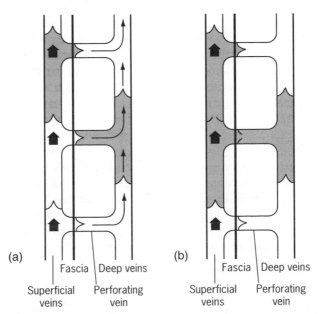

Figure 17.13 (a) Venous valves. (b) An incompetent valve effectively creates a much longer column of blood.

If the varicosities fill within a few seconds, the fault lies with the incompetent perforating veins. However, if the varicosities do not fill within 20 seconds, the tourniquet is released and filling of the great saphenous vein from above the tourniquet site demonstrates incompetence of the valves of the greater saphenous system.

Green and Wickenden (1984) reported that varicose veins can be caused by:

- Proximal venous obstruction caused by chronic constipation or pregnancy.
- Hormonal influence that causes smooth muscle relaxation, such as occurs in pregnancy.
- Maintaining a stationary upright position for long periods, as in shop assistants.
- Obesity.

Hereditary weakness of the vein wall may contribute to the development of varicosities. Gage and Gage (1987) suggested that if both parents have varicose veins then the children are likely to develop the condition.

Patient Problems

Varicose veins can cause venous stasis, local pain, oedema, recurrent superficial phlebitis, pigmentation of the skin over the ankle, leakage of red cells into the tissues, eczema, and gravitational ulceration. They can be very large and unsightly and may cause the patient considerable embarrassment or distress. The patient may complain of ache and fatigue of the leg muscles accompanied by cramp, particularly at night. Oedema will tend to accumulate at the ankles, which may progressively swell over the course of the day. The oedema may resolve overnight when the body is in a supine position. If thrombosis occurs in the deep veins, the leg may become oedematous, painful, and pigmented; dermatitis and ulceration may also occur.

Patient Education

If a possible cause or contributing factor can be identified, for example chronic constipation, it should be treated. Obese patients will need encouragement and support to lose weight. Suitable exercise should be advised such as walking or swimming, and the patient should be encouraged to change position frequently and sit with the legs elevated whenever possible. Constricting clothing should be avoided, but support hose may relieve the ache and tiredness of the legs.

Treatment

Elastic support stockings may be the treatment of choice for pregnant women, elderly patients, or patients who represent a poor surgical or anaesthetic risk. However, surgical treatment is usual for symptom relief and cosmetic considerations. The two main approaches to treatment are sclerotherapy and ligation. If the varicosities are present below the knee only they can be treated by schlerotherapy and compression. Injection of an irritating chemical (sclerosant) produces localized phlebitis and fibrosis, thereby obliterating the lumen of the vein. Following this procedure, elastic compression bandages are applied to the leg for six weeks and the patient is advised to walk at least six miles a day. However, the value of sclerotherapy is debated. Some authorities do not recommend sclerotherapy due to its disadvantages, a high recurrence rate, and effective surgical alternatives (Flye, 1991).

Surgical interventions include:

- Ligation of the great saphenous vein in the groin.
- Ligation of the small saphenous vein at the junction with the popliteal vein.
- Stripping of the great and small saphenous veins.
- Ligation of any incompetent communicator veins missed by the stripping procedure.

Nursing Management

The patient is admitted the day before surgery and given an explanation of what is to happen. Vital signs are checked, an electrocardiogram (ECG) and chest radiograph are obtained, and urinalysis is recorded. The patient's groin area may be shaved and a bath or shower taken. The affected veins are usually marked with the patient in the standing position as the varicosities tend to subside once the patient lies down. A general anaesthetic is usual and requires pre-operative fasting and usually a premedication. Postoperative care follows the usual pattern, but care of the leg wounds represents a specific challenge. The wounds are usually closed with steristrips and the patient is advised to observe the groin wound carefully as it is prone to infection. Blueline bandages and crepe bandages are applied firmly to the leg from the ankle to the thigh. Pain can be kept to a minimum by infiltrating the wound with bupivacaine at the time of surgery. Paracetamol can be prescribed to relieve the pain, and nausea can be prevented by the use of oral metoclopramide before surgery. The dressings and bandages are replaced by thrombo-embolic-deterrent (TED) stockings the day after the operation, and the patient is given written instructions to keep the stockings on day and night for the first week to prevent bleeding or thrombophlebitis in the remaining veins. The nurse must emphasize the importance of exercise and avoidance of the stationary upright position. By the second week, the patient may remove the stockings to go to the bath, but other than that, the stockings should be worn night and day for the next three weeks. Carrington (1991) describes a scheme for day care surgery for patients for varicose vein surgery. The preassessment clinic ensures the patient is prepared physically and psychologically and close liaison with the community team enables the benefits of the scheme to prove very satisfactory for most patients.

CHEST DRAINS

Chest drains are used in both surgical and medical practice to remove pathological collections of air or fluid from the pleural space. Air or fluid in the pleural space impedes lung expansion and the aim of drainage is to restore complete expansion of the lung as quickly as possible. *Box 17.3* lists the main indications for inserting a chest drain. The pleurae of the lung (*Figure 17.14*) are formed from two membranes, the parietal and visceral pleura. The parietal

---

Box 17.3 Indications for chest drains (adapted from Soni and Riley, 1993).

- Pneumothorax (spontaneous, tension, iatrogenic)
- Haemothorax
- Chylothorax
- Penetrating chest injuries, thoracic trauma
- Post-thoracic surgery drainage
- Empyema
- Pleural effusion (usually associated with malignancy)

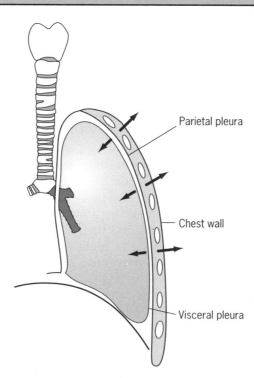

Parietal pleura

Chest wall

Visceral pleura

Figure 17.14 The pleura of the lung.

pleura lines the pleural cavity and the visceral pleura covers the lung. A thin film of serous fluid provides lubrication between the two layers allowing the visceral pleura to glide easily over the parietal pleura during inspiration and expiration. The potential space between the pleurae is called the pleural space or cavity. However, it does not actually exist in the healthy lung: it is only a potential space. The pleural fluid exerts an extremely strong surface tension between the two pleural layers that keeps the lung expanded. This effect can best be demonstrated by taking two glass slides and placing one on top of the other. They are easily pulled apart. However, if a drop of water is placed between the slides they slide easily over each other, but it is difficult to pull them apart. If air or fluid collects between the pleura the surface tension is lost, the elasticity of the lungs will tend to pull the pleura apart, and that part of the lung will collapse. Collapse of the lung is a potentially life-threatening condition requiring immediate treatment. *Box 17.4* lists and defines the terms used to describe air or fluid within the pleural space.

Treatment usually involves insertion of a drain into the pleural space. Chest drains need to incorporate non-return valves or underwater seal drainage to prevent air entering the pleural space.

Managing Chest Drains

Chest drains may be inserted during operations on the thorax or to treat conditions such as spontaneous pneumothorax. Location of the drain will depend on the nature of the drainage. They are usually located in the fifth or sixth intercostal space. Air tends to rise in the pleural space so drains inserted for pneumothorax are sometimes located in the second intercostal space in the midclavicular line.

Box 17.4 Pneumothorax and related terminology.

Pneumothorax
- Collection of air or gas within the pleural space

Tension pneumothorax
- Collection of air or gas under positive pressure within the pleural space

Haemothorax
- Collection of blood within the pleural space

Hydrothorax
- Collection of fluid within the pleural space

Chylothorax
- Collection of chyle (from lymphatics) within the pleural space

However, Appleton (1994) does not recommend this location because of the risk of damaging the subclavian vessels. Once the drain is inserted it must be connected to a one-way valve. Mechanical valves such as the Heimlich flutter valve or special chest drain bags, which incorporate a one-way flutter valve may be used, but the most common approach is to use underwater seal drainage. In underwater seal drainage the chest drain is connected to a sealed bottle containing water, as shown in *Figure 17.15a*. The water acts as a seal, preventing air from entering the drainage tube. If heavy drainage is expected a two-bottle system may be used (*Figure 17.15b*), and if suction is used a three-bottle system (*Figure 17.15c*) will help regulate the force of suction.

With appropriate management the incidence of complications with chest drains is low. However, complications, which are usually associated with insertion, can occur and include:

- Lung laceration, pulmonary oedema, and empyema.
- Heart and great vessel trauma, exsanguination, and tamponade.
- Damage to the stomach, spleen, or liver.
- Blockage, usually with blood. (Large-bore tubes are preferred for haemothorax.)
- Infection (tends to be a longer-term consequence).
- Discomfort, pain, and restricted mobility.

The chest drain will be sutured to secure it to the skin, and the puncture wound may be covered by a small non-adherent dressing. In addition a loose 'purse-string' suture will be inserted. Heavy dressings or strapping are best avoided as they can restrict chest expansion and serve little practical purpose. The wound is observed for signs of inflammation and drainage is recorded. If the chest drain is inserted to treat a pneumothorax, bubbles should be observed rising through the

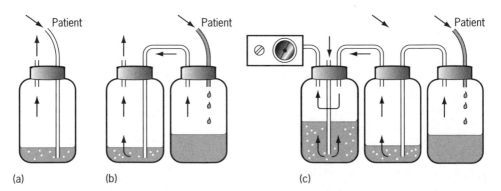

Figure 17.15 Underwater seal drainage. (a) One-bottle system. (b) Two-bottle system. (c) Three-bottle system. (Reproduced with kind permission of *British Journal of Nursing*, Mark Allen Publishing Ltd.)

water. When observing the drain a rise and fall of water in the drainage tube in time with ventilation will indicate that it is patent and effective. The key aspects of the nurse's role have been identified by Welch (1993) as:

- Observation for potential complications.
- Ensuring the integrity and safety of the system.
- Maintaining patency and free drainage of air or fluid.

To ensure patency and integrity all connections must be tight and should be checked frequently. Taping of the joints will not be required with correctly assembled systems and may conceal disconnections. A coil of tubing may be secured to the edge of the bed, but it is best to avoid dependent loops or kinks. The drainage bottle must always be positioned below the level of the chest to prevent air or fluid from entering the pleural space. If the drain is raised above chest level fluid can flow into the pleural space creating a hydrothorax. It is not generally recommended that drains are clamped because of the risk of tension pneumothorax, but clamps should be available in case of accidental disconnection. Some surgeons prefer that the system is clamped 12–24 hours before removal of the drain to ensure all air or fluid has been evacuated. The length of tube under the water dictates the pressure required to expel air or fluid from the pleural space. This length should be as short as possible while maintaining a seal. Generally 2–3 cm of water is recommended. Deep breathing, coughing, and mobilization should be encouraged to promote drainage. Pain relief may be necessary to facilitate these activities. Milking or stripping of the drains to promote drainage and avoid clot formation is a controversial procedure of uncertain value. There is little evidence that milking drains is beneficial and it can create negative pressure within the drainage tube and possibly result in fragile lung tissue being drawn into the tube. If milking is required, twisting or squeezing the tube to mobilize the clot is probably better than using a mechanical roller.

When drainage has stopped and radiography indicates that the lungs are fully expanded the drain can be removed. The patient should be given a bolus dose of analgesia and assisted into an upright position. Sometime Entonox analgesia is prescribed for chest drain removal.The insertion site is cleaned and the retaining suture removed. The patient is asked to take and hold a deep breath and the tube is withdrawn in a single smooth movement. The purse-string suture is tightened to close the puncture site and the wound is covered with a simple dressing. The patient's general condition and respiratory function are observed for the next 24 hours and a chest radiograph is ordered to check lung inflation.

References

Akwari OE (1991) Pilonidal cysts and sinuses. In *Textbook of Surgery*. Sabiston DC (ed.). pp. 1399–1402. WB Saunders, Philadephia.
Appleton SG (1994) Chest drains: placement and management. *Surgery* **12(11)**:247–248.

Brunner L, Suddarth D (1992) *Textbook of Adult Nursing*, 1st edition, pp. 1132–1138. Chapman and Hall, London.

Burkitt HG, Quick CRG, Gatt D (1990) *Essential Surgery: Problems, Diagnosis and Management*. Churchill Livingstone, Edinburgh.

Campbell WB (1990) Acute limb ischaemia. *Surgery* 81:1937–1941.

Carrington S (1991) A waiting list initiative for varicose vein surgery in Bristol. *Br J Theatre Nurs* 1(5):23–25.

Cullimore E (1993) Magnetic resonance imaging. *Surg Nurse* 6(1):18–22.

Devlin HB (1993) Groin hernias. *Surgery* 11(5):385–396.

Duncan JL, Rogers K (1991) Umbilical and epigastric hernias. *Surgery* 97:2326–2329.

Edwards MH (1992) Pilonidal sinus. *Surgery* 10(12):283–285.

Ellis H, Calne R (1993a) *Lecture Notes on General Surgery*. 8th edition, p. 147. Blackwell Scientific Publications, London.

Ellis H, Calne R (1993b) *Lecture Notes on General Surgery*. 8th edition, pp. 224–232. Blackwell Scientific Publications, London.

Farquharson EL (1955) Early ambulation with special reference to herniorrhaphy as an out-patient procedure. *Lancet* ii:517–519.

Flye MW (1991) Venous disorders. In *Textbook of Surgery. The Biological Basis of Modern Surgical Practice*, 14th edition. Sabiston DC (ed.). pp. 1490–1501. WB Saunders, Philadephia.

Gage AM, Gage AA (1987) Evaluation and treatment of varicose veins. *Hosp Med* 9:93–120.

Gannon MX, Crowson MC, Fielding JWL (1988) Periareolar pilonidal disease in a hairdresser. *Br Med J* 297:1641.

Green F, Wickenden A (1984) Varicose veins. *Nursing* 2(26):779–781.

Nyhus LM, Bombeck CT, Klein M (1991) In *Textbook of Surgery. The Biological Basis of Modern Surgical Practice*, Sabiston D (ed.). 14th edition, p. 1134. WB Saunders, Philadephia.

Sailors DM, Layman TS, Burns RP, Chandler KE, Russell WL (1993) Laparoscopic hernia repair: a preliminary report. *Am Surg* 59(2):85–89.

Sheehan AL, Shepherd NA (1994) Degenerative vascular diseases. *Surgery* 12(1):19–22.

Skinner DB (1991) Hiatal hernia and gastroesophageal reflux. In *Textbook of Surgery*, Sabiston DC (ed.). pp. 704–715. WB Saunders, Philadephia.

Soni N, Riley B (1993) Insertion of a chest drain. *Curr Anaesth Crit Care* 4:46–52.

Welch J (1993) Chest drains – chest tubes and pleural drainage. *Surg Nurse* 8(5):7–12.

Ziffren SE, Hartford CE (1972) Comparative mortality for various surgical operations in older versus younger age groups. *J Am Geriatr Soc* 20:485–489.

Index

Numbers in *italic* refer to illustrations; numbers in **bold** refer to tables and boxes